500
400-Calorie
Recipes

**Delicious and Satisfying Meals That Keep You to a Balanced
1200-Calorie Diet So You Can Lose Weight without Starving Yourself**

DICK LOGUE

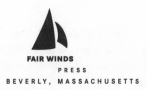

FAIR WINDS
PRESS
BEVERLY, MASSACHUSETTS

Text © 2011 Dick Logue
Design © 2011 Fair Winds Press

First published in the USA in 2011 by
Fair Winds Press, a member of
Quayside Publishing Group
100 Cummings Center
Suite 406-L
Beverly, MA 01915-6101
www.fairwindspress.com

15 14 13 12 11   1 2 3 4 5

ISBN-13: 978-1-59233-462-9
ISBN-10: 1-59233-462-8

Digital edition published in 2011
eISBN-13: 978-1-61058-058-8

Library of Congress Cataloging-in-Publication Data available

Cover and Book design by Kathie Alexander

Printed and bound in Canada

*The information in this book is for educational purposes only. It is not intended
to replace the advice of a physician or medical practitioner. Please see your
healthcare provider before beginning any new health program.*

To my wife, Ginger,
my greatest helper and biggest fan

Contents

Introduction

Why 400-Calorie Recipes?

N o doubt that is the first question that came to your
mind when you saw this book. The answer is simple,
a 400-calorie meal is just what you need to lose weight, a
meal that satisfies you and keeps your hunger at bay until
the next meal but only contains 400 calories. You might
call them "mega." Of course, there is more to it than that.
The goal of our meals is to help you be healthier, lose
weight, and do it all without feeling deprived or hungry.

Does this sound too good to be true? It's not! The key is to eat foods that contain
all the nutrients you need and that stick with you until the next meal. Each meal
we offer here is approximately 400 calories, so you can eat three of these filling
meals, or even four, and still only get 1200 to 1600 calories per day. In the next
chapter, we'll explore in detail how all this works, talking about calories, nutrient
density, and the kind of foods you should and should not be eating. But for now
all you need to know is that it does work.

This is not something that I created. It is based on the research of a number of
doctors and nutritional experts. One of the most important is Dr. Barbara Rolls, a
professor of nutrition at the University of Pennsylvania. Dr. Rolls has published a
number of articles and research papers on the subject of diet and weight loss.
She says that people feel full because of the amount of food they eat not
because of the number of calories or the grams of fat, protein, or carbohydrates.
So the trick is to fill up on foods that aren't full of calories. She has done a
number of experiments to confirm her findings. She found that given free choice,
people tended to eat the same *amount* of food each day. By varying the amount
of high volume, low calorie foods compared to high calorie, low volume foods,

people were able to eat the same amount and feel just as satisfied while eating as much as 400 fewer calories per day. She uses the term *energy density* to describe the number of calories in a given quantity of food.

In order to see how significant this is, let's take a quick look at how people lose weight. There are lots of different diets and lots of different theories, but the bottom line is that if we burn more calories than we take in, we lose weight. If we eat more calories than our bodies use, we gain weight. About 3500 calories is equivalent to a pound. So in order to lose a pound a week, we need to keep our calorie intake to about 500 calories a day less than our bodies use. So Dr. Rolls' findings mean that people could lose almost a pound a week not even watching how *much* they eat, just replacing some of the foods with high energy density with other foods with lower energy density. An example is a pasta salad. If it contains a lot of pasta compared to vegetables, it will have a high energy density. If you replace some of the pasta with additional vegetables you will still have the same volume of food and feel just as satisfied but with fewer calories. That is one of the main concepts that went into creating these recipes.

So the obvious question is how many calories we burn in a day. There isn't any simple answer. It depends on a number of factors including age, gender, activity level, and your current weight and height. There are a number of sites online that contain a calorie needs calculator that will do your specific calculation. But I can tell you this, no matter what I put into them I didn't come up with anything less than 1500 calories per day. That figure was for a small, older, sedentary woman. For my own calculation, I came up with more than 2200 per day to maintain my weight.

So how does all that relate to this book? I'm suggesting that if you want to lose weight, you can eat three satisfying meals a day of about 400 calories each, maybe throw in a healthy snack or two, and end up with a total daily calorie count of less than 1500 calories. In my case, that would translate to a weight loss of about a pound and a half (0.68 kg) a week. Of course as the auto commercials used to say "your mileage may vary". Your answers to the calorie calculator are going to be different than mine and your expected weight loss will be different. But unless you are a person already so thin that you don't need to lose weight, you will almost certainly be eating fewer calories than you burn.

Of course it isn't quite that simple. Since I came to create recipes because of a need to eat heart healthy food, I have some ideas about how we should structure these mega meals for maximum health, not just weight loss. In the next section, we'll discuss some of those.

Our Approach to Weight Loss

I've identified six key areas that I looked at as I created these recipes. As I said, the goal is a healthy diet that will help you to lose weight. We'll look at each of those areas in more detail in the next chapter.

Low Energy Density

We can eat the healthiest diet imaginable, but if we eat too many calories we aren't going to lose weight. That statement isn't quite true. The other concepts of healthy eating actually support this goal also. High fat foods are generally unhealthy to eat. They also provide more calories for a given quantity of food. Fiber contains few calories, so high fiber foods are not only good for you, but they are also a way to speed your weight loss.

High Nutrient Density

This is in some ways the opposite of energy density. What it measures is the amount of nutrients in a specific quantity of a given food. A system of rating nutrient density called the Aggregate Nutrient Density Index (ANDI) was developed by Dr. Joel Fuhrman, a New Jersey physician who specializes in preventing and reversing disease through nutrition. The rankings are based not only on vitamins and minerals but also phytochemicals, compounds that are thought to promote good health but have not been established as essential nutrients. This includes things that you have probably heard of like antioxidants and beta carotene.

Focus on Fresh, Minimally Processed Foods

There has been an increased focus on avoiding processed foods in recent years. This has resulted in things like the caveman diet and Paleolithic diets. I'm not going to go so far as to suggest that, but I will say that I believe processing reduces natural nutrients and replaces them with chemicals, some of questionable safety. The Canyon Ranch spa cookbook I own suggests "Don't eat anything your great-grandmother didn't," and that seems like a reasonable approach to me. That being said, I do use artificial sweeteners to help hold down the calories in some recipes with significant amounts of sugar, so I do make compromises.

Low Sodium

Some of you may know (especially if you've skipped ahead to the next section) that I got started creating recipes and eventually writing books because I was on a low sodium diet for congestive heart failure and I was dissatisfied with the kind of food I could eat. Not all of the recipes here are as strictly low in sodium as my personal diet. I've used regular baking powder and cheese and included a few recipes with ham and other high sodium ingredients. But I'm still convinced that most people get more sodium in their diet than they really need.

Low Saturated Fat

To a large degree I've tried to hold down the total fat level in these recipes as much as is practical. But all fat is not created equal. Fats such as those found in olive and canola oil and vegetables like avocados may actually be beneficial. But it is pretty much universally accepted that both saturated and trans fats represent health risks and I have tried to limit them as much as possible.

High Fiber

Eating foods high in fiber is another of those things that has multiple positive effects. In the first place, it's healthy from both the heart and digestive point of view. But it also plays a part in our attempts to lower the energy density of meals. Fiber-rich foods such as legumes and whole grains tend to have a lower energy density and a higher nutrient density, so that's good all around.

How This Book Came About

Some of you may already know about me, either from my website at www.lowsodiumcooking.com or from the other books I've written. If so, you know that I have focused primarily on heart healthy cooking. I started thinking about low sodium cooking after being diagnosed with congestive heart failure in 1999. One of the first and biggest things I had to deal with was the doctor's insistence that I follow a low sodium diet . . . 1200 mg a day or less. At first, like many people, I found it easiest to just avoid the things that had a lot of sodium in them. But I was bored. And I was convinced that there had to be a way to create low sodium versions of the food I missed. So I learned all kinds of new ways to cook things. I researched where to get low sodium substitutes for the things that I couldn't have any more, bought cookbooks, and basically redid my whole diet.

Along the way, I learned some things. And I decided to try to share this information with others who were in the same position I had been in. I started a website, www.lowsodiumcooking.com, to share recipes and information. I sent out an email newsletter with recipes that now has over 20,000 subscribers. And I wrote my first book, *500 Low Sodium Recipes*.

By that time I had progressed to other areas of interest in healthy cooking. When my cholesterol became too high to please my cardiologist, I had to learn about low cholesterol cooking. When I was told that my blood sugar levels indicated that I was a borderline diabetic, I became interested in the role of carbohydrates in your diet. I became more aware of the work that had been done on glycemic index and glycemic load and began incorporating these concepts into the food we prepared and ate. Both of these interests turned into another 500 recipes book.

But I was also concerned about my weight. And so was my wife. I was following the exercise plan my doctor had given me, but I wasn't able to lose those last 10 pounds or so that I wanted to, even though I thought I was cooking healthy meals. So once more, I went back to the research. And there I discovered the work of Dr. Rolls and others with similar ideas. So we began incorporating these concepts into our cooking. It turns out it was easy to maintain a heart healthy diet while looking at nutrient density. Many of the same things that made food heart healthy also made it a good choice for these meals. And as we began to pay more attention to these ideas and began to lose that weight that had been so stubborn, the idea of another book developed. And here it is, 500 mega meals to get you started on losing weight and feeling better.

How Is the Nutritional Information Calculated?

The nutritional information included with these recipes was calculated using the AccuChef program. It calculates the values using the latest U.S. Department of Agriculture Standard reference nutritional database. I've been using this program since I first started trying to figure out how much sodium was in the recipes I've created. It's inexpensive, easy to use, and has a number of really handy features. For instance, if I go in and change the nutrition figures for an ingredient, it remembers those figures whenever I use that ingredient. AccuChef is available online from www.accuchef.com. They offer a free trial version if you want to try it out, and the full version costs less than $20US.

Of course, that implies that these figures are estimates. Every brand of tomatoes or any other product is a little different in nutritional content. These figures were calculated using products that I buy in southern Maryland. If you use a different brand, your nutrition figures may be different. Use the nutritional analysis as a guideline in determining whether a recipe is right for your diet.

Where's the Salt?

One question that may occur to some people looking over the recipes in this book is "Why is there no salt in any of the ingredient lists?" That's a fair question and deserves an answer. As I said in the Introduction, I first got involved with healthy cooking because my doctor put me on a low sodium diet. It took some time and lots of experimentation, but I learned how to cook things that both taste good and are easy to prepare that are still low in sodium. Along the way we literally threw away our saltshaker. There's one shaker of light salt, which is half salt and half salt substitute, on the table. My wife uses that occasionally. Two of my children have given up salt completely, not because they need to for medical reasons, but because they are convinced like I am that it's the healthy thing to do. When I started looking at creating 400-calorie meal recipes, going back to using salt wasn't even something I considered.

Most Americans get far more than the 2300 mg of sodium a day recommended for a healthy adult. This happens without our even thinking about it. In creating these recipes, I was not as strict about the amount of sodium as I usually am. But I also didn't add any salt. I think if you try the recipes you'll find that they taste good without it. If you are tempted to add some salt because you think it's needed, I'd suggest you check with your doctor first. I believe that most of them will agree that in the interest of total health, you are better off without the salt.

Changing the Way You Think about What You Eat

To a large degree, this book is a starting point. In this chapter, I'm going to describe what I think constitutes a healthy diet. Then I'm going to give you recipes for 500 complete meals that are samples of those concepts. At the end of the book, we are going to talk about how you can pick and choose different items to make up your own 400-calorie meals. So the goal is not just to give you some recipes. You'd probably get pretty tired of those same things after the first couple of times through the book. So I'm also going to try to show you in this chapter a little bit about how those recipes were created so you can go forth and create more on your own. To do that, we are going to look at each of the six areas we talked about in the introduction in more detail.

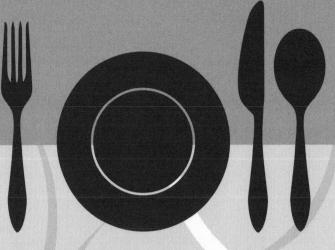

Energy Density

Let's look in a little more detail at the idea of energy density that we introduced previously. Energy density is defined as the number of calories in a gram of food. Dr. Rolls introduces a simple way to estimate that for items containing a nutrition label. The label contains both the number of calories and the number of grams in a serving, making a comparison relatively easy. If the number of calories is less than the number of grams in a serving, that food in general has a low energy density and can be eaten freely. This category includes many fruits and vegetables, nonfat dairy products, and soups. If the number of calories is between 1 and 2 times the number of grams, you should be aware of the amount you eat and be strict about portion control. This group includes starchy vegetables, low fat meats, and many bean and grain products. The closer the ratio is to 2, the more careful you should be. If the number of calories is more than twice the number of grams, you should limit how much you eat. This includes fried foods, butter and oil, and candies.

Here are some samples of foods that fall into those different categories. These are in approximate order of lower to higher.

Low:
   Broth and broth-based soups
   Nonstarchy vegetables
      Lettuce
      Greens such as spinach and kale
      Tomatoes
      Asparagus
      Mushrooms
      Broccoli and cauliflower
      Peppers
      Carrots
   Fruits
      Strawberries
      Citrus fruits
      Melons
      Peaches
      Apples and pears
   Fat-free dairy products
   Fat-free salad dressings
   Fat-free mayonnaise
   Dried beans
   Corn

Medium
  Fish and seafood
  Sweet potatoes
  Low fat and regular dairy products
  Potatoes
  Rice
  Pasta
  Avocados
  Chicken and turkey
  Canned tuna
  Lean beef
High
  Bread
  Cheese
  Full fat dressings
  Baked goods
  Regular mayonnaise
  Fried foods (French fries, chips, onion rings)
  Nuts and nut butters
  Bacon
  Butter
  Oil

Another way to look at this is in terms of the basic food building blocks and how many calories they contain. At the top end are fats, which contain 9 calories per gram. We obviously want to limit those. Carbohydrates contain about 4 calories per gram, less than half that of fat. Fiber contains only 2 calories per gram. Water contains none at all. This is why many of the recipes in this book contain lots of vegetables that contain a high percentage of water like zucchini and eggplant. This is free volume for your diet; it helps to fill you up without providing any calories.

Nutrient Density

Nutrient density was a key element in creating these recipes. If we are going to reduce the number of calories we take in, we want to make sure that we still get all the nutrition we need. In many cases, the same foods that have low energy density have high nutrient density, so that is a help. In looking at nutrient density, one of the things I looked at was the information that was published by Dr. Fuhrman. His ANDI scale calculates nutrient density based on a number of vitamins, minerals, and other nutrients in food, coming up with a way of comparing different foods to see which have the most nutrients for a specific quantity. His general recommendation is to focus on bright colored plant products. Green leafy vegetables rate near the top of the list, as do things like carrots, tomatoes, and strawberries. The bottom of the list contains things like oils, processed grain products like bread and pasta, dairy products, and meats.

The U.S. Department of Agriculture also supports the concept of nutrient density on its www.mypyramid.gov site, stating "Smart choices are the foods with the lowest amounts of solid fats or added sugars: for example, fat-free (skim) milk instead of whole milk and unsweetened rather than sweetened applesauce."

In general, both of these sets of recommendations correspond with what we saw for reducing energy density, so that makes creating recipes that contain high nutritional content easier. In order to help attain the desired level to nutrient density, we've tried to adhere to the following guidelines:

• Brightly colored fruits
• Brightly colored vegetables and potatoes
• Whole grain and fiber-rich grain foods
• Low-fat and fat-free milk, cheese, and yogurt
• Lean meat, skinless poultry, fish, eggs, and beans

Focus on Fresh Foods

What we have to say here mirrors much of the other things we've said in this chapter. The idea is that processing takes away the nutrient content of food. So the best thing you can do for both the nutrient density of food and the freshness is to process it as little as possible. A couple of quick guidelines:

• Eat foods as close to the way they grow as possible. Fresh is better than frozen. Whole is better than juice. Real potatoes are better than fried chips. It's really a simple rule to that can make a lot of difference.
• Avoid refined and processed food as much as possible. Eat whole grains rather than white flour. Eat natural sweeteners rather than white sugar and high fructose corn syrup.
• Avoid things that contain added chemicals as much as possible. It may not help you lose weight, but it has to be healthier.

Sodium

To me this is obvious and second nature. After 11 years on a low sodium diet I can't imagine eating any other way. The fact that I feel so much better now than I did when I first started it is enough proof for me. But you don't have to rely on my word alone:

- The U.S. Food and Drug Administration recommends 2300 milligrams (mg) of sodium daily for healthy adults.
- The U.S. Department of Agriculture recommends that individuals with hypertension, African Americans, and adults 50 and above should consume no more than 1500 mg of sodium per day.
- The United Kingdom Recommended Nutritional Intake (RNI) is 1600 mg daily.
- The National Research Council of the National Academy of Sciences recommends 1100 to 1500 mg daily for adults.
- Many experts recommend less than 1500 mg daily for anyone with a history of heart trouble, high blood pressure, or other risk factors for heart disease.
- It's estimated that the average daily intake consumed in the United States and Western Europe is 3 to 5 times these recommendations.

I've tried not to be a fanatic about sodium content in these recipes. There are a couple that have almost as much sodium as I'm allowed daily. I don't eat those. But I'm not going to tell you that you shouldn't. But as I said in the Where's the Salt section in the introduction, I don't add salt to things. Ever. So if you feel the need to, you'll have to do that on your own.

Fats

Another of those areas that are good news for multiple reasons is the reduction of fats. There are two main types of fats we want to limit: saturated fat and trans fats.

In general, saturated fats are fats that are solid at room temperature. There are several categories of saturated fats. In each case, there are better alternatives or things we can do to reduce the fat. The recipes in this book are designed with that in mind.

- Red Meats—Beef, pork, and lamb have been mentioned often as being the worse in terms of saturated fat. It's true that they tend to have more than fish or poultry. But how much they have is very dependent on which cut you choose. Some high fats cuts of beef may contain 5 times the amount of saturated fat as a lean cut.
- Poultry Skin—While not containing as much saturated fat as red meat, poultry skin does have a significant amount. A chicken thigh with the skin has more than 2 grams additional saturated fat, compared to the meat only. And this is a case where eliminating that fat is really easy, just don't eat the skin.
- Whole Milk Dairy Foods—Dairy products are another area where making smart choices can significantly reduce the amount of saturated fat. Avoid using products made from whole milk or cream. Choose skim milk, reduced fat cheeses, and fat-free versions of sour cream and cream cheese. Use fat-free evaporated milk in place of cream.

- Tropical Oils—Some plant oils in the category typically called tropical oil also contain saturated fats. These include palm, palm kernel, and coconut oils and cocoa butter. They are generally easy to avoid, but be aware that some commercial baked goods and processed foods may contain them.

Trans fats are also called trans-fatty acids. They are produced by adding hydrogen to vegetable oil through a process called hydrogenation. This makes the fat more solid and less likely to spoil. Although increased awareness of their health risks have started to reduce their use, trans fat are still a common ingredient in commercial baked goods and fried foods. Food manufacturers are required to list trans fat content on nutrition labels.

- Margarine and Other Hydrogenated Oils—Avoid margarine and solid shortening containing hydrogenated or partially hydrogenated oils.
- Commercial Baked Goods and Fried Foods—These are bad news for our 400-calorie diet anyway, so they aren't really a concern.

There are also some positive fat choices you can make.

- Olive and Canola Oils—While we want to limit the amount of fats in our diet to help us maintain our ideal weight, oils like olive and canola oil contain polyunsaturated fat, which is the most healthful kind. All of the recipes in this book that contain oil specify either olive or canola.
- Fish—The oils contained in fish contain a compound called omega-3 fatty acids that actually help to reduce blood vessel blockages and clots. It's often recommended that you eat fish at least twice a week.

Fiber

As we already saw, foods that are high in fiber are generally lower in energy density, so that a good thing for us right out of the gate. But there are some other health benefits of increasing the fiber in your diet.

- Reduce the Risk of Certain Cancers—A major benefit is the role that fiber has been shown to have in reducing cancer. Studies have shown that people who eat a high fiber diet have less incidents of colon cancer. Studies done in England have shown not only that women who eat a high fiber diet are less likely to develop breast cancer, but also that women who already had breast cancer had a longer life expectancy on a high fiber diet. And finally, studies have also shown a significant reduction in uterine cancer in women who ate a high fiber diet.
- Help the Heart and Circulatory System—Fiber has also been shown to have positive effects in fighting heart disease by helping to reduce cholesterol levels.
- Help Control Blood Pressure—Another way that fiber contributes to heart and overall health is by reducing high blood pressure. High fiber diets have been

shown to reduce blood pressure by 3 to 7 points, enough to reduce the risk of heart disease by up to 9%.

- Help Fight Diabetes—Finally, a high fiber diet can reduce your risk of developing Type 2 diabetes. It slows the absorption of sugar into the bloodstream. Research has found that a high fiber meal can reduce blood sugar levels by as much as 28%.

These recipes contribute to meeting the recommended daily fiber intake by including the following kinds of ingredients:

- Legumes—Beans and other legumes are the poster child for high fiber foods. A single serving can provide 15 grams or more of fiber. They also have been proven to be one of the foods that is effective at keeping you from feeling hungry the longest and have been linked to reduced risk of heart disease, diabetes, and certain kinds of cancer.
- Whole Grains—Whole grains are a great source of fiber and one that's included in many of these recipes Whole grains contribute to that full feeling that keep you from overeating and have been shown to slow the absorption of sugar into the blood. They also contain many other minerals and nutrients that are removed from processed grains.

Things We Want More of In Our Healthy Diet
Based on the above can list, a couple of general guidelines for things that we want to see more of in our diet:

- Whole foods such as produce and fresh meats
- Brightly colored fruits and vegetables
- Whole grains
- Legumes, including lentils, soybeans, dried peas, and beans

Things We Want Less of
We can also come up with a high level list of those things that we want to limit:

- Refined, processed foods such as white flour and sugar
- Packaged foods, which often contain ingredients you would be better off without
- Saturated fats and trans fats
- Empty calories, such as sweetened beverages and alcohol

Comments on Ingredients Used in the Recipes
- Butter vs. Margarine—The recipes in this book call for unsalted butter. I've been back and forth over the years about butter or margarine, but my current thinking is that the amount of cholesterol in the butter does not outweigh the possible health effects of the trans fats in margarine.

- Eggs—Unless a recipe specific needs a whole egg for something like poached or deviled eggs all the recipes call for egg substitute. It contains fewer calories and less cholesterol than whole eggs and is essentially a *real* product, being primarily colored egg whites.
- Milk and Dairy Products—The recipes call for skim milk and nonfat dairy products when they are readily available, reduced fat ones when they are not. This is another area where I thought I couldn't stand the taste of things like skim milk, but I found after using it that it really was just fine. I use fat-free evaporated milk in place of cream wherever it is called for. This is a great product for reducing fat and calories while still allowing you the taste and feel of the original.
- Canned Tomato Products, Vegetables, and Beans—I use no-salt-added products wherever possible. It's gotten easier to find them for many products, and it really does help to hold down the sodium level.
- Soups, Broth, and Bouillon—Like other products, low sodium versions of these are available but not as widely as might be hoped. I personally make a point of finding them and that is what the nutritional calculations are based on.
- Alcohol—There are some recipes in this book that contain beer, wine, or other alcohol. I realize that these will not be right for everyone. There are some alternatives that will still let you enjoy the recipes. Nonalcoholic beers and wines have had most of the alcohol removed. Typically they contain about one half of one percent alcohol. I've seen it stated that this is about the same as what occurs naturally in orange juice, but I've never seen any conclusive proof of this. You'll have to decide if that is acceptable to you or not. Many of the recipes made with beer or white wine could have chicken broth substituted with no ill effects. For recipes made with red wine, you could replace it with grape juice, adding a few tablespoons of vinegar to counteract the sweetness, although the final flavor may be a little different. In some recipes, you may also choose to omit the alcohol. One note—if you decide to use wine in cooking, do not buy the cooking wine in the supermarket. It is poor quality and contains added salt, which will affect the taste of the recipe. You'd be better off leaving it out. The rule I follow is if you wouldn't drink it, don't cook with it.
- Drinks—Very few of the recipes here contain drinks or drink recommendations. But our usual guidelines apply here too. Regular soft drinks with empty sugar (or more likely corn syrup) calories will ruin your diet. One regular soda a day is the equivalent of more than 10 pounds (4.5 kg) more of calories in a year. Artificially sweetened ones have fewer calories … and more chemicals. Water is the best possible drink. Unsweetened tea is good. However, contrary to many recommendations, it appears that drinking water before a meal does not make you more full at the start and cause you to eat less. Studies by Dr. Rolls and others have found that people who drank water before a meal ate the

same amount as they did when they didn't drink the water. You body is smart enough to know the difference between filling your stomach with water and filling your stomach with high volume, low calorie food.

A Few Final Thoughts

Hopefully the information in this chapter has gotten you thinking about some of the ways that you can be satisfied with the quantity and taste of your food, yet still hold down the calorie count to a level that allows you to lose weight. The rest of this book contains recipes to help you do just that. Most of them are a complete meal with around 400 calories. There are meals for breakfast, lunches, and light dinners and more traditional dinners. At the end of the book are a couple of chapters of mix and match ideas to let you create your own meals.

A Few Basic Building Blocks

This chapter doesn't really contain meals. What it does contain are some basic ingredients that are used multiple times in making the meals in the rest of the book. So it seemed to make sense to pull them out here, rather than repeating the same ingredients over and over. Some of them are the kind of things that you might want to make ahead and have on your pantry shelf or in your refrigerator. But you don't have to do that if you don't want to. You can always make them when you are making the meal that requires them.

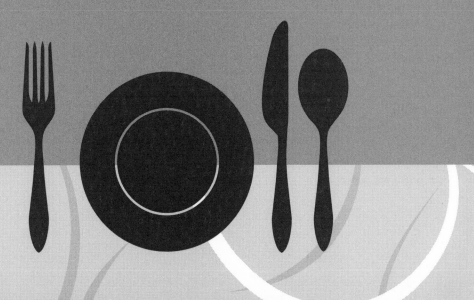

A Peppercorn Ranch Dressing That You Can Actually Eat

This is my favorite dressing recipe. It's similar to a ranch dressing, but with a little extra pop from the peppercorns. By using the low fat mayonnaise and buttermilk, you hold the calories to 25 per serving, rather than the 80 in commercial ranch dressing. If you can't find low fat buttermilk, you can use buttermilk powder and skim milk and only end up with a few more calories.

1 cup (225 g) low fat mayonnaise
1 cup (235 ml) low fat buttermilk
2 teaspoons dried parsley
1 teaspoon onion powder
¼ teaspoon garlic powder
¼ teaspoon dill weed
1 teaspoon black peppercorns,
   coarsely cracked

Mix all ingredients together well. Refrigerate overnight before using.

16 SERVINGS

Each with: 25 Calories (27% from Fat, 12% from Protein, 61% from Carb); 1 g Protein; 1 g Total Fat; 0 g Saturated Fat; 0 g Monounsaturated Fat; 0 g Polyunsaturated Fat; 3 g Carb; 0 g Fiber; 2 g Sugar; 19 mg Phosphorus; 20 mg Calcium; 136 mg Sodium; 36 mg Potassium; 34 IU Vitamin A; 1 mg ATE Vitamin E; 0 mg Vitamin C; 2 mg Cholesterol

Creamy Asian Salad Dressing

Asian-inspired salads are a great deal for diets. Many Asian vegetables are very low in calories and this creamy salad dressing with Asian flavorings complements them well. Try it with our *Super Asian Side Salad* in chapter 14, but you may find that you like it well enough to use every day.

8 ounces (225 g) tofu
¼ teaspoon dried oregano
¼ teaspoon marjoram
1 teaspoon garlic, minced
3 tablespoons (45 ml) balsamic
   vinegar
2 tablespoons (28 ml) low sodium
   soy sauce
¼ cup (25 g) green onion,
   chopped
2 tablespoons (28 ml) lemon juice
¼ cup (60 ml) water

Place tofu slices in a blender or a food processor fitted with the metal blade. Add remaining ingredients and only as much water as needed to make desired consistency. Process until smooth.

16 SERVINGS

Each with: 11 Calories (31% from Fat, 30% from Protein, 39% from Carb); 1 g Protein; 0 g Total Fat; 0 g Saturated Fat; 0 g Monounsaturated Fat; 0 g Polyunsaturated Fat; 1 g Carb; 0 g Fiber; 0 g Sugar; 12 mg Phosphorus; 7 mg Calcium; 68 mg Sodium; 40 mg Potassium; 18 IU Vitamin A; 0 mg ATE Vitamin E; 1 mg Vitamin C; 0 mg Cholesterol

Fruity Orange Yogurt Dressing

This dressing is great on fruit salads like our *MaxiFruit Salad* in chapter 14,
but it's also great on plain veggie salads.

1 cup (230 g) low fat plain yogurt
¼ cup (60 ml) orange juice
1 tablespoon (20 g) honey

Mix until well blended. Refrigerate any unused portion.

10 SERVINGS

Each with: 25 Calories (14% from Fat, 21% from Protein, 65% from Carb);
1 g Protein; 0 g Total Fat; 0 g Saturated Fat; 0 g Monounsaturated Fat; 0 g
Polyunsaturated Fat; 4 g Carb; 0 g Fiber; 3 g Sugar; 36 mg Phosphorus; 46 mg
Calcium; 17 mg Sodium; 70 mg Potassium; 17 IU Vitamin A; 3 mg ATE Vitamin E;
2 mg Vitamin C; 1 mg Cholesterol

Lower Fat Balsamic Vinaigrette

Most vinaigrette dressings have oil as their main ingredient. This one has only just enough to
hold everything together. It has a more distinct flavor than many of the Balsamic dressings sold
commercially, possibly because of the lemon juice and the mustard.

2 tablespoons (22 g) Dijon
  mustard
½ cup (120 ml) balsamic vinegar
¼ cup (60 ml) water
¼ cup (60 ml) fresh lemon juice
½ teaspoon black pepper
½ teaspoon dried tarragon
1 teaspoon garlic, minced
¼ cup (60 ml) olive oil

In a jar, combine the mustard, vinegar, water, lemon juice,
black pepper, tarragon, and garlic. Shake well to combine.
Add oil and shake again. Chill before serving.

11 SERVINGS

Each with: 49 Calories (87% from Fat, 1% from Protein, 11% from Carb);
0 g Protein; 5 g Total Fat; 1 g Saturated Fat; 4 g Monounsaturated Fat; 1 g
Polyunsaturated Fat; 1 g Carb; 0 g Fiber; 1 g Sugar; 4 mg Phosphorus; 4 mg Calcium;
32 mg Sodium; 24 mg Potassium; 10 IU Vitamin A; 0 mg ATE Vitamin E; 3 mg
Vitamin C; 0 mg Cholesterol

No Fat at All Balsamic Sun-Dried Tomato Dressing

Ok, I lied. There actually is 1 gram of fat, probably from the tofu, but it's very close to being fat-free. And that means that a typical 2 tablespoon (28 g) serving of this tasty, creamy dressing contains only 21 calories. What better dressing could you find to top your *Mega Starter Side Salad* in chapter 14, giving you a good tasting and filling start to a meal for about 50 calories?

¼ cup (60 ml) balsamic vinegar

2 tablespoons (7 g) sun-dried tomatoes, dried

6 ounces (170 g) tofu

8 ounces (225 g) no-salt-added tomato sauce

¼ teaspoon onion powder

½ teaspoon dried basil

¼ teaspoon garlic powder

Combine all ingredients in a blender or food processor and process until smooth. Transfer to a covered jar and refrigerate.

10 SERVINGS

Each with: 21 Calories (20% from Fat, 22% from Protein, 57% from Carb); 1 g Protein; 1 g Total Fat; 0 g Saturated Fat; 0 g Monounsaturated Fat; 0 g Polyunsaturated Fat; 3 g Carb; 1 g Fiber; 2 g Sugar; 23 mg Phosphorus; 11 mg Calcium; 21 mg Sodium; 162 mg Potassium; 125 IU Vitamin A; 0 mg ATE Vitamin E; 3 mg Vitamin C; 0 mg Cholesterol

Reduced Fat Italian Dressing

You may find this dressing a little more sour than commercial Italian dressing because it has a higher percentage of vinegar. So you may want to use a little less. But even if you use the full two tablespoons (28 ml), you are getting a lot of taste for not many calories.

1 tablespoon (15 ml) olive oil

½ cup (120 ml) cider vinegar

2 tablespoons (22 g) Dijon mustard

½ teaspoon garlic powder

½ teaspoon black pepper

½ teaspoon sugar substitute, such as Splenda

1 teaspoon dried basil

1 teaspoon dried oregano

½ teaspoon dried rosemary

Combine all ingredients in a jar with a tight fitting lid. Shake well.

6 SERVINGS

Each with: 28 Calories (70% from Fat, 4% from Protein, 26% from Carb); 0 g Protein; 2 g Total Fat; 0 g Saturated Fat; 2 g Monounsaturated Fat; 0 g Polyunsaturated Fat; 2 g Carb; 0 g Fiber; 1 g Sugar; 9 mg Phosphorus; 12 mg Calcium; 59 mg Sodium; 40 mg Potassium; 31 IU Vitamin A; 0 mg ATE Vitamin E; 0 mg Vitamin C; 0 mg Cholesterol

Yes You Can Have Blue Cheese Dressing

You can have it, but you'll want to be more careful about this dressing than the others. It does have more calories, but if you are like me, every once in a while it is what you really want. So here is a version that has about one-third the calories of the last one I picked up on a grocery shelf.

2 ounces (55 g) blue cheese
1 cup (225 g) low fat mayonnaise
½ cup (115 g) fat-free sour cream
½ cup (120 ml) low fat buttermilk

Combine ingredients and chill overnight.

20 SERVINGS

Each with: 61 Calories (82% from Fat, 7% from Protein, 11% from Carb); 1 g Protein; 6 g Total Fat; 2 g Saturated Fat; 0 g Monounsaturated Fat; 0 g Polyunsaturated Fat; 2 g Carb; 0 g Fiber; 1 g Sugar; 29 mg Phosphorus; 29 mg Calcium; 144 mg Sodium; 31 mg Potassium; 68 IU Vitamin A; 12 mg ATE Vitamin E; 0 mg Vitamin C; 9 mg Cholesterol

Low Fat, Low Calorie Cream Cheese Substitute

Have you ever thought of making your own cheese? Neither had I until I came across this suggestion. The idea is really simple, drain the extra liquid out of plain yogurt until it is thick and use it in place of cream cheese. The great news is it has all the nutrition (probably more, because it also contains the healthy active bacteria cultures) and only a little more than half the calories of fat-free cream cheese. And I challenge you to taste both this and fat-free cream cheese and tell me you don't think this tastes better. The nutrition figures below are probably a little high since it's hard to account for what drains off, so if anything it has even fewer calories than listed.

2 cups (460 g) low fat plain yogurt

Place a strainer with feet into a larger bowl with low sides. Line the strainer with a double layer of cheesecloth. Put the yogurt into the cheesecloth. Place into the refrigerator for at least 24 hours. Stir occasionally to help the liquid to drain. After 24 hours, remove the thickened yogurt from the strainer and store in a covered container in the refrigerator. Use in place of cream cheese or as a spread instead of mayonnaise.

8 SERVINGS

Each with: 39 Calories (22% from Fat, 33% from Protein, 45% from Carb); 3 g Protein; 1 g Total Fat; 1 g Saturated Fat; 0 g Monounsaturated Fat; 0 g Polyunsaturated Fat; 4 g Carb; 0 g Fiber; 4 g Sugar; 88 mg Phosphorus; 112 mg Calcium; 43 mg Sodium; 143 mg Potassium; 31 IU Vitamin A; 9 mg ATE Vitamin E; 0 mg Vitamin C; 4 mg Cholesterol

Reduced Fat Baking Mix

This makes a mix similar to the Reduced Fat Bisquick, but it's even lower in fat.
Use it in any recipes that call for baking mix.

4 cups (500 g) all purpose flour

2 cups (240 g) whole wheat pastry flour

3 tablespoons (41.5) baking powder

⅓ cup (75 g) unsalted butter

Stir flour and baking powder together. Cut in butter with pastry blender or 2 knives until mixture resembles coarse crumbs. Store in a container with a tight fitting lid.

12 SERVINGS

Each with: 267 Calories (20% from Fat, 10% from Protein, 70% from Carb); 7 g Protein; 6 g Total Fat; 3 g Unsaturated Fat; 1 g Monounsaturated Fat; 1 g Polyunsaturated Fat; 47 g Carb; 4 g Fiber; 0 g Sugar; 191 mg Phosphorus; 217 mg Calcium; 368 mg Sodium; 128 mg Potassium; 159 IU Vitamin A; 42 mg ATE Vitamin E; 0 mg Vitamin C; 14 mg Cholesterol

Reduced Fat Pesto

This makes a fairly typical pesto, but it's lower in fat and sodium than commercial ones. This is accomplished by lowering the amount of oil and leaving out the salt. It's not a really difficult thing, but one that doesn't seem to occur to commercial pesto makers.

2 cups (80 g) fresh basil, packed

3 tablespoons (27 g) pine nuts

1 teaspoon garlic, finely minced

¼ cup (25 g) Parmesan cheese

¼ cup (60 ml) olive oil

 Tip: Serve over pasta or on toasted bread.

Place basil leaves in small batches in food processor and whip until well chopped (do about ¾ cup [60 g] at a time). Add about ⅓ the nuts and garlic and blend again. Add about ⅓ of the Parmesan cheese; blend while slowly adding about ⅓ of the olive oil, stopping to scrape down sides of container. Process basil pesto until it forms a thick smooth paste. Repeat until all ingredients are used; mix all batches together well. Basil pesto keeps in refrigerator one week or freeze for a few months.

12 SERVINGS

Each with: 77 Calories (73% from Fat, 9% from Protein, 18% from Carb); 2 g Protein; 7 g Total Fat; 1 g Unsaturated Fat; 4 g Monounsaturated Fat; 1 g Polyunsaturated Fat; 4 g Carb; 2 g Fiber; 0 g Sugar; 55 mg Phosphorus; 142 mg Calcium; 34 mg Sodium; 208 mg Potassium; 535 IU Vitamin A; 2 mg ATE Vitamin E; 4 mg Vitamin C; 2 mg Cholesterol

Traditional Breakfasts

Are you a big breakfast fan (like me!)? And are you thinking that breakfast is going to be changed completely as you follow our new meal plan? Think again. Breakfast is just as important as any other meal in our new way of eating. In fact, it may be more important because it's the meal that gets you started on your path of feeling satisfied on fewer calories each day. And there are lots of recipes that contain eggs and other traditional breakfast foods but still adhere to our principles.

Fill Yourself Up but Not Out Breakfast Casserole

This is a fairly traditional breakfast casserole. Well, except for the chilies, which do add a little flavor and heat. Along with those, it contains a generous helping of other vegetables to keep you going through the morning.

24 ounces (680 g) frozen hash browns
1 cup (233 ml) skim milk
1 cup (235 ml) egg substitute
½ cup (80 g) onion, diced
½ cup (75 g) red bell pepper
4 ounces (115 g) diced green chilies
¾ cup (83 g) Swiss cheese, grated
6 slices low sodium bacon, cooked and crumbled

Spray a 9 × 13 inch (23 × 33 cm) pan with nonstick vegetable oil spray. Add hash browns. Cook in 350°F (180°C, or gas mark 4) oven for 20 minutes. Mix all remaining ingredients, pour over potatoes, and cook for 30 more minutes.

6 SERVINGS

Each with: 414 Calories (48% from Fat, 17% from Protein, 35% from Carb); 18 g Protein; 23 g Total Fat; 9 g Saturated Fat; 9 g Monounsaturated Fat; 3 g Polyunsaturated Fat; 37 g Carb; 3 g Fiber; 3 g Sugar; 322 mg Phosphorus; 234 mg Calcium; 3 mg Iron; 230 mg Sodium; 811 mg Potassium; 763 IU Vitamin A; 61 mg ATE Vitamin E; 24 mg Vitamin C; 25 mg Cholesterol

Ham and Egg Casserole

This is a fairly typical ham and egg bake, except for the addition of the zucchini and mushrooms. They take the place of the more typical potatoes, which have significantly more calories.

2 tablespoons (28 g) unsalted butter, melted

1 pound (455 g) low fat Monterey Jack cheese, shredded

2½ cups (570 ml) egg substitute, beaten

2 tablespoons (16 g) all purpose flour

16 ounces (455 g) fat-free cottage cheese

2 cups (300 g) ham, cubed

⅛ teaspoon Tabasco sauce

1 teaspoon baking powder

1 cup (120 g) zucchini, shredded

8 ounces (225 g) mushrooms, sliced

1 cup (150 g) red bell pepper, chopped

Preheat oven to 400°F (200°C, or gas mark 6). Put butter in 9-inch (23 cm) pan and melt in oven. Combine all other ingredients and put in pan. Bake at 400°F (200°C, or gas mark 6) for 15 minutes and then at 350°F (180°C, or gas mark 4) degrees for 15 to 20 minutes more.

6 SERVINGS

Each with: 413 Calories (39% from Fat, 51% from Protein, 10% from Carb); 52 g Protein; 18 g Total Fat; 8 g Unsaturated Fat; 6 g Monounsaturated Fat; 3 g Polyunsaturated Fat; 10 g Carb; 1 g Fiber; 5 g Sugar; 764 mg Phosphorus; 471 mg Calcium; 1540 mg Sodium; 853 mg Potassium; 1503 IU Vitamin A; 85 mg ATE Vitamin E; 52 mg Vitamin C; 49 mg Cholesterol

Asparagus Omelet and Citrus Salad

This breakfast exemplifies what mega meals are all about. You get a large quantity of great tasting food without going over your calorie goals.

Omelet

10 ounces (280 g) asparagus, cut into ⅓-inch (8 mm) pieces

1½ cups (355 ml) egg substitute

⅓ cup (33 g) Parmesan cheese, finely grated

¼ teaspoon black pepper

¼ cup (25 g) scallion, thinly sliced

Salad

6 ounces (170 g) mandarin oranges

2 grapefruits, cut into sections

3 cups (165 g) Bibb lettuce

6 tablespoons (90 g) poppy seed dressing

Steam the asparagus until crisp/tender, about 5 minutes, and drain. Whisk the egg substitute, grated Parmesan cheese, and black pepper in a large bowl to blend well. Spray a skillet with nonstick vegetable oil spray. Sauté sliced scallions for 3 minutes or until softened. Add cooked asparagus and sauté until heated through. Reduce heat to medium; spread the asparagus mixture in a single layer in the skillet. Pour the egg mixture over the asparagus. Cook until the eggs are softly set, tilting skillet and gently running a rubber spatula around the edge to allow uncooked egg to flow underneath, about 4 minutes. Slide the omelet out onto a plate, folding in half. Cut omelet into wedges and serve. While the omelet is cooking, combine mandarin oranges, grapefruit sections, and lettuce in a large salad bowl; toss lightly with dressing and divide onto salad plates.

3 SERVINGS

Each with: 388 Calories (43% from Fat, 24% from Protein, 32% from Carb); 24 g Protein; 19 g Total Fat; 4 g Saturated Fat; 2 g Monounsaturated Fat; 2 g Polyunsaturated Fat; 32 g Carb; 6 g Fiber; 25 g Sugar; 331 mg Phosphorus; 272 mg Calcium; 6 mg Iron; 906 mg Sodium; 1167 mg Potassium; 5667 IU Vitamin A; 13 mg ATE Vitamin E; 105 mg Vitamin C; 11 mg Cholesterol

Ready to Ride the Range Breakfast

This is a fairly spicy Southwestern breakfast that's full of flavor but within the limits of your diet. So enjoy yourself before saddling up and going off to work.

1 large potato
¾ pound (340 g) turkey sausage
1 small onion, chopped
1 teaspoon chili powder
¼ teaspoon cayenne pepper
¾ cup (175 ml) egg substitute
6 whole wheat tortillas, 8-inch (20 cm)
½ cup (58 g) reduced fat Monterey Jack cheese
½ cup (130 g) salsa

Cook the potato in boiling water 35 minutes until tender. (I cooked mine in the microwave.) When cool, peel and cut into cubes. Brown sausage in frying pan. Add chopped onion, chili powder, and cayenne pepper. Cook for 10 minutes. Drain and discard any fat. Add cubed, cooked potato. Beat egg substitute and add to pan. Stir until eggs are set. Spoon mixture into center of warmed tortilla, top with shredded cheese, and roll up tortilla to enclose mixture. Serve topped with salsa.

6 SERVINGS

Each with: 409 Calories (40% from Fat, 21% from Protein, 39% from Carb); 21 g Protein; 18 g Total Fat; 7 g Saturated Fat; 6 g Monounsaturated Fat; 3 g Polyunsaturated Fat; 40 g Carb; 3 g Fiber; 3 g Sugar; 297 mg Phosphorus; 191 mg Calcium; 767 mg Sodium; 640 mg Potassium; 502 IU Vitamin A; 21 mg ATE Vitamin E; 28 mg Vitamin C; 44 mg Cholesterol

Breakfast Enchiladas for Family and Guests

A make-ahead breakfast, you can assemble this the night before and then just bake it in the morning. This and the large number of servings make it a great choice when you have company staying overnight. Or just freeze the extras so you'll have it ready the next time you want it.

12 ounces (340 g) ham, finely chopped
½ cup (50 g) green onion, chopped
2 cups (300 g) green bell pepper, chopped
1 cup (160 g) onion, chopped
1½ cups (180 g) low fat cheddar cheese, grated
8 whole wheat tortillas, 8-inch (20 cm)
1½ cups (355 ml) egg substitute
2 cups (475 g) skim milk
1 tablespoon (8 g) all purpose flour
¼ teaspoon garlic powder
1 teaspoon Tabasco sauce
1 avocado

Preheat oven to 350°F (180°C, or gas mark 4). Mix together ham, onion, green bell pepper, and cheese. Divide mixture among tortillas and roll up. Place seam side down in a greased 12 × 7 × 2-inch (30 × 18 × 5 cm) pan. In separate bowl, beat egg substitute, skim milk, flour, garlic, and Tabasco sauce. Pour over enchiladas. Place in refrigerator overnight if desired. Cover with foil and bake for 30 minutes. Uncover for last 10 minutes. Top with slices of avocado to serve.

8 SERVINGS

Each with: 385 Calories (32% from Fat, 29% from Protein, 38% from Carb); 28 g Protein; 14 g Total Fat; 4 g Saturated Fat; 7 g Monounsaturated Fat; 2 g Polyunsaturated Fat; 37 g Carb; 4 g Fiber; 3 g Sugar; 425 mg Phosphorus; 291 mg Calcium; 951 mg Sodium; 716 mg Potassium; 587 IU Vitamin A; 52 mg ATE Vitamin E; 35 mg Vitamin C; 24 mg Cholesterol

Easy, Tasty, Filling Breakfast Strata

The title says it all. What more could you want? This is a great fix-head breakfast.
We usually have some variation of this on holidays when there is a lot to do
in the morning, but we want a special family breakfast.

1 pound (455 g) turkey sausage

2 cups (475 ml) egg substitute

10 slices whole wheat bread,
cubed

3 cups (700 ml) skim milk

1 cup (115 g) low fat cheddar
cheese, shredded

1 cup (160) onion, chopped

1 cup (150 g) red bell pepper,
chopped

10 ounces (280 g) frozen chopped
broccoli, thawed

2 tablespoons (28 g) unsalted
butter, melted

2 tablespoons (16 g) all purpose
flour

1 tablespoon (9 g) dry mustard

2 teaspoons dried basil

In large skillet, brown sausage. Drain. In large bowl, beat egg
substitute. Add remaining ingredients and mix well. Spoon into
greased 13 × 9-inch (33 × 23 cm) baking pan. Cover and
refrigerate 8 hours or overnight. Preheat oven to 350°F (180°C,
or gas mark 4). Bake 60 to 70 minutes or until knife inserted
near center comes out clean.

8 SERVINGS

Each with: 391 Calories (42% from Fat, 29% from Protein, 29% from Carb);
29 g Protein; 18 g Total Fat; 7 g Saturated Fat; 5 g Monounsaturated Fat; 3 g
Polyunsaturated Fat; 28 g Carb; 3 g Fiber; 4 g Sugar; 442 mg Phosphorus; 308 mg
Calcium; 857 mg Sodium; 691 mg Potassium; 1534 IU Vitamin A; 90 mg ATE Vitamin
E; 69 mg Vitamin C; 48 mg Cholesterol

Breakfast Quesadilla

This is a fairly traditional breakfast quesadilla, but it has the increased nutrition of added vegetables.

1 slice low sodium bacon
¼ cup (40 g) onion, chopped
½ cup (75 g) red bell pepper, chopped
¼ cup (60 ml) egg substitute
2 tablespoons (22 g) black beans
1 ounce (28 g) fat-free sour cream, divided
3 tablespoons (49 g) salsa, divided
1 whole wheat tortilla, 6-inch (15 cm)
¾ ounce (21 g) Swiss cheese

Cook bacon according to package directions, either in a pan with nonstick vegetable oil spray or in the microwave. Once cool enough to handle, roughly chop and set aside. Bring a medium large pan (at least the size of the tortilla) sprayed with nonstick vegetable oil spray to medium heat. Add the red bell pepper and onion and cook until softened, about 3 minutes. Add egg substitute and scramble until fully cooked. Transfer mixture to a bowl and set pan aside to cool. Add bacon, beans, 1 tablespoon (15 g) sour cream and 1 tablespoon (16 g) salsa to the egg scramble bowl. Lightly mix and set aside. Clean and dry the pan, spray with nonstick vegetable oil spray, and bring to medium-high heat. Place tortilla flat in the pan and sprinkle evenly with cheese. Spoon egg mixture over one half of the tortilla, fold the other half over the mixture to form the quesadilla, and then press down with a spatula to seal. Cook until both sides are crispy, about 2 minutes per side. Top with remaining salsa and sour cream.

1 SERVING

Each with: 400 Calories (34% from Fat, 22% from Protein, 44% from Carb); 22 g Protein; 15 g Total Fat; 7 g Unsaturated Fat; 5 g Monounsaturated Fat; 2 g Polyunsaturated Fat; 45 g Carb; 6 g Fiber; 9 g Sugar; 380 mg Phosphorus; 362 mg Calcium; 786 mg Sodium; 788 mg Potassium; 3168 IU Vitamin A; 73 mg ATE Vitamin E; 152 mg Vitamin C; 31 mg Cholesterol

Cheese and Vegetable Frittata

This is one of those recipes that ended up being quite a bit fewer than 400 calories. But if we put any more vegetables in it, it wouldn't fit in the pan. As low as it is, I guarantee you won't go away hungry.

2 cups (200 g) fresh green beans
1 cup (130) carrot, chopped
1 cup (100 g) cauliflower florets
¼ cup (80 g) onion, chopped
8 ounces (225 g) spinach
½ cup (75 g) green bell pepper, diced
½ cup (120 ml) egg substitute
1 cup (235 ml) fat-free evaporated milk
¼ cup (60 ml) water
1¾ cups (205 g) low fat cheddar cheese, shredded
⅛ teaspoon black pepper

Steam the vegetables for about 5 minutes, just to soften a little. In a mixing bowl, beat the egg substitute with the evaporated milk and water. Add ¾ cup (90 g) cheese and black pepper and mix well. Place the vegetables in an 8 × 8-inch (20 × 20 cm) glass baking dish. Cool slightly and then pour the liquid over. Sprinkle with remaining cheese. Bake for about 35 minutes at 375°F (190°C, or gas mark 5).

4 SERVINGS

Each with: 234 Calories (22% from Fat, 44% from Protein, 35% from Carb); 26 g Protein; 6 g Total Fat; 3 g Unsaturated Fat; 2 g Monounsaturated Fat; 1 g Polyunsaturated Fat; 21 g Carb; 5 g Fiber; 12 g Sugar; 519 mg Phosphorus; 538 mg Calcium; 559 mg Sodium; 979 mg Potassium; 10 108 IU Vitamin A; 110 mg ATE Vitamin E; 57 mg Vitamin C; 15 mg Cholesterol

Tortillas for Breakfast

And why not have tortillas for breakfast? These are made in a style like enchiladas. Extra lean ground beef adds a flavor boost while allowing the calories to stay low. Lots of veggies and eggs provide the bulk and the nutrition.

2 teaspoons olive oil
1 cup (160 g) onion, chopped
¾ pound (340 g) extra lean ground beef
1 cup (150 g) green bell pepper, chopped
¼ teaspoon black pepper
1½ cups (355 ml) egg substitute
6 whole wheat tortillas, 8-inch (20 cm)
½ cup (115 g) fat-free sour cream
½ cup (130 g) salsa

Heat oil in large fry pan. Add chopped onion, beef, green bell pepper, and black pepper. Stir-fry until tender. Pour egg substitute over onion mix and cook until half-cooked. Spoon into tortilla shells and roll. Bake at 350°F (180°C, or gas mark 4) for 25 minutes. Top with sour cream and salsa and bake 5 to 10 minutes longer.

6 SERVINGS

Each with: 397 Calories (44% from Fat, 24% from Protein, 32% from Carb); 23 g Protein; 19 g Total Fat; 7 g Unsaturated Fat; 8 g Monounsaturated Fat; 2 g Polyunsaturated Fat; 32 g Carb; 3 g Fiber; 3 g Sugar; 250 mg Phosphorus; 130 mg Calcium; 470 mg Sodium; 583 mg Potassium; 538 IU Vitamin A; 20 mg ATE Vitamin E; 25 mg Vitamin C; 48 mg Cholesterol

Chile Relleno Casserole

Chili relleno is not a dish that we usually associate with breakfast, but adding extra egg turns it into a breakfast full of flavor and nutrition.

4 ounces (115 g) green chili peppers, whole

8 ounces (225 g) low fat cheddar cheese, grated

4 ounces (115 g) low fat Monterey Jack cheese, grated

1 cup (235 ml) egg substitute

2 tablespoons (16 g) all purpose flour

14 ounces (425 ml) fat-free evaporated milk

Rinse chilies and remove seeds. Place half the chilies in a greased casserole dish. Sprinkle half of both cheeses on top and add remaining chilies. Top with remaining cheese. Beat egg substitute, flour, and evaporated milk until smooth. Pour over top and bake about 45 minutes in 350°F (180°C, or gas mark 4) oven.

3 SERVINGS

Each with: 397 Calories (26% from Fat, 50% from Protein, 24% from Carb); 48 g Protein; 11 g Total Fat; 6 g Unsaturated Fat; 3 g Monounsaturated Fat; 2 g Polyunsaturated Fat; 23 g Carb; 1 g Fiber; 16 g Sugar; 918 mg Phosphorus; 913 mg Calcium; 1144 mg Sodium; 838 mg Potassium; 1105 IU Vitamin A; 224 mg ATE Vitamin E; 15 mg Vitamin C; 30 mg Cholesterol

Not Exactly Eggs Benedict

This will remind you of Eggs Benedict, but it's easier to fix. Eggs are baked in cheese until well enough done, then served on English muffins in a breakfast that is filling as well as tasty.

½ cup (115 g) low fat cheddar cheese, shredded

4 eggs

¼ cup (60 g) fat-free sour cream

3 tablespoons (45 ml) skim milk

½ teaspoon prepared mustard

⅛ teaspoon black pepper

¼ teaspoon Worcestershire sauce

1½ tablespoons (12 g) all purpose flour

2 English muffins, split and toasted

Sprinkle half the cheese evenly over the bottom of greased baking dish. Break and slip eggs onto cheese in dish. Beat together remaining ingredients except remaining cheese and muffins. Pour over eggs, sprinkle with remaining cheese. Bake in a 325°F (170°C, or gas mark 3) oven until whites are set and yolks are soft and creamy, about 25 to 30 minutes. Serve over toasted muffin halves.

2 SERVINGS

Each with: 412 Calories (41% from Fat, 29% from Protein, 30% from Carb); 29 g Protein; 19 g Total Fat; 7 g Unsaturated Fat; 6 g Monounsaturated Fat; 2 g Polyunsaturated Fat; 30 g Carb; 2 g Fiber; 3 g Sugar; 512 mg Phosphorus; 363 mg Calcium; 659 mg Sodium; 342 mg Potassium; 795 IU Vitamin A; 225 mg ATE Vitamin E; 2 mg Vitamin C; 510 mg Cholesterol

Fancy Baked Egg Scramble

Here's a great company breakfast that no one will suspect is low calorie and full of nutrition (unless you want to brag about it of course). Eggs and vegetables are baked in a cheesy, creamy sauce with a crunchy topping that really makes this something special.

Eggs

2 tablespoons (28 g) unsalted butter

¼ cup (40 g) onion, chopped

¼ cup (38 g) green bell pepper, chopped

2 cups (300 g) ham, cubed

3 cups (700 ml) egg substitute

8 ounces (225 g) mushrooms, sliced

Sauce

2 tablespoons (16 g) all purpose flour

1 tablespoon (14 g) unsalted butter

1½ cups (355 ml) skim milk

2 ounces (55 g) Swiss cheese, shredded

¼ cup (25 g) Parmesan cheese, grated

Topping

1 cup (115 g) bread crumbs

¼ cup (25 g) Parmesan cheese, grated

2 tablespoons (8 g) fresh parsley, chopped

Preheat oven to 350°F (180°C, or gas mark 4). Grease a 2-quart (1.9 L) baking dish. Melt 2 tablespoons (28 g) butter in large skillet. Cook and stir onion and green bell pepper until onion is crisp-tender. Add ham and egg substitute; cook over medium heat until eggs are firm but moist, stirring occasionally. Fold in mushrooms. Remove from heat. Melt 1 tablespoon (14 g) butter in medium saucepan. Blend in flour; cook until smooth and bubbly. Gradually add skim milk; cook until mixture boils and thickens, stirring constantly. Add Swiss cheese and ¼ cup (25 g) Parmesan cheese; stir until smooth. Fold scrambled eggs into sauce. Pour into greased pan. Combine all topping ingredients and sprinkle over eggs. Bake at 350°F (180°C, or gas mark 4) for 25 to 30 minutes or until light golden brown.

6 SERVINGS

Each with: 424 Calories (43% from Fat, 36% from Protein, 21% from Carb); 37 g Protein; 20 g Total Fat; 9 g Unsaturated Fat; 6 g Monounsaturated Fat; 3 g Polyunsaturated Fat; 22 g Carb; 2 g Fiber; 3 g Sugar; 512 mg Phosphorus; 381 mg Calcium; 1021 mg Sodium; 897 mg Potassium; 996 IU Vitamin A; 115 mg ATE Vitamin E; 9 mg Vitamin C; 53 mg Cholesterol

Fiesta Eggs

Green chilies and taco seasoning provide the Southwestern flavor of this beef, egg, and cheese bake. It's as good for lunch and dinner as breakfast, but that is when we usually have it.

½ pound (225 g) extra lean ground beef

2 tablespoons (6 g) taco seasoning mix

¾ cup (86 g) low fat Monterey Jack cheese, shredded

1 cup (115 g) low fat cheddar cheese, shredded

4 ounces (115 g) green chilies, diced

1½ cups (355 ml) skim milk

⅓ cup (42 g) all purpose flour

2 cups (475 ml) egg substitute

½ cup (130 g) salsa

In medium skillet, brown ground beef; drain off excess fat. Stir in taco seasoning mix. In 12 × 8-inch (30 × 20 cm) baking dish, toss beef mixture with cheese and chilies. In large bowl, blend a small amount of skim milk into flour until smooth. Stir in remaining skim milk and egg substitute. Pour milk mixture over mixture in dish. Bake at 350°F (180°C, or gas mark 4) for 40 to 50 minutes or until knife inserted in center comes out clean. Let stand 10 minutes before cutting into serving pieces. Spoon salsa over servings.

4 SERVINGS

Each with: 429 Calories (39% from Fat, 43% from Protein, 17% from Carb); 45 g Protein; 18 g Total Fat; 7 g Unsaturated Fat; 7 g Monounsaturated Fat; 3 g Polyunsaturated Fat; 18 g Carb; 1 g Fiber; 2 g Sugar; 637 mg Phosphorus; 464 mg Calcium; 921 mg Sodium; 893 mg Potassium; 1011 IU Vitamin A; 91 mg ATE Vitamin E; 15 mg Vitamin C; 54 mg Cholesterol

Breakfast in a Pocket

This breakfast sandwich starts with hard boiled eggs so it's really quick to make if you have the eggs cooked ahead of time. We then add cheese and vegetables to up the nutrition level, ending up with a filling meal for around 350 calories.

3 eggs, hard boiled

2 ounces (55 g) low fat cheddar cheese, grated

2 whole wheat pita breads, 6-inch (15 cm)

1 cup (180 g) tomato, chopped

½ cup (52 g) sprouts

Peel and slice hard boiled eggs. Grate cheese. Divide cheese and egg between pocket bread halves and microwave approximately 25 seconds or until cheese is melted. Add tomato and sprouts.

2 SERVINGS

Each with: 358 Calories (29% from Fat, 28% from Protein, 43% from Carb); 24 g Protein; 12 g Total Fat; 4 g Unsaturated Fat; 4 g Monounsaturated Fat; 2 g Polyunsaturated Fat; 38 g Carb; 2 g Fiber; 4 g Sugar; 385 mg Phosphorus; 225 mg Calcium; 621 mg Sodium; 390 mg Potassium; 1116 IU Vitamin A; 138 mg ATE Vitamin E; 10 mg Vitamin C; 374 mg Cholesterol

Spinach and Bacon Special

Here's another baked omelet kind of a dish. This one has the nutrition kicked into high gear with spinach, one of the green leafy vegetables right at the top of the ANDI index of nutrient density. But even more important, it tastes good.

16 ounces (455 g) fat-free cottage cheese

20 ounces (570 g) frozen spinach, drain well

4 ounces (115 g) low fat cheddar cheese, grated

5 tablespoons (40 g) all purpose flour

1½ cups (355 ml) egg substitute

2 tablespoons (28 ml) lemon juice

⅛ teaspoon black pepper

12 slices low sodium bacon, fried very crisp

Thaw spinach in colander; drain very well. Mix all together except bacon. Put in 9-inch (23 cm) greased pan. Bake at 325°F (170°C, or gas mark 3) for 1½ hours. Break bacon into bits. Sprinkle evenly on top. Return to oven for a few minutes. Remove and let set before slicing.

4 SERVINGS

Each with: 410 Calories (37% from Fat, 45% from Protein, 17% from Carb); 46 g Protein; 17 g Total Fat; 6 g Unsaturated Fat; 6 g Monounsaturated Fat; 3 g Polyunsaturated Fat; 18 g Carb; 3 g Fiber; 5 g Sugar; 612 mg Phosphorus; 382 mg Calcium; 1161 mg Sodium; 1374 mg Potassium; 13 749 IU Vitamin A; 32 mg ATE Vitamin E; 44 mg Vitamin C; 38 mg Cholesterol

Spinach and Mushroom Quiche with Spinach Salad

This versatile dish can work for breakfast, lunch, or dinner. We like it for weekend breakfasts to get the day off to a great start.

Quiche

4 slices low sodium bacon

1 cup (160 g) onion, chopped

1 cup (235 ml) egg substitute, beaten

1 cup (235 ml) fat-free evaporated milk

1 cup (235 ml) skim milk

1 tablespoon (8 g) all purpose flour

⅛ teaspoon nutmeg

12 ounces (340 g) spinach, thawed and chopped

12 ounces (340 g) mushrooms, sliced, divided

1 cup (115 g) Monterey Jack cheese, shredded

1 cup (115 g) low fat cheddar cheese, shredded

1 pie crust

Salad

1 pound (455 g) fresh spinach

5 ounces (140 g) water chestnuts

2 oranges, sectioned

2 tablespoons (28 ml) orange juice

1 tablespoon (15 ml) reduced sodium soy sauce

¼ teaspoon dry mustard

⅛ teaspoon black pepper

Sauté bacon and onion. Crumble bacon. Mix together the egg substitute, evaporated milk, skim milk, flour, nutmeg, thawed frozen spinach, mushrooms, and cheeses. Add the bacon and onion. Pour into pie crust in quiche baking dish. Bake at 325°F (170°C, or gas mark 3) for 50 minutes. Let stand 10 minutes before serving. Assemble the salad. Combine the fresh spinach, water chestnuts, and orange sections. Whisk together the orange juice, soy sauce, dry mustard, and black pepper. Arrange the salad on each plate and drizzle with dressing. Serve with a wedge of quiche alongside.

8 SERVINGS

Each with: 305 g Water ; 384 Calories (39% from Fat, 25% from Protein, 36% from Carb); 25 g Protein; 17 g Total Fat; 7 g Saturated Fat; 6 g Monounsaturated Fat; 3 g Polyunsaturated Fat; 36 g Carb; 7 g Fiber; 11 g Sugar; 437 mg Phosphorus; 527 mg Calcium; 4 mg Iron; 474 mg Sodium; 991 mg Potassium; 12 539 IU Vitamin A; 99 mg ATE Vitamin E; 32 mg Vitamin C; 25 mg Cholesterol

Apple Strata

We often have a strata for Christmas morning breakfast. It's great because you can make it the night before and all you need to do in the morning is put it in the oven. Of course, that also works any other night when you want a good hot breakfast.

---

6 slices whole wheat bread, cubed
4 cups (440 g) apples, peeled and sliced
1 cup (150 g) ham, cubed
4 ounces (115 g) cheddar cheese, shredded
1 cup (235 ml) egg substitute
¼ cup (60 ml) skim milk

Cube bread and place in 9-inch (23 cm) square pan sprayed with nonstick vegetable oil spray. Slice apples over bread. Sprinkle with ham and cheese. Combine egg substitute and skim milk and pour over. Cover with plastic wrap and refrigerate overnight. Preheat oven to 350°F (180°C, or gas mark 4). Bake uncovered for 40 to 45 minutes or until top is lightly browned and center is set.

4 SERVINGS

Each with: 208 g Water ; 384 Calories (37% from Fat, 28% from Protein, 35% from Carb); 27 g Protein; 16 g Total Fat; 8 g Saturated Fat; 5 g Monounsaturated Fat; 2 g Polyunsaturated Fat; 34 g Carb; 3 g Fiber; 14 g Sugar; 386 mg Phosphorus; 321 mg Calcium; 3 mg Iron; 865 mg Sodium; 554 mg Potassium; 583 IU Vitamin A; 83 mg ATE Vitamin E; 5 mg Vitamin C; 45 mg Cholesterol

Baked French Toast

This makes an easy make-ahead breakfast for a weekend or holiday.

---

8 slices whole wheat bread, cubed

¾ cup (175 ml) egg substitute

3 tablespoons (27 g) sugar

1 teaspoon vanilla

2¼ cups (535 ml) skim milk

¼ cup (31 g) all purpose flour

6 tablespoons (6 g) brown sugar substitute, such as Splenda

½ teaspoon cinnamon, packed

2 tablespoons (28 g) unsalted butter

2 cups blueberries, fresh (290 g) or frozen (310 g)

 Tip: You can substitute strawberries or raspberries or use some combination of fruit, if you prefer.

Cut bread into cubes and place in a greased 9 × 13-inch (23 × 33 cm) baking dish. In a medium bowl, lightly beat egg substitute, sugar, and vanilla. Stir in the skim milk until well blended. Pour over bread, turning pieces to coat well. Cover and refrigerate overnight. Preheat oven to 375°F (190°C, or gas mark 5). In a small bowl, combine the flour, brown sugar substitute, and cinnamon. Cut in butter until mixture resembles coarse crumbs. Turn bread over in baking dish. Cover with blueberries. Sprinkle evenly with crumb mixture. Bake about 40 minutes until golden brown.

6 SERVINGS

Each with: 391 Calories (16% from Fat, 12% from Protein, 71% from Carb); 12 g Protein; 7 g Total Fat; 3 g Saturated Fat; 2 g Monounsaturated Fat; 1 g Polyunsaturated Fat; 70 g Carb; 3 g Fiber; 39 g Sugar; 202 mg Phosphorus; 217 mg Calcium; 131 mg Sodium; 416 mg Potassium; 450 IU Vitamin A; 88 mg ATE Vitamin E; 2 mg Vitamin C; 13 mg Cholesterol

Strawberry Dream Pancakes

These taste and look like they contain a lot of calories, but they don't. Thanks to fat-free ingredients, the creamy rich topping contributes well under 100 calories. The strawberries up the nutrition, as does the whole wheat flour, providing a satisfying breakfast that doesn't look like diet food.

Topping

4½ ounces (130 g) fat-free frozen whipped topping, thawed

⅓ cup (77 g) fat-free sour cream

16 ounces (455 g) frozen strawberries, thawed

Pancakes

2 cups (240 g) whole wheat pastry flour

¼ cup (50 g) sugar

2 tablespoons baking powder

½ teaspoon baking soda

½ cup (120 ml) egg substitute

1½, cups (355 ml) skim milk

8 ounces (225 g) fat-free sour cream

2 tablespoons (28 ml) canola oil

Thoroughly drain strawberries. Chop ½ cup (64 g) drained strawberries; reserve remainder for topping. Combine reserved strawberries, whipped topping, and ⅓ cup (77 g) sour cream. Set aside. In a medium bowl, mix flour, sugar, baking powder, and baking soda. In another medium bowl, mix egg substitute, skim milk, sour cream, and oil. Add to flour mixture. Add ½ cup (64 g) chopped strawberries. Stir only until combined; the batter will still be lumpy. Preheat griddle. Brush preheated griddle with oil. Using ¼ cup (55 g) batter for each pancake, cook over medium-high heat 2 to 3 minutes or until underside is golden brown and surface is bubbly. Turn and cook 2 to 3 minutes more or until other side is golden brown. Keep warm. Place a pancake on each of 6 serving plates. Spread with about ⅓ cup (85 g) of topping. Place remaining pancakes on top. Garnish with an additional dollop of topping and a fresh strawberry if desired.

6 SERVINGS

Each with: 389 Calories (34% from Fat, 12% from Protein, 54% from Carb); 13 g Protein; 15 g Total Fat; 7 g Unsaturated Fat; 5 g Monounsaturated Fat; 2 g Polyunsaturated Fat; 55 g Carb; 6 g Fiber; 20 g Sugar; 409 mg Phosphorus; 452 mg Calcium; 694 mg Sodium; 531 mg Potassium; 419 IU Vitamin A; 89 mg ATE Vitamin E; 45 mg Vitamin C; 22 mg Cholesterol

Strawberry Banana Three Ways Breakfast

If you are a strawberry and banana fan, this is the breakfast for you. Start with strawberry–banana muffins. But make them healthier by using whole wheat flour and holding down the amount of oil. Then don't make the huge muffins you think you need to fill you up. Instead, fill up on fresh strawberries and bananas topped with—what else—strawberry–banana yogurt.

Muffins

¾ cup (90 g) whole wheat pastry flour

2 tablespoons (3 g) sugar substitute, such as Splenda

¼ cup (29 g) wheat germ

1¼ teaspoon baking powder

¼ teaspoon baking soda

2 tablespoons (28 ml) egg substitute

½ cup (120 ml) skim milk

¼ cup (60 ml) canola oil

½ cup (113 g) banana, mashed

½ cup (75 g) strawberries, chopped

Fruit

4 cups (580 g) strawberries

3 cups (450 g) banana, sliced

8 ounces (225 g) low fat strawberry–banana yogurt

Stir together the dry ingredients. Mix together the rest of the ingredients and stir into dry, stirring until just moistened. Spoon into 6 greased or paper lined muffin tins. Bake at 350°F (180°C, or gas mark 4) for 20 to 25 minutes or until done. While muffins are baking, slice fruit into a bowl and top with yogurt.

6 SERVINGS

Each with: 352 Calories (27% from Fat, 9% from Protein, 64% from Carb); 8 g Protein; 11 g Total Fat; 1 g Saturated Fat; 6 g Monounsaturated Fat; 3 g Polyunsaturated Fat; 60 g Carb; 8 g Fiber; 28 g Sugar; 246 mg Phosphorus; 168 mg Calcium; 198 mg Sodium; 877 mg Potassium; 177 IU Vitamin A; 13 mg ATE Vitamin E; 79 mg Vitamin C; 4 mg Cholesterol

Breakfast Fruit (with Some Cereal)

A big helping of warm, lightly spiced fruit tops granola in this breakfast that is perfect for cool mornings. Almost fat free and full of natural fiber and nutrition, it will warm you up and keep you going.

3 apples, peeled and thickly sliced
½ cup (88 g) prunes, pitted
¾ cup (110 g) raisins
1 orange, peeled and sectioned
3¼ cups (765 ml) water, divided
½ cup (12 g) sugar substitute
½ teaspoon ground cinnamon
2 tablespoons (16 g) cornstarch
4 cups (500 g) granola

 Tip: This will keep well in the refrigerator for up to a week.

In a saucepan, combine apples, prunes, raisins, orange, and 3 cups (700 ml) water. Bring to boil, reduce heat, and simmer 10 minutes. Stir in sugar substitute and cinnamon. Combine cornstarch and remaining water. Stir into saucepan. Cook for 2 minutes. Serve over granola.

6 SERVINGS

Each with: 352 Calories (7% from Fat, 6% from Protein, 87% from Carb); 6 g Protein; 3 g Total Fat; 1 g Unsaturated Fat; 1 g Monounsaturated Fat; 1 g Polyunsaturated Fat; 80 g Carb; 6 g Fiber; 45 g Sugar; 189 mg Phosphorus; 54 mg Calcium; 212 mg Sodium; 488 mg Potassium; 165 IU Vitamin A; 0 mg ATE Vitamin E; 20 mg Vitamin C; 0 mg Cholesterol

Hot Fruit and Nut Cereal

A sweet and satisfying breakfast for those chilly mornings, it's full of nutrition from all the fruit as well as the cholesterol-fighting oats.

4 apples, peeled and quartered
1 orange, peeled and chopped
1 cup (80 g) rolled oats
¼ cup (29 g) wheat germ
½ cup (89 g) dates
½ cup (55 g) slivered almonds
2 tablespoons (40 g) honey

Chop fruit. Cook oats according to package directions. Add wheat germ and mix. Then add fruit and nuts. Drizzle honey over top.

4 SERVINGS

Each with: 386 Calories (25% from Fat, 10% from Protein, 65% from Carb); 10 g Protein; 11 g Total Fat; 1 g Unsaturated Fat; 6 g Monounsaturated Fat; 3 g Polyunsaturated Fat; 68 g Carb; 10 g Fiber; 42 g Sugar; 296 mg Phosphorus; 94 mg Calcium; 2 mg Sodium; 616 mg Potassium; 162 IU Vitamin A; 0 mg ATE Vitamin E; 30 mg Vitamin C; 0 mg Cholesterol

Stuffed Cantaloupe

Well it IS stuffed, but it's stuffed with fruit, not the usual kind of stuffing. This raises the question of how anything that tastes this good can have so much nutrition and be this low in calories. The answer of course is that's exactly why fruit is so good for us.

2 cantaloupes, halved and cleaned

16 ounces (455 g) strawberries, cleaned and halved

16 ounces (455 g) seedless green grapes

2 bananas, sliced

4 apricots, pitted and chopped in quarters

12 ounces (340 g) low fat blackberry yogurt

1 cup (125 g) granola

fresh mint, for garnish

Mix all fruit except cantaloupe. Heap everything into the cantaloupe center, spoon yogurt on top of fruit mixture, top with granola, and garnish with sprig of mint.

4 SERVINGS

Each with: 363 Calories (6% from Fat, 7% from Protein, 86% from Carb); 7 g Protein; 3 g Total Fat; 1 g Unsaturated Fat; 1 g Monounsaturated Fat; 0 g Polyunsaturated Fat; 84 g Carb; 7 g Fiber; 59 g Sugar; 199 mg Phosphorus; 167 mg Calcium; 129 mg Sodium; 920 mg Potassium; 855 IU Vitamin A; 9 mg ATE Vitamin E; 60 mg Vitamin C; 4 mg Cholesterol

Cherry Parfait

This is really more like a dessert than a breakfast, with sweet cherries added into a creamy mixture that is layered with shredded wheat cereal for crunch (and fiber).

1½ cups (233 g) cherries, pitted and cut into halves

½ cup (115 g) plain low fat yogurt

1 teaspoon honey

½ teaspoon vanilla extract

1 cup (49 g) shredded wheat, crumbled

In a bowl, combine the first 4 ingredients, mixing until blended. Layer into parfait glasses with cereal.

2 SERVINGS

Each with: 379 Calories (4% from Fat, 8% from Protein, 87% from Carb); 9 g Protein; 2 g Total Fat; 1 g Unsaturated Fat; 0 g Monounsaturated Fat; 0 g Polyunsaturated Fat; 90 g Carb; 10 g Fiber; 65 g Sugar; 229 mg Phosphorus; 169 mg Calcium; 58 mg Sodium; 1365 mg Potassium; 3545 IU Vitamin A; 9 mg ATE Vitamin E; 1 mg Vitamin C; 4 mg Cholesterol

Breakfast in Paradise Smoothies

This smoothie will whisk you away to the islands, with its bananas, melons, and papaya. Smoothies make a great quick breakfast, but if you aren't careful when building them, you'll be hungry again before noon. This one solves that problem with a generous amount of fruit and a boost from tofu for added protein.

8 ounces (225 g) soft tofu
2 cups (280 g) papaya, peeled and chopped
2 cups (300 g) banana, sliced
1 cup (160 g) cantaloupe, peeled and cubed
½ cup (120 ml) skim milk
½ cup (120 ml) orange juice

Place all ingredients in blender and process until smooth.

2 SERVINGS

Each with: 400 Calories (9% from Fat, 12% from Protein, 79% from Carb); 12 g Protein; 4 g Total Fat; 1 g Saturated Fat; 1 g Monounsaturated Fat; 2 g Polyunsaturated Fat; 85 g Carb; 9 g Fiber; 44 g Sugar; 216 mg Phosphorus; 182 mg Calcium; 63 mg Sodium; 1836 mg Potassium; 4842 IU Vitamin A; 38 mg ATE Vitamin E; 160 mg Vitamin C; 1 mg Cholesterol

Dreamcicle Smoothie

Low fat buttermilk and orange juice concentrate provide the flavor here as well as the nutrition. Oat bran gives it a nice fiber boost.

1 cup (235 ml) low fat buttermilk
⅓ cup (95 g) orange juice concentrate
2 tablespoons (30 g) brown sugar
1 teaspoon vanilla
¼ cup (24 g) oat bran
½ cup (115 g) crushed ice

In a blender container, combine low fat buttermilk, orange juice concentrate, brown sugar, vanilla, and oat bran. Cover and blend until smooth. With blender running, add ice slowly through the opening in lid. Blend until smooth and frothy.

1 SERVING

Each with: 407 Calories (6% from Fat, 12% from Protein, 82% from Carb); 12 g Protein; 3 g Total Fat; 1 g Saturated Fat; 1 g Monounsaturated Fat; 0 g Polyunsaturated Fat; 84 g Carb; 2 g Fiber; 76 g Sugar; 337 mg Phosphorus; 364 mg Calcium; 4 mg Iron; 317 mg Sodium; 1159 mg Potassium; 532 IU Vitamin A; 50 mg ATE Vitamin E; 134 mg Vitamin C; 10 mg Cholesterol

Mixed Fruit Smoothie

Smoothies make a quick and easy breakfast, and they are packed with nutrition. The protein from the yogurt will help to keep you from being hungry as the morning goes on.

2 cups (460 g) low fat peach
  yogurt
1 cup (145 g) blueberries
2 cups (300 g) banana, sliced

Mix all ingredients in a blender and then serve.

2 SERVINGS

Each with: 382 Calories (3% from Fat, 11% from Protein, 86% from Carb); 14 g Protein; 1 g Total Fat; 1 g Saturated Fat; 0 g Monounsaturated Fat; 0 g Polyunsaturated Fat; 108 g Carb; 8 g Fiber; 81 g Sugar; 350 mg Phosphorus; 388 mg Calcium; 145 mg Sodium; 1337 mg Potassium; 213 IU Vitamin A; 5 mg ATE Vitamin E; 28 mg Vitamin C; 5 mg Cholesterol

Full of Fruit Healthy Shake

This smoothie is quick to fix and eat, but it provides a huge amount of nutrients like antioxidants, as well as the bulk and protein to keep you from being hungry before lunch.

2 bananas
1 cup (160 g) cantaloupe
1 cup (145 g) blueberries
2 cups (460 g) nonfat vanilla
  yogurt

Place all of the ingredients into blender and blend until smooth. Thaw fruit if frozen.

2 SERVINGS

Each with: 413 Calories (8% from Fat, 14% from Protein, 78% from Carb); 15 g Protein; 4 g Total Fat; 2 g Unsaturated Fat; 1 g Monounsaturated Fat; 0 g Polyunsaturated Fat; 86 g Carb; 6 g Fiber; 66 g Sugar; 386 mg Phosphorus; 439 mg Calcium; 178 mg Sodium; 1366 mg Potassium; 3234 IU Vitamin A; 29 mg ATE Vitamin E; 55 mg Vitamin C; 12 mg Cholesterol

Tropical Smoothie

There's protein from the yogurt, nutrition and bulk from the fruit, the "carry me away to the islands" taste, and all for less than 350 calories. That's the kind of breakfast I like.

½ cup (113 g) frozen strawberries
½ cup (80 g) crushed pineapple, drained
½ cup (115 g) plain low fat yogurt
¼ cup (60 ml) pineapple juice, unsweetened
1 banana

Blend all ingredients together in a blender for a great breakfast drink or after school snack. This recipe may easily be doubled or tripled.

1 SERVING

Each with: 336 Calories (7% from Fat, 10% from Protein, 83% from Carb); 9 g Protein; 3 g Total Fat; 1 g Unsaturated Fat; 1 g Monounsaturated Fat; 0 g Polyunsaturated Fat; 74 g Carb; 7 g Fiber; 55 g Sugar; 241 mg Phosphorus; 272 mg Calcium; 90 mg Sodium; 1156 mg Potassium; 219 IU Vitamin A; 17 mg ATE Vitamin E; 75 mg Vitamin C; 7 mg Cholesterol

New Ways to Think about Breakfast

Breakfast, it's not just for eggs anymore. This chapter is an attempt to get you to think differently about the things you eat. There are some recipes here that have eggs in them. There are also recipes with eggplant, curry powder, black beans, and things that aren't the first foods that come to most people's minds when they think about breakfast. But there's no reason these things can't be part of healthy, tasty filling meals at the start of the day as well as the end. You just need to think about it in the right way.

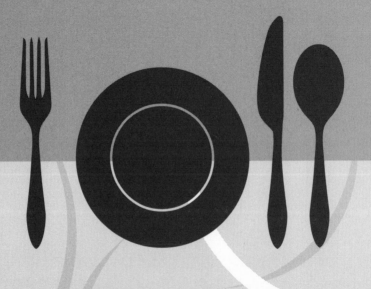

And Why Not Shrimp for Breakfast?

Of course, you could also have it for lunch or dinner, but why not try a shrimp quiche for breakfast. It is kind of an egg dish, and it has the kind of ingredients that will get you out of bed to begin with and keep you going all morning once you've eaten it.

Pastry

⅓ cup (60 ml) olive oil

1⅓ cups (160 g) whole wheat pastry flour

2 tablespoons (28 ml) cold water

Filling

½ cup (80 g) onion, chopped

8 ounces (225 g) mushrooms, chopped

1 tablespoon (15 ml) olive oil

¾ cup (175 ml) egg substitute

1½ cups (355 ml) skim milk

1 tablespoon (8 g) all purpose flour

¼ teaspoon black pepper

6 ounces (170 g) shrimp, cooked, thawed

1½ cups (107 g) broccoli florets

6 ounces (170 g) low fat Swiss cheese, shredded

Cut the oil into the flour until the pieces are the size of peas. Add the water, one tablespoon (15 ml) at a time, tossing with a fork, until all the dough is moistened. Form into a ball. Roll out to ⅛-inch (3 mm) thickness. Line a 9-inch (23 cm) pie plate with dough, trimming off any that extends over the edge. Line pastry with double layer of foil and fill with dry beans. Bake in 450°F (230°C, or gas mark 8) oven for 5 minutes. Remove from oven and remove beans and foil. Reduce oven temperature to 325°F (170°C, or gas mark 3). In a skillet, sauté the onion and mushrooms in oil until soft. Combine the egg substitute, skim milk, flour, and black pepper with a whisk. Stir in onion–mushroom mixture, shrimp, broccoli, and cheese. Pour into the hot pastry shell. Bake at 325°F (170°C, or gas mark 3) for 30 to 35 minutes until a knife inserted near center comes out clean. Cover edge of pastry with foil if necessary to prevent over browning. Let stand 10 minutes before slicing.

6 SERVINGS

Each with: 371 Calories (43% from Fat, 27% from Protein, 30% from Carb); 26 g Protein; 18 g Total Fat; 3 g Saturated Fat; 11 g Monounsaturated Fat; 2 g Polyunsaturated Fat; 28 g Carb; 4 g Fiber; 2 g Sugar; 458 mg Phosphorus; 411 mg Calcium; 238 mg Sodium; 605 mg Potassium; 880 IU Vitamin A; 68 mg ATE Vitamin E; 20 mg Vitamin C; 67 mg Cholesterol

California Breakfast Sandwich

As sort of California version of Eggs Benedict, this is a great weekend breakfast. This is the kind of meal you could serve to guests and everyone would be happy and full and never know that it is low in calories.

½ cup (58 g) low fat cheddar cheese
1 cup (160 g) onion, chopped
1½ cups (225 g) green bell pepper, chopped
6 ounces (170 g) mushrooms, sliced
1 tablespoon (14 g) unsalted butter
1 avocado, sliced
1½ cups (270 g) tomato, chopped
1 cup (150 g) ham, chopped
1½ cups (355 ml) egg substitute
6 whole wheat English muffins

Grate cheese; chop vegetables. Beat egg substitute. Brown chopped onion and green bell pepper until limp in large skillet with butter. Add mushrooms, avocado, tomato, and ham. Stir. Add egg substitute. Cook until almost set; add grated cheese. Spoon onto toasted English muffins.

6 SERVINGS

Each with: 360 Calories (37% from Fat, 24% from Protein, 38% from Carb); 22 g Protein; 15 g Total Fat; 5 g Saturated Fat; 6 g Monounsaturated Fat; 3 g Polyunsaturated Fat; 35 g Carb; 6 g Fiber; 5 g Sugar; 309 mg Phosphorus; 234 mg Calcium; 654 mg Sodium; 833 mg Potassium; 888 IU Vitamin A; 44 mg ATE Vitamin E; 40 mg Vitamin C; 27 mg Cholesterol

Broccoli for Breakfast?

Eggs and veggies are a favorite breakfast combination around our house. But you may not think of broccoli first when you think of breakfast. Let me tell you that you should. This makes a great breakfast that's low in calories and high in nutrition and bulk.

24 ounces (680 g) low fat cottage cheese
8 ounces (225 g) mushrooms, sliced
20 ounces (570 g) frozen broccoli, thawed and drained
2½ cups (283 g) low fat cheddar cheese, shredded, divided
1½ cups (355 ml) egg substitute
⅓ cup (42 g) all purpose flour
¼ cup (55 g) unsalted butter, melted
3 tablespoons (30 g) onion, finely chopped

In a large bowl, combine all ingredients, reserving ½ cup (58 g) of the cheddar cheese. Pour into a 2-quart (1.9 L) casserole and bake at 350°F (180°C, or gas mark 4) until eggs are set, about 40 minutes. Sprinkle remaining cheese on top and return to oven just long enough to melt cheese.

6 SERVINGS

Each with: 380 Calories (38% from Fat, 43% from Protein, 19% from Carb); 41 g Protein; 16 g Total Fat; 9 g Saturated Fat; 4 g Monounsaturated Fat; 2 g Polyunsaturated Fat; 18 g Carb; 4 g Fiber; 3 g Sugar; 603 mg Phosphorus; 376 mg Calcium; 1157 mg Sodium; 622 mg Potassium; 1721 IU Vitamin A; 120 mg ATE Vitamin E; 39 mg Vitamin C; 42 mg Cholesterol

Fill Up on Crustless Bacon Quiche

Cut back on the carbs while keeping the flavor and nutrition with this crustless quiche.
Two kinds of cheese team with bacon and vegetables to give it great flavor and the power to
keep you from getting hungry mid-morning.

1 cup (235 ml) skim milk
½ cup (60 g) whole wheat pastry
  flour
1½ cups (355 ml) egg substitute
16 ounces (455 g) cottage cheese
1 cup (115 g) low fat Monterey
  Jack cheese, shredded
12 slices low sodium bacon,
  cooked and crumbled
8 ounces (225 g) mushrooms,
  sliced
1 cup (150 g) red bell pepper,
  chopped
1 cup (160 g) onion, chopped
2 tablespoons (28 g) unsalted
  butter

Preheat oven to 350°F (180°C, or gas mark 4). Mix all
ingredients thoroughly except butter. Melt butter and pour half
of butter into an 8 × 12-inch (20 × 30 cm) glass pan. Pour
remaining butter into batter and pour batter into pan. Bake for
50 minutes.

6 SERVINGS

Each with: 352 Calories (38% from Fat, 42% from Protein, 20% from Carb);
37 g Protein; 15 g Total Fat; 6 g Saturated Fat; 5 g Monounsaturated Fat; 2 g
Polyunsaturated Fat; 17 g Carb; 3 g Fiber; 5 g Sugar; 474 mg Phosphorus; 222 mg
Calcium; 449 mg Sodium; 662 mg Potassium; 1280 IU Vitamin A; 79 mg ATE Vitamin
E; 50 mg Vitamin C; 39 mg Cholesterol

Full of Veggies Frittata

For those of you not familiar with frittatas, they are like omelets except that they cook in the oven rather than on the stove, meaning you don't have to watch them as closely. This one is meatless, but it contains a great assortment of vegetables baked into the eggs.

¼ cup (60 ml) olive oil

2 baking potatoes, peeled and thinly sliced

1 cup (160 g) onion, thinly sliced

2 cups (240 g) zucchini, thinly sliced

1 cup (150 g) red bell pepper, cut in ½-inch (1.3 cm) cubes

8 ounces (225 g) mushrooms, sliced

2 cups (360 g) plum tomato, coarsely chopped

1 cup (150 g) green bell pepper, cut in ½-inch (1.3 cm) cubes

3 cups (700 ml) egg substitute

2 tablespoons (8 g) fresh parsley, chopped

Preheat oven to 450°F (230°C, or gas mark 8). Pour oil into 12-inch (30 cm) square or round baking dish. Heat oil in oven for 5 minutes and then remove. Place potatoes and onions over bottom of dish and bake until potatoes are just tender, 20 minutes. Arrange zucchini slices over potatoes and onions and then sprinkle red and green bell pepper, mushrooms, and tomatoes over all. Beat egg substitute and season with black pepper, if desired. Add chopped parsley to eggs. Pour eggs over vegetables. Bake until eggs are set and sides are puffy, about 25 minutes. The top should be golden brown. Serve hot or at room temperature.

6 SERVINGS

Each with: 327 Calories (37% from Fat, 24% from Protein, 39% from Carb); 20 g Protein; 14 g Total Fat; 2 g Saturated Fat; 8 g Monounsaturated Fat; 3 g Polyunsaturated Fat; 32 g Carb; 6 g Fiber; 7 g Sugar; 301 mg Phosphorus; 105 mg Calcium; 241 mg Sodium; 1418 mg Potassium; 1926 IU Vitamin A; 0 mg ATE Vitamin E; 109 mg Vitamin C; 1 mg Cholesterol

Quiche Mexican Style

These individual sausage and egg dishes can be easily made in whatever quantity is needed.
This is good for breakfast or for a light dinner, providing both great taste and filling portion size.

4 whole wheat tortillas, 8-inch (20 cm)

2 ounces (55 g) low fat Monterey Jack cheese

8 ounces (225 g) turkey sausage

½ cup (80 g) onion, chopped

½ cup (75 g) green bell pepper, chopped

1 cup (235 ml) egg substitute

1 cup (235 ml) skim milk

Heat tortillas and place in small dish such as a soup bowl that has been sprayed with nonstick vegetable oil spray. Top with half of the cheese. Cook sausage, onion, and green bell pepper and add to dish. Mix together remaining ingredients and pour over top. Top with rest of cheese. Bake at 350°F (180°C, or gas mark 4) for 30 to 35 minutes until eggs are set.

4 SERVINGS

Each with: 396 Calories (39% from Fat, 27% from Protein, 34% from Carb); 26 g Protein; 17 g Total Fat; 6 g Saturated Fat; 5 g Monounsaturated Fat; 3 g Polyunsaturated Fat; 33 g Carb; 2 g Fiber; 2 g Sugar; 384 mg Phosphorus; 261 mg Calcium; 785 mg Sodium; 561 mg Potassium; 449 IU Vitamin A; 46 mg ATE Vitamin E; 34 mg Vitamin C; 39 mg Cholesterol

Fried Rice Omelet

Fried rice often has egg in it. But in this case, the egg takes center stage and the rice just filler.
The result is a breakfast that will satisfy your taste buds and keep you satisfied all morning.

1 cup (195 g) brown rice, uncooked

2 tablespoons (28 ml) olive oil

½ cup (80 g) onion, chopped

½ cup (75 g) red bell pepper, chopped

½ cup (75 g) green bell pepper, chopped

1½ cups (355 ml) egg substitute

¾ cup (86 g) low fat cheddar cheese, gated

⅛ teaspoon black pepper

Cook rice as directed. Sauté vegetables in oil in frying pan until softened. Add cooked rice and pour egg substitute over the top. Add cheese and black pepper. Scramble until egg is done.

4 SERVINGS

Each with: 370 Calories (32% from Fat, 23% from Protein, 45% from Carb); 22 g Protein; 13 g Total Fat; 3 g Unsaturated Fat; 7 g Monounsaturated Fat; 3 g Polyunsaturated Fat; 41 g Carb; 3 g Fiber; 3 g Sugar; 402 mg Phosphorus; 171 mg Calcium; 323 mg Sodium; 532 mg Potassium; 1043 IU Vitamin A; 15 mg ATE Vitamin E; 52 mg Vitamin C; 6 mg Cholesterol

Eggplant Omelet

And why NOT eggplant in an omelet? It also includes some of the more normal fillings like onion, ham, and tomato, but the eggplant adds bulk and nutrition in addition to taste. And it's all still so low in calories that you can have a slice of toast with it.

2 tablespoons (28 ml) olive oil

1 cup (82 g) eggplant, peeled and diced

½ cup (80 g) onion, diced

½ cup (75 g) ham, diced

¼ teaspoon black pepper

¼ teaspoon dried oregano

¼ cup (45 g) tomato, diced

1 cup (235 ml) egg substitute

2 slices whole wheat bread, toasted

Heat olive oil in a small skillet. Add the eggplant, onion, and ham. Sauté in the hot oil. Season lightly with black pepper and oregano. Add the tomatoes. Adjust to medium heat. Add the egg substitute. Place a cover on the skillet for several minutes. Remove the lid and turn the omelet when the egg begins to thicken on top. When cooked, remove from the skillet.

2 SERVINGS

Each with: 379 Calories (52% from Fat, 27% from Protein, 21% from Carb); 26 g Protein; 22 g Total Fat; 4 g Unsaturated Fat; 13 g Monounsaturated Fat; 4 g Polyunsaturated Fat; 20 g Carb; 3 g Fiber; 5 g Sugar; 293 mg Phosphorus; 112 mg Calcium; 732 mg Sodium; 786 mg Potassium; 640 IU Vitamin A; 0 mg ATE Vitamin E; 7 mg Vitamin C; 16 mg Cholesterol

Eggplant Frittata

Eggplant may not be something you think of for breakfast, but this frittata, which is an oven cooked omelet, will fill you up as well as please your taste buds. It's meatless, but it contains a great variety of vegetables and will provide a big, puffy wedge of goodness.

¼ cup (60 ml) olive oil

2 medium potatoes, peeled and thinly sliced

1 cup (160 g) onion, peeled and thinly sliced

2 cups (240 g) zucchini, thinly sliced

2 small eggplants, thinly sliced

2 cups (300 g) red bell pepper, minced

3 cups (700 ml) egg substitute

Preheat oven to 450°F (230°C, or gas mark 8). Pour the olive oil into a 12-inch (30 cm) baking dish. Heat the oil in the oven for 5 minutes and remove. Arrange the potato and onion slices in the baking dish and bake for 20 minutes or until potatoes are slightly tender. Arrange the zucchini and eggplant slices on top of the potatoes and bake for 5 minutes. Sprinkle the red bell pepper over the other vegetables. Pour the egg substitute over the vegetables. Bake until the eggs are set and the sides have puffed, about 20 minutes. The top will become golden brown and a knife inserted in the middle should come out clean.

6 SERVINGS

Each with: 349 Calories (35% from Fat, 23% from Protein, 42% from Carb); 20 g Protein; 14 g Total Fat; 2 g Unsaturated Fat; 8 g Monounsaturated Fat; 3 g Polyunsaturated Fat; 38 g Carb; 9 g Fiber; 8 g Sugar; 297 mg Phosphorus; 114 mg Calcium; 239 mg Sodium; 1565 mg Potassium; 2141 IU Vitamin A; 0 mg ATE Vitamin E; 119 mg Vitamin C; 1 mg Cholesterol

Egg Muffins

A Southwestern egg mixture is baked in muffin cups for a quick grab-and-go breakfast that is also nutritious.

3 cups (585 g) brown rice, cooked

4 ounces (115 g) low fat cheddar cheese, shredded, divided

4 ounces (115 g) green chilies, diced

2 ounces (55 g) pimentos, drained

⅓ cup (80 ml) skim milk

½ cup (120 ml) egg substitute

½ teaspoon ground cumin

½ teaspoon ground black pepper

 Tip: If you have a pan for large muffins, you can make six of those, increasing the baking time to 25 minutes.

Combine rice, ½ cup (58 g) cheese, green chilies, pimentos, skim milk, egg substitute, cumin, and black pepper in large bowl. Evenly divide mixture into 12 muffin cups coated with nonstick vegetable oil spray. Sprinkle with remaining cheese. Bake at 400°F (200°C, or gas mark 6) for 15 minutes or until set.

6 SERVINGS

Each with: 405 Calories (11% from Fat, 15% from Protein, 74% from Carb); 15 g Protein; 5 g Total Fat; 2 g Unsaturated Fat; 2 g Monounsaturated Fat; 1 g Polyunsaturated Fat; 74 g Carb; 4 g Fiber; 1 g Sugar; 445 mg Phosphorus; 140 mg Calcium; 244 mg Sodium; 354 mg Potassium; 420 IU Vitamin A; 20 mg ATE Vitamin E; 15 mg Vitamin C; 4 mg Cholesterol

"Did You Say Fish Omelet?"

Fish isn't usually thought of as a breakfast food, but it has a lot to offer. It's much lower in calories than more traditional breakfast meat, as well as being low in sodium and high in omega-3 fatty acids. This baked omelet shows how well it can be incorporated into breakfast dishes.

2 tablespoons (28 g) unsalted butter

3 tablespoons (24 g) all purpose flour

1 cup (235 ml) skim milk

4 ounces (115 g) halibut fillets, cooked, or other white fish

½ cup (75 g) green bell pepper, chopped

½ teaspoon onion powder

¼ teaspoon black pepper

½ cup (105 g) frozen hash brown potatoes

1 cup (235 ml) egg substitute

Melt the butter in a saucepan. Stir in flour until combined. Add skim milk and cook and stir until thickened. Add fish, vegetables, and seasonings. Beat egg substitute and mix lightly with fish. Pour into 1½-quart (1.4 L) baking dish. Bake at 350°F (180°C, or gas mark 4) until set, about ½ an hour.

2 SERVINGS

Each with: 416 Calories (39% from Fat, 34% from Protein, 27% from Carb); 35 g Protein; 18 g Total Fat; 9 g Unsaturated Fat; 5 g Monounsaturated Fat; 3 g Polyunsaturated Fat; 28 g Carb; 2 g Fiber; 2 g Sugar; 466 mg Phosphorus; 286 mg Calcium; 340 mg Sodium; 1133 mg Potassium; 1284 IU Vitamin A; 197 mg ATE Vitamin E; 36 mg Vitamin C; 52 mg Cholesterol

Curried Eggs

Are you looking for something a little different for a weekend breakfast? How about curried eggs over brown rice? If you are a person like me who likes the taste of curry, this should be right up your alley.

1 cup (190 g) brown rice
½ cup (50 g) green onion, chopped
1 cup (150 g) green bell pepper, chopped
1 tablespoon (15 ml) olive oil
2 tablespoons (16 g) all purpose flour
1 tablespoon (6 g) curry powder
2 cups (475 ml) skim milk
1½ cups (204 g) eggs, hard boiled and diced
⅛ teaspoon black pepper

Cook rice according to package directions. Sauté onion and green bell pepper in oil. Remove from heat and blend in flour and curry. Return to heat, stir until smooth, and gradually add skim milk, stirring until thickened. Add eggs and season with black pepper. Serve over rice.

4 SERVINGS

Each with: 361 Calories (27% from Fat, 18% from Protein, 55% from Carb); 16 g Protein; 11 g Total Fat; 3 g Unsaturated Fat; 5 g Monounsaturated Fat; 2 g Polyunsaturated Fat; 50 g Carb; 3 g Fiber; 2 g Sugar; 401 mg Phosphorus; 233 mg Calcium; 143 mg Sodium; 520 mg Potassium; 827 IU Vitamin A; 161 mg ATE Vitamin E; 34 mg Vitamin C; 219 mg Cholesterol

Couscous with Egg and Cheese

This is a simple breakfast, but it's one that will keep you going all morning.

½ cup (88 g) whole wheat couscous
1 tablespoon (15 ml) olive oil
1 cup (235 ml) egg substitute
3 tablespoons (15 g) Parmesan cheese, grated

Cook couscous according to directions. Then add oil. Beat egg substitute and pour in. Slowly cook over low heat to cook egg. Add cheese. Stir and serve warm.

2 SERVINGS

Each with: 368 Calories (35% from Fat, 27% from Protein, 39% from Carb); 24 g Protein; 14 g Total Fat; 3 g Unsaturated Fat; 7 g Monounsaturated Fat; 3 g Polyunsaturated Fat; 35 g Carb; 2 g Fiber; 1 g Sugar; 294 mg Phosphorus; 181 mg Calcium; 370 mg Sodium; 498 mg Potassium; 493 IU Vitamin A; 11 mg ATE Vitamin E; 0 mg Vitamin C; 10 mg Cholesterol

Corned Beef Hash Pie

We don't eat corned beef very often because of the high sodium count, but this baked pie with a corned beef crust and a creamy egg filling is a hit whenever we do fix it.

32 ounces (905 g) corned beef hash

¾ cup (175 ml) egg substitute, divided

1 cup (160 g) onion, chopped

1 tablespoon (15 ml) olive oil

4 ounces (115 g) low fat cheddar cheese, grated

10 ounces (280 g) frozen mixed vegetables

½ cup (120 ml) fat-free evaporated miik

1 tablespoon (8 g) all purpose flour

½ teaspoon dry mustard

⅛ teaspoon garlic powder

⅛ teaspoon black pepper

Spray a 9-inch (23 cm) pie plate with nonstick vegetable oil spray. Mix the corned beef hash and ¼ cup (60 ml) egg substitute. Press into plate to form a crust. Bake at 375°F (190°C, or gas mark 5) for 10 minutes. Sauté onion in oil. Layer cheese, sautéed onion, and vegetables in crust. Beat remaining egg substitute, evaporated milk, flour, mustard, garlic powder, and black pepper. Pour over mixture in crust. Bake at 350°F (180°C, or gas mark 4) for 30 to 40 minutes until filling is set. Let stand 10 minutes before serving.

6 SERVINGS

Each with: 391 Calories (47% from Fat, 26% from Protein, 28% from Carb); 25 g Protein; 20 g Total Fat; 8 g Unsaturated Fat; 10 g Monounsaturated Fat; 1 g Polyunsaturated Fat; 27 g Carb; 4 g Fiber; 6 g Sugar; 204 mg Phosphorus; 204 mg Calcium; 856 mg Sodium; 569 mg Potassium; 2258 IU Vitamin A; 37 mg ATE Vitamin E; 5 mg Vitamin C; 54 mg Cholesterol

Black Bean and Spinach Breakfast Burrito

Almost as quick as fast food, this will get your day off to a good start with something a little different. It's high in nutrition and fiber, but not in calories.

6 tablespoons (90 ml) egg substitute
1 cup (30 g) fresh spinach
¼ cup (45 g) tomato, diced
¼ cup (43 g) black beans, drained
1 tablespoon (8 g) low fat cheddar cheese, grated
1 tablespoon (16 g) salsa
1 whole wheat tortilla, 8-inch (20 cm)

Preheat the oven to 350°F (180°C, or gas mark 4). Scramble the egg substitute quickly in a small frying pan. Fold in all the other ingredients. Place this mixture in the middle of the tortilla. Wrap the two sides over tightly and place the roll seam side down on a lightly oiled cookie sheet. Bake at 350°F (180°C, or gas mark 4) for about 6 minutes until the tortilla is crisp and the filling is heated through.

1 SERVING

Each with: 370 Calories (19% from Fat, 30% from Protein, 50% from Carb); 29 g Protein; 8 g Total Fat; 2 g Saturated Fat; 3 g Monounsaturated Fat; 3 g Polyunsaturated Fat; 49 g Carb; 13 g Fiber; 3 g Sugar; 379 mg Phosphorus; 452 mg Calcium; 692 mg Sodium; 1225 mg Potassium; 23 693 IU Vitamin A; 5 mg ATE Vitamin E; 11 mg Vitamin C; 3 mg Cholesterol

Break Your Fast Vegetable Pie

Full of nutritious vegetables in a creamy sauce, this pie could also be used for lunch or dinner. But if you are looking for something a little different from eggs, it may also be just the ticket for breakfast.

4 tablespoons (55 g) unsalted butter

8 ounces (225 g) mushrooms, sliced

¼ cup (31 g) all purpose flour

1 cup (235 ml) skim milk

2 ounces (55 g) part skim mozzarella, grated

1 tablespoon (11 g) Dijon mustard

½ teaspoon dried thyme

2 cups (244 g) carrot, sliced

2 cups (142) broccoli florets

1 teaspoon dill weed

½ teaspoon black pepper

1 teaspoon garlic powder

1 pie crust, baked

Preheat oven to 350°F (180°C, or gas mark 4). Heat butter in medium saucepan and sauté mushrooms, carrot, and broccoli. Add flour and stir until browned. Gradually add skim milk and cook until sauce thickens. Add cheese, mustard, and spices. Steam broccoli and carrots until just beginning to soften. Spoon cooked vegetables into the pie crust and pour sauce over top. Bake 35 minutes or until sauce bubbles.

5 SERVINGS

Each with: 412 Calories (55% from Fat, 13% from Protein, 33% from Carb); 14 g Protein; 25 g Total Fat; 11 g Unsaturated Fat; 9 g Monounsaturated Fat; 4 g Polyunsaturated Fat; 34 g Carb; 5 g Fiber; 4 g Sugar; 279 mg Phosphorus; 299 mg Calcium; 442 mg Sodium; 580 mg Potassium; 6908 IU Vitamin A; 134 mg ATE Vitamin E; 36 mg Vitamin C; 40 mg Cholesterol

Black Bean Burrito

Black beans add flavor and fiber to a quick-to-fix breakfast burrito.

1½ cups (355 ml) egg substitute

1 cup (172 g) black beans, rinsed and drained

½ cup (130 g) salsa

½ cup (115 g) low fat cheddar cheese, shredded

4 whole wheat tortillas, 8-inch (20 cm)

Scramble egg substitute, black beans, salsa, and cheese. Fill tortillas with egg mixture.

4 SERVINGS

Each with: 386 Calories (17% from Fat, 30% from Protein, 53% from Carb); 29 g Protein; 7 g Total Fat; 2 g Unsaturated Fat; 2 g Monounsaturated Fat; 2 g Polyunsaturated Fat; 51 g Carb; 9 g Fiber; 3 g Sugar; 413 mg Phosphorus; 200 mg Calcium; 563 mg Sodium; 1152 mg Potassium; 590 IU Vitamin A; 10 mg ATE Vitamin E; 5 mg Vitamin C; 4 mg Cholesterol

Herbed Cheese and Tomato Bagel

This is low in calories compared to many of the recipes here. And if it were just the bagel it would be the kind of calorie dense meal that will leave you hungry in a couple of hours. But the protein of the cheese and the thick slices of tomato help to prevent that, giving you a good-tasting meal that will stick with you.

1 cup (225 g) low fat cottage cheese

1 tablespoon (3 g) fresh chives

4 teaspoons (5 g) fresh parsley

4 teaspoons (3 g) fresh basil

¼ teaspoon black pepper

2 bagels, toasted

4 tomato slices, ½-inch (1.3 cm) thick

Blend cottage cheese with hand blender. Stir in fresh herbs and black pepper. Spread on toasted bagel and top with tomato.

2 SERVINGS

Each with: 279 Calories (10% from Fat, 32% from Protein, 58% from Carb); 23 g Protein; 3 g Total Fat; 2 g Unsaturated Fat; 1 g Monounsaturated Fat; 1 g Polyunsaturated Fat; 42 g Carb; 5 g Fiber; 5 g Sugar; 278 mg Phosphorus; 135 mg Calcium; 757 mg Sodium; 595 mg Potassium; 1743 IU Vitamin A; 24 mg ATE Vitamin E; 24 mg Vitamin C; 9 mg Cholesterol

Asparagus and Poached Eggs on Toast

This is a little different variation on poached eggs or Eggs Benedict. There's no meat here, but the asparagus more than makes up for it in flavor and nutrition.

4 slices whole wheat bread

1 pound (455 g) asparagus, tough ends trimmed

2 tablespoons (28 ml) olive oil

½ teaspoon black pepper

8 eggs

¼ cup (25 g) Parmesan cheese

 Tip: If you have a microwave or stove top egg poacher, that is an easier option than poaching them in water.

Preheat the broiler. Place the bread and asparagus on a baking sheet. Drizzle with the oil and season with black pepper. Broil until the bread is toasted, 1 to 2 minutes per side; transfer the bread to plates. Continue broiling the asparagus, tossing once, until tender, 4 to 8 minutes more. Meanwhile, bring a large saucepan of water to a boil. Carefully lower the eggs into the water. Reduce heat and gently simmer for 6 minutes. Cool under running water and peel. Divide the asparagus among the toast, sprinkle on the Parmesan cheese, and top with the eggs.

4 SERVINGS

Each with: 345 Calories (55% from Fat, 25% from Protein, 20% from Carb); 22 g Protein; 21 g Total Fat; 6 g Unsaturated Fat; 10 g Monounsaturated Fat; 3 g Polyunsaturated Fat; 18 g Carb; 4 g Fiber; 4 g Sugar; 364 mg Phosphorus; 185 mg Calcium; 393 mg Sodium; 446 mg Potassium; 1451 IU Vitamin A; 169 mg ATE Vitamin E; 6 mg Vitamin C; 496 mg Cholesterol

Zucchini Quiche

With enough vegetables to satisfy anyone, including a nutritionist, this is still a very low calorie breakfast. Cooking it without a crust greatly reduces the fat and the calories.

3 cups (360 g) zucchini, grated
1 cup (160 g) onion, grated
1 cup (70 g) mushrooms, sliced
1 cup (150 g) green bell pepper
1 cup (125 g) reduced fat baking
  mix, see recipe in chapter 2
1 cup (235 ml) egg substitute
¼ cup (60 ml) canola oil
½ cup (58 g) low fat cheddar
  cheese, grated
½ teaspoon dried parsley
¼ teaspoon black pepper
8 ounces (225 g) ham, finely
  diced

Mix all ingredients and put in a greased 9-inch (23 cm) pie plate. Bake at 350°F (180°C, or gas mark 4) for 30 minutes until set.

6 SERVINGS

Each with: 308 Calories (48% from Fat, 26% from Protein, 26% from Carb); 19 g Protein; 15 g Total Fat; 3 g Unsaturated Fat; 8 g Monounsaturated Fat; 4 g Polyunsaturated Fat; 19 g Carb; 2 g Fiber; 6 g Sugar; 344 mg Phosphorus; 123 mg Calcium; 637 mg Sodium; 592 mg Potassium; 395 IU Vitamin A; 7 mg ATE Vitamin E; 33 mg Vitamin C; 19 mg Cholesterol

Zucchini Pancakes

Zucchini patties become a healthy, lower calorie, version of pancakes here, providing a generous amount of food without many calories.

6 cups (720 g) zucchini, grated
1 cup (235 ml) egg substitute
½ cup (63 g) all purpose flour
⅛ teaspoon black pepper
¼ teaspoon garlic powder
¼ cup (15 g) fresh parsley,
  chopped
3 tablespoons (45 ml) olive oil
6 ounces (170 g) ham steaks

Squeeze the grated zucchini until it is dry. In a bowl, combine the zucchini and all the other ingredients except the oil and ham. Heat 3 tablespoons (45 ml) of oil in a heavy skillet over medium heat. Drop zucchini mixture by heaping tablespoons into hot oil. Flatten them a little and fry until golden brown on bottom. Turn and brown the second side. Drain on paper towels. Serve with ham steaks.

3 SERVINGS

Each with: 363 Calories (42% from Fat, 30% from Protein, 28% from Carb); 27 g Protein; 17 g Total Fat; 3 g Unsaturated Fat; 10 g Monounsaturated Fat; 3 g Polyunsaturated Fat; 26 g Carb; 3 g Fiber; 5 g Sugar; 347 mg Phosphorus; 96 mg Calcium; 782 mg Sodium; 1178 mg Potassium; 1222 IU Vitamin A; 0 mg ATE Vitamin E; 49 mg Vitamin C; 24 mg Cholesterol

Spinach Soufflé

It may sound like a strange thing to have for breakfast, but it is similar to other quiches and baked egg dishes. And with the spinach, it is incredibly full of the kind of nutrition that will get you through the morning.

2 ounces (55 g) low fat cheddar
cheese
2 tablespoons (28 g) unsalted butter
20 ounces (570 g) frozen spinach,
drained and squeezed dry
16 ounces (455 g) fat-free cottage
cheese
7 tablespoons (56 g) all purpose
flour
¼ cup (40 g) onion, chopped
1 tablespoon (4 g) fresh parsley
1¾ cups (425 ml) egg substitute
⅛ teaspoon black pepper

Preheat oven to 350°F (180°C, or gas mark 4). Cut cheddar cheese and butter into small pieces. In large bowl, combine with spinach, cottage cheese, flour, onion, and parsley. In separate bowl, beat egg substitute with black pepper; fold into spinach mixture. Pour into well buttered 9 × 13 × 2-inch (23 × 33 × 5 cm) baking dish. Bake about 1 hour or until brown and bubbly. Cool slightly; cut into squares.

4 SERVINGS

Each with: 373 Calories (32% from Fat, 44% from Protein, 24% from Carb); 41 g Protein; 13 g Total Fat; 6 g Unsaturated Fat; 3 g Monounsaturated Fat; 2 g Polyunsaturated Fat; 23 g Carb; 6 g Fiber; 5 g Sugar; 512 mg Phosphorus; 468 mg Calcium; 967 mg Sodium; 938 mg Potassium; 17 775 IU Vitamin A; 77 mg ATE Vitamin E; 4 mg Vitamin C; 27 mg Cholesterol

Scrambled Eggs and Corn with Bacon

Corn and other vegetables enliven what we otherwise be fairly bland scrambled eggs. They also add significantly to the nutrition and filling power of the dish.

12 slices low sodium bacon
1 cup (164 g) frozen corn
1 cup (160 g) onion, chopped
1 cup (150 g) red bell pepper,
chopped
1½ cups (355 ml) egg substitute
¼ cup (60 ml) skim milk
⅛ teaspoon black pepper

 Tip: Add a little garlic and cumin to give it a southwestern flavor.

Fry bacon. Cut in pieces and set aside. Cook corn, onion and red bell pepper in same pan. Add egg substitute beaten with skim milk and black pepper. Stir and cook until partly set. Add bacon and continue cooking until eggs are set. Do not overcook.

3 SERVINGS

Each with: 367 Calories (45% from Fat, 33% from Protein, 22% from Carb); 30 g Protein; 18 g Total Fat; 5 g Unsaturated Fat; 7 g Monounsaturated Fat; 4 g Polyunsaturated Fat; 21 g Carb; 3 g Fiber; 7 g Sugar; 419 mg Phosphorus; 116 mg Calcium; 575 mg Sodium; 954 mg Potassium; 2062 IU Vitamin A; 16 mg ATE Vitamin E; 102 mg Vitamin C; 37 mg Cholesterol

Potato Pancakes

These are sort of like latkes and served the traditional way with sour cream and applesauce but including the very untraditional bacon. This makes a nice weekend breakfast to relax with over with a cup of coffee.

2 large potatoes, grated
⅛ teaspoon black pepper
½ cup (120 ml) egg substitute
2 tablespoons (16 g) all purpose flour
1 tablespoon (10 g) onion, finely chopped
½ cup (115 g) fat-free sour cream
2 cups (490 g) applesauce
8 slices low sodium bacon

Combine the first five ingredients in a bowl. Drop by spoonfuls into a lightly oiled hot skillet. Fry until brown on one side and then turn and brown on other side. Serve topped with sour cream with bacon and applesauce on the side.

4 SERVINGS

Each with: 411 Calories (26% from Fat, 15% from Protein, 60% from Carb); 15 g Protein; 12 g Total Fat; 5 g Unsaturated Fat; 4 g Monounsaturated Fat; 2 g Polyunsaturated Fat; 62 g Carb; 5 g Fiber; 21 g Sugar; 272 mg Phosphorus; 83 mg Calcium; 249 mg Sodium; 1142 mg Potassium; 261 IU Vitamin A; 32 mg ATE Vitamin E; 22 mg Vitamin C; 30 mg Cholesterol

Potato Pancake Breakfast

Potatoes add nutrition to these pancakes, which are teamed with ham and applesauce for a complete breakfast.

1 cup (125 g) reduced fat baking mix, see recipe in chapter 2
½ cup (120 ml) skim milk
1 cup (235 ml) egg substitute
3 cups (630 g) frozen hash brown potatoes
1 cup (160 g) onion, finely chopped
2 cups (490 g) applesauce
1 pound (455 g) ham slices

Beat baking mix, skim milk, and egg substitute until smooth. Stir in frozen potatoes and onion for each pancake. Pour ¼ cup (55 g) batter into greased hot griddle, spreading batter slightly to make 4-inch (10 cm) pancakes. Cook until pancakes are dry around the edges, turn, and cook until golden brown. Serve with applesauce and ham.

6 SERVINGS

Each with: 413 Calories (21% from Fat, 26% from Protein, 53% from Carb); 26 g Protein; 9 g Total Fat; 3 g Unsaturated Fat; 4 g Monounsaturated Fat; 2 g Polyunsaturated Fat; 52 g Carb; 3 g Fiber; 18 g Sugar; 414 mg Phosphorus; 111 mg Calcium; 1003 mg Sodium; 861 mg Potassium; 203 IU Vitamin A; 13 mg ATE Vitamin E; 12 mg Vitamin C; 32 mg Cholesterol

Not What You Are Thinking Zucchini Casserole

Full of zucchini, this breakfast bake offers great nutrition as well as the ability to keep you full.
It's delicious served hot, warm, or cold and works equally well for breakfast, lunch, or dinner.

3 cups (360 g) zucchini, finely
diced

1 cup (160 g) onion, diced

1 cup (115 g) low fat Monterey
Jack cheese, grated

1 cup (125 g) reduced fat baking
mix, see recipe in chapter 2

¾ cup (175 ml) egg substitute

2 tablespoons (28 ml) olive oil

¼ teaspoon black pepper

In large bowl gently mix zucchini, onion, ¾ cup (86 g) of
cheese, and the baking mix. In smaller bowl, beat together
egg substitute, oil, and black pepper until frothy. Blend the
mixtures together thoroughly. Spread in a well greased
9 × 13-inch (23 × 33 cm) pan. Sprinkle with remaining ¼ cup
(29 g) of cheese. Bake at 350°F (180°C, or gas mark 4) for 40
to 45 minutes until set and golden brown on top.

3 SERVINGS

Each with: 414 Calories (38% from Fat, 25% from Protein, 37% from Carb);
23 g Protein; 16 g Total Fat; 4 g Unsaturated Fat; 9 g Monounsaturated Fat; 3 g
Polyunsaturated Fat; 35 g Carb; 3 g Fiber; 9 g Sugar; 573 mg Phosphorus; 315 mg
Calcium; 561 mg Sodium; 702 mg Potassium; 569 IU Vitamin A; 27 mg ATE Vitamin
E; 25 mg Vitamin C; 11 mg Cholesterol

Mexican Egg Breakfast

This is a sort of a Mexican quiche, mildly flavored except for the addition of chili peppers.
Creamy and rich with cheese, it makes a great company breakfast.

½ cup (112 g) unsalted butter

2½ cups (570 ml) egg substitute

½ cup (63 g) all purpose flour

1 teaspoon baking powder

4 ounces (115 g) green chilies,
chopped

16 ounces (455 g) fat-free cottage
cheese

2 cups (230 g) low fat Monterey
Jack cheese

Melt butter. Beat egg substitute; add flour and baking powder.
Add butter. Then add chilies, cottage cheese, and Monterey
Jack cheese. Put into a 9-inch (23 cm) pan. Bake at 400°F
(200°C, or gas mark 6) for 15 minutes and then bake 35 to
40 minutes at 350°F (180°C, or gas mark 4).

6 SERVINGS

Each with: 396 Calories (52% from Fat, 35% from Protein, 13% from Carb);
34 g Protein; 23 g Total Fat; 13 g Unsaturated Fat; 6 g Monounsaturated Fat; 2 g
Polyunsaturated Fat; 13 g Carb; 1 g Fiber; 3 g Sugar; 475 mg Phosphorus; 342 mg
Calcium; 920 mg Sodium; 476 mg Potassium; 995 IU Vitamin A; 162 mg ATE Vitamin
E; 6 mg Vitamin C; 54 mg Cholesterol

Italian Eggs

Eggs poached in an Italian sauce provide a little something different for breakfast, with the added nutrition boost of the tomatoes and other veggies.

4 tablespoons (60 ml) olive oil

1 teaspoon garlic, minced

1 cup (150 g) green bell pepper, chopped

1 cup (160 g) onion, minced

16 ounces (455 g) no-salt-added tomato sauce

½ teaspoon dried thyme

½ teaspoon dried basil

1 teaspoon dried parsley

⅛ teaspoon black pepper

8 eggs

4 slices French bread, ½-inch (1.3 cm) thick

Heat oil in saucepan that has a tight cover. Split garlic lengthwise and run a toothpick through each piece. Brown slowly in oil. Add minced onion and green bell pepper and cook slowly for 10 minutes. Add tomato sauce and add seasonings and herbs. Cook 15 minutes, stirring often. When done, remove garlic and toothpicks and discard. Break eggs into sauce, spacing evenly. Spoon sauce over them. Cover loosely and cook slowly for 20 minutes or until eggs are cooked through. Serve over French bread, dry toasted in oven.

4 SERVINGS

Each with: 358 Calories (64% from Fat, 19% from Protein, 17% from Carb); 17 g Protein; 25 g Total Fat; 5 g Unsaturated Fat; 14 g Monounsaturated Fat; 3 g Polyunsaturated Fat; 15 g Carb; 3 g Fiber; 8 g Sugar; 278 mg Phosphorus; 96 mg Calcium; 178 mg Sodium; 709 mg Potassium; 1137 IU Vitamin A; 161 mg ATE Vitamin E; 48 mg Vitamin C; 491 mg Cholesterol

Paris Sidewalk Cafe Quiche Lorraine

Transport yourself to a cafe along the Seine with this recipe. But don't worry about how bad French food is for you. This version of the classic quiche has had the fat reduced by using low fat dairy products and the nutrition increased with more than the usual vegetables.

1 pie crust
6 slices low sodium bacon, chopped and sautéed
¼ cup (40 g) onion, chopped and sautéed
½ cup (75 g) red bell pepper, chopped
12 ounces (340 g) shrimp
¼ cup (28 g) low fat Swiss cheese, shredded
1 teaspoon Parmesan cheese
¼ teaspoon baking powder
1 teaspoon all purpose flour
1¾ cups (403 g) fat-free sour cream
1 cup (235 ml) egg substitute

Bake the pie crust at 400°F (200°C, or gas mark 6) for 20 minutes. In the baked pie crust, place in layers the bacon, onion, red bell pepper, shrimp, and cheeses. In a mixing bowl, combine the baking powder, flour, sour cream, and egg substitute. Beat the mixture well and pour over the layers in the pie crust. Bake at 400°F (200°C, or gas mark 6) for 40 minutes.

6 SERVINGS

Each with: 405 Calories (55% from Fat, 25% from Protein, 20% from Carb); 25 g Protein; 25 g Total Fat; 10 g Unsaturated Fat; 9 g Monounsaturated Fat; 4 g Polyunsaturated Fat; 20 g Carb; 1 g Fiber; 1 g Sugar; 342 mg Phosphorus; 199 mg Calcium; 466 mg Sodium; 441 mg Potassium; 917 IU Vitamin A; 105 mg ATE Vitamin E; 26 mg Vitamin C; 125 mg Cholesterol

Salmon Asparagus Deluxe

I know it doesn't sound like breakfast, but it tastes great, provides great nutrition, and besides, there's that toast, which is a traditional breakfast food.

20 ounces (570 g) salmon
20 ounces (570 g) low sodium cream of mushroom soup
¼ cup (60 ml) fat-free evaporated milk
¼ cup (60 ml) dry white wine
24 spears asparagus, steamed
4 slices whole wheat bread, toasted

Tip: You could serve it for lunch or dinner too.

Remove skin and bones from salmon. Place soup, evaporated milk, and wine in saucepan. Beat over heat until smooth and heated through. Add asparagus and drained and flaked salmon. Serve over toast.

4 SERVINGS

Each with: 375 Calories (28% from Fat, 41% from Protein, 31% from Carb); 37 g Protein; 11 g Total Fat; 3 g Unsaturated Fat; 4 g Monounsaturated Fat; 3 g Polyunsaturated Fat; 28 g Carb; 3 g Fiber; 7 g Sugar; 682 mg Phosphorus; 463 mg Calcium; 802 mg Sodium; 1216 mg Potassium; 705 IU Vitamin A; 47 mg ATE Vitamin E; 4 mg Vitamin C; 60 mg Cholesterol

Quesadillas with Fruit Salsa

A sweet fruit salsa makes these quesadillas both a treat and full of excellent nutrition.

1 pint (357 g) strawberries, hulled and diced

1 pear, cored and diced

1 tablespoon (1 g) fresh cilantro, chopped

1 tablespoon (20 g) honey

4 ounces (115 g) part skim mozzarella

4 whole wheat tortillas, 8-inch (20 cm)

2 teaspoons olive oil

2 tablespoons (30 g) fat-free sour cream

 Tip: You can save the turning by using a contact grill.

To make fruit salsa, combine strawberries, pear, cilantro, and honey in medium bowl; set aside. Sprinkle 2 tablespoons (14 g) cheese on one half of each tortilla. Top with ⅓ cup (83 g) salsa (drain and discard any liquid that has formed from the fruit) and another 2 tablespoons (14 g) cheese on each tortilla. Fold tortillas in half. Brush top of each folded tortilla with some of the oil. Grill folded tortillas, oiled side down, in dry preheated skillet until light golden brown and crisp, about 2 minutes. Brush tops with remaining oil; turn and brown other sides. Remove to serving plate or platter. Cut each tortilla in half. Serve with remaining fruit falsa. Garnish with sour cream. Serve immediately.

4 SERVINGS

Each with: 336 Calories (29% from Fat, 14% from Protein, 57% from Carb); 12 g Protein; 11 g Total Fat; 5 g Unsaturated Fat; 5 g Monounsaturated Fat; 1 g Polyunsaturated Fat; 49 g Carb; 5 g Fiber; 15 g Sugar; 216 mg Phosphorus; 310 mg Calcium; 400 mg Sodium; 325 mg Potassium; 270 IU Vitamin A; 43 mg ATE Vitamin E; 48 mg Vitamin C; 21 mg Cholesterol

Baked Stuffed Peaches

Serve these stuffed peaches warm. The coconut flavor of the macaroons just seems to go with the peach flavor.

6 peaches, peeled and halved

½ cup (12 g) sugar substitute, such as Splenda

2 cups (220 g) macaroons, crushed

1 cup (235 ml) egg substitute

 Tip: You could offer cream for those who don't count calories—or not.

Scoop out about 1 teaspoon of the center pulp of each peach half. Mash pulp; mix with sugar substitute, macaroon crumbs, and egg substitute. Place halves close together, cut side up, in greased baking dish (about 8 × 12-inch [20 × 30 cm]). Spoon macaroon mixture into center of each. Bake at 300°F (150°C, or gas mark 3) for 30 minutes or until peaches are tender.

6 SERVINGS

Each with: 387 Calories (24% from Fat, 9% from Protein, 67% from Carb); 9 g Protein; 11 g Total Fat; 8 g Unsaturated Fat; 1 g Monounsaturated Fat; 1 g Polyunsaturated Fat; 67 g Carb; 4 g Fiber; 64 g Sugar; 113 mg Phosphorus; 37 mg Calcium; 252 mg Sodium; 549 mg Potassium; 662 IU Vitamin A; 0 mg ATE Vitamin E; 10 mg Vitamin C; 0 mg Cholesterol

Cinnamon Apple Omelet

This is a little different version of an omelet. I remember years ago there were often recipes for omelets with jelly or other sweet fillings, but you don't see them much anymore. This one makes me think they are still a good idea. This is a delightfully sweet yet highly nutritious breakfast or lunch idea.

1 tablespoon (14 g) unsalted butter, divided

2 apples, peeled and sliced thin

½ teaspoon cinnamon

½ cup (105 g) frozen hash brown potatoes, thawed

1 tablespoon (1 g) brown sugar substitute, such as Splenda

1¼ cups (285 ml) egg substitute

1 tablespoon (15 ml) skim milk

¼ cup (60 g) fat-free sour cream

Melt 2 teaspoons butter in a skillet. Add apples, cinnamon, potatoes, and brown sugar substitute. Sauté until tender. Set aside. Whip egg substitute and skim milk until fluffy; set aside. Clean skillet. Melt remaining butter, spread around pan, and pour in egg mixture. Cook as you would for an omelet. When eggs are ready to flip, turn them. Then add the sour cream to the center of the eggs and the apple mixture on top of that. Fold it onto a plate.

2 SERVINGS

Each with: 375 Calories (45% from Fat, 23% from Protein, 32% from Carb); 22 g Protein; 19 g Total Fat; 9 g Saturated Fat; 6 g Monounsaturated Fat; 3 g Polyunsaturated Fat; 30 g Carb; 3 g Fiber; 15 g Sugar; 271 mg Phosphorus; 147 mg Calcium; 309 mg Sodium; 860 mg Potassium; 920 IU Vitamin A; 83 mg ATE Vitamin E; 8 mg Vitamin C; 29 mg Cholesterol

Fill Yourself for Fall Apple and Sausage Quiche

Apples and sausage are a great combination, but it may not be one that we think about for breakfast. This crustless quiche will cure that. We especially seem to go to it in the fall when apples are plentiful, and it provides the kind of breakfast you want on a cool morning. It can also be used for dinner.

½ cup (115 g) low fat mayonnaise

½ cup (120 ml) skim milk

2 tablespoons (16 g) all purpose flour

½ cup (120 ml) egg substitute

3 apples, peeled, cored, and sliced

1 cup (110 g) Swiss cheese, shredded

6 ounces (170 g) hash brown potatoes, thawed

8 ounces (225 g) sausage links, cooked and thinly sliced

Preheat oven to 350°F (180°C, or gas mark 4). Combine mayonnaise, skim milk, flour, and egg substitute in a bowl. Stir in apples, cheese, potatoes, and sausage. Pour the ingredients into a pie pan. Bake 60 minutes or until top is nicely browned. Cool in pan for 10 minutes before serving.

6 SERVINGS

Each with: 363 Calories (54% from Fat, 22% from Protein, 24% from Carb); 18 g Protein; 20 g Total Fat; 7 g Saturated Fat; 4 g Monounsaturated Fat; 1 g Polyunsaturated Fat; 19 g Carb; 1 g Fiber; 8 g Sugar; 286 mg Phosphorus; 272 mg Calcium; 707 mg Sodium; 419 mg Potassium; 358 IU Vitamin A; 59 mg ATE Vitamin E; 6 mg Vitamin C; 59 mg Cholesterol

Bacon and Eggs . . . and Apples?

Similar to the Bisquick impossible pies which make their own crust, the dish has a crusty bottom surrounding apples and bacon, topped with an egg mixture.

4 apples, peeled and thinly sliced

2 tablespoons (3 g) sugar substitute, such as Splenda

1 cup (115 g) low fat cheddar cheese, shredded

4 slices low sodium bacon, fried and crumbled

1½ cups (188 g) reduced fat baking mix, see recipe in chapter 2

1½ cups (355 ml) skim milk

1 cup (235 ml) egg substitute

Combine apples and sugar substitute. Mix well. Spread evenly in a lightly greased 13 × 9-inch (33 × 23 cm) baking dish. Sprinkle bacon and cheese on top. Combine remaining ingredients and beat at medium speed until smooth. Pour over cheese and bacon. Bake at 375°F (190°C, or gas mark 5) for 30 to 35 minutes or until golden brown. Serve warm.

4 SERVINGS

Each with: 435 Calories (23% from Fat, 27% from Protein, 51% from Carb); 26 g Protein; 10 g Total Fat; 4 g Unsaturated Fat; 4 g Monounsaturated Fat; 2 g Polyunsaturated Fat; 50 g Carb; 3 g Fiber; 18 g Sugar; 646 mg Phosphorus; 386 mg Calcium; 638 mg Sodium; 627 mg Potassium; 536 IU Vitamin A; 78 mg ATE Vitamin E; 6 mg Vitamin C; 19 mg Cholesterol

Colorful Fruit Salad

This salad is cool and colorful! And that's not even the best part. It's also tasty and nutritious.

16 ounces (455 g) pineapple chunks, in juice

16 ounces (455 g) fruit cocktail, in juice

2 cups (290 g) strawberries

2 bananas, sliced

4 tablespoons (32 g) instant orange drink mix, sugar free

1 small sugar-free instant vanilla pudding mix

Drain fruit, reserving liquid. In mixing bowl, blend reserved juice, drink mix, and vanilla pudding for 2 minutes until thickened. Add fruit; toss and chill.

3 SERVINGS

Each with: 364 Calories (2% from Fat, 3% from Protein, 95% from Carb); 3 g Protein; 1 g Total Fat; 0 g Unsaturated Fat; 0 g Monounsaturated Fat; 0 g Polyunsaturated Fat; 92 g Carb; 7 g Fiber; 75 g Sugar; 306 mg Phosphorus; 60 mg Calcium; 485 mg Sodium; 853 mg Potassium; 595 IU Vitamin A; 0 mg ATE Vitamin E; 84 mg Vitamin C; 0 mg Cholesterol

Banana Breakfast Splits

It's hard to believe that anything this good and this rich looking could be less than 300 calories. But it is. And they are not empty calories. Loaded with fruit and yogurt, with enough granola to provide a good helping of fiber, it's the kind of thing that looks and tastes special but won't ruin your diet.

8 pancakes, warm

16 ounces (455 g) low fat vanilla yogurt

4 bananas, cut into chunks

2 cups (330 g) pineapple chunks, unsweetened

1½ pounds (680 g) strawberries, halved

1 cup (125 g) granola

Place 1 pancake on a plate. Spoon on yogurt, then the bananas, strawberries, and pineapple. Sprinkle with granola.

8 SERVINGS

Each with: 297 Calories (8% from Fat, 9% from Protein, 82% from Carb); 7 g Protein; 3 g Total Fat; 1 g Unsaturated Fat; 1 g Monounsaturated Fat; 1 g Polyunsaturated Fat; 64 g Carb; 5 g Fiber; 34 g Sugar; 286 mg Phosphorus; 152 mg Calcium; 286 mg Sodium; 655 mg Potassium; 175 IU Vitamin A; 19 mg ATE Vitamin E; 47 mg Vitamin C; 6 mg Cholesterol

Dessert for Breakfast Ambrosia

We usually think of ambrosia as a dessert, but fruit makes a wonderful choice for breakfast too. We've added apples and melon to the usual recipe. You get a huge 2 cup (455 g) serving with a creamy orange dressing and it still doesn't quite come to our 400 calories.

4 cups (640 g) cantaloupe, cubed

4 cups (740 g) orange sections

4 cups (600 g) bananas, sliced

4 cups (600 g) apples, peeled and cubed

1 cup (110 g) pecans, coarsely chopped

2 ounces (55 g) coconut

¼ cup (60 ml) orange juice

8 ounces (225 g) low fat vanilla yogurt

In a large bowl, arrange layers of cantaloupe, orange sections, bananas, apples, pecans, and coconut. Combine orange juice and yogurt and pour over. Chill before serving.

8 SERVINGS

Each with: 352 Calories (31% from Fat, 6% from Protein, 63% from Carb); 6 g Protein; 13 g Total Fat; 3 g Saturated Fat; 6 g Monounsaturated Fat; 3 g Polyunsaturated Fat; 60 g Carb; 8 g Fiber; 39 g Sugar; 141 mg Phosphorus; 112 mg Calcium; 35 mg Sodium; 1007 mg Potassium; 3314 IU Vitamin A; 3 mg ATE Vitamin E; 95 mg Vitamin C; 1 mg Cholesterol

Oat Baked Apples

Call it inside out oatmeal. In this case, healthy oats and oat bran are put inside an apple, along with other good tasting things. The apple is baked until tender and then served with milk poured over it.

4 ounces (115 g) low fat cheddar cheese

6 tablespoons (30 g) quick cooking oats, uncooked

2 tablespoons (2 g) brown sugar substitute, such as Splenda

2 tablespoons (12 g) oat bran

2 tablespoons (14 g) pecans, coarsely chopped

2 tablespoons (18 g) raisins

¼ teaspoon cinnamon

2 apples, cored

½ cup (120 ml) cold water

1 cup (235 ml) skim milk

Preheat oven to 375°F (190°C, or gas mark 5). Cut half of the cheddar cheese into small cubes and shred the remainder. Mix cheese cubes, oats, brown sugar substitute, oat bran, pecans, raisins, and cinnamon until well blended. Place baking apples in 8-inch (20 cm) square pan; fill with oat mixture. Pour water in bottom of pan. Cover with foil; bake 30 minutes. Uncover and continue baking 15 minutes or until tender. Sprinkle with shredded cheese and continue baking until cheese is melted. Serve each apple with skim milk poured over top of it.

2 SERVINGS

Each with: 358 Calories (26% from Fat, 25% from Protein, 50% from Carb); 23 g Protein; 11 g Total Fat; 3 g Unsaturated Fat; 4 g Monounsaturated Fat; 2 g Polyunsaturated Fat; 46 g Carb; 5 g Fiber; 20 g Sugar; 543 mg Phosphorus; 446 mg Calcium; 433 mg Sodium; 549 mg Potassium; 448 IU Vitamin A; 117 mg ATE Vitamin E; 7 mg Vitamin C; 14 mg Cholesterol

Get You through the Morning Couscous Cereal with Fruit

I get bored sometimes. This is a little different take on hot breakfast cereal. The fruit adds to the nutrition, and the volume will definitely keep you going until lunch.

1½ cups (355 ml) apple juice
1 cup (175 g) whole wheat couscous
½ cup (75 g) raisins
½ cup (60 g) dried cranberries
1 tablespoon (20 g) honey
½ teaspoon cinnamon
1 cup (235 ml) skim milk

Bring apple juice to a boil. Add the couscous, stir, cover, remove from heat, and let stand for 5 min. Stir in the remaining ingredients except skim milk. Serve with skim milk.

4 SERVINGS

Each with: 355 Calories (2% from Fat, 10% from Protein, 88% from Carb); 9 g Protein; 1 g Total Fat; 0 g Saturated Fat; 0 g Monounsaturated Fat; 0 g Polyunsaturated Fat; 81 g Carb; 4 g Fiber; 36 g Sugar; 171 mg Phosphorus; 119 mg Calcium; 50 mg Sodium; 461 mg Potassium; 126 IU Vitamin A; 38 mg ATE Vitamin E; 2 mg Vitamin C; 1 mg Cholesterol

Peach Melba Smoothie

Here's another great tasting smoothie, with the classic peach and raspberry combination. The raspberries give this one a special boost in fiber as well as flavor.

3 cups (375 g) fresh raspberries
2 cups (475 ml) skim milk
¼ cup (60 g) vanilla yogurt, low fat
1 tablespoon (20 g) honey
3 cups (510 g) peaches, sliced

Combine all ingredients in a blender or food processor and process until smooth.

2 SERVINGS

Each with: 394 Calories (4% from Fat, 13% from Protein, 82% from Carb); 14 g Protein; 2 g Total Fat; 1 g Saturated Fat; 0 g Monounsaturated Fat; 1 g Polyunsaturated Fat; 88 g Carb; 17 g Fiber; 55 g Sugar; 393 mg Phosphorus; 421 mg Calcium; 162 mg Sodium; 1212 mg Potassium; 1989 IU Vitamin A; 150 mg ATE Vitamin E; 65 mg Vitamin C; 5 mg Cholesterol

Cranberry Orange Smoothie

OK, this probably could have gone in the traditional breakfast chapter with the other smoothies, but do you REALLY think of cranberry sauce when you think of breakfast. This tasty smoothie is a great way to use up that leftover cranberry sauce and works as well with either the jellied or whole berry kind.

¾ cup (208 g) cranberry sauce
1 cup (235 ml) orange juice
1 cup (230 g) plain nonfat yogurt
1 cup (150 g) banana, sliced
½ cup (235 ml) skim milk

Combine all ingredients in blender and process until smooth.

2 SERVINGS

Each with: 406 Calories (3% from Fat, 11% from Protein, 86% from Carb); 12 g Protein; 1 g Total Fat; 0 g Saturated Fat; 0 g Monounsaturated Fat; 0 g Polyunsaturated Fat; 91 g Carb; 4 g Fiber; 63 g Sugar; 306 mg Phosphorus; 354 mg Calcium; 163 mg Sodium; 1091 mg Potassium; 346 IU Vitamin A; 40 mg ATE Vitamin E; 55 mg Vitamin C; 4 mg Cholesterol

Peanut Butter Banana Milk Shake

It may sound a little strange, but it tastes great. And it provides the kind of nutrition that will carry you through the morning.

1¼ cups (285 ml) skim milk
½ cup (40 g) quick cooking oats, uncooked
1 banana, cut in chunks
3 tablespoons (48 g) peanut butter
1 teaspoon honey
¼ teaspoon vanilla
¼ cup (55 g) ice cubes

Combine skim milk, oats, banana, peanut butter, honey, and vanilla in blender container. Cover; blend 1 minute on medium speed or until smooth and creamy. Add ice cubes; cover. Blend 1 minute on high speed or until frothy.

2 SERVINGS

Each with: 362 Calories (33% from Fat, 17% from Protein, 50% from Carb); 16 g Protein; 14 g Total Fat; 3 g Unsaturated Fat; 6 g Monounsaturated Fat; 4 g Polyunsaturated Fat; 47 g Carb; 6 g Fiber; 14 g Sugar; 362 mg Phosphorus; 244 mg Calcium; 97 mg Sodium; 803 mg Potassium; 360 IU Vitamin A; 94 mg ATE Vitamin E; 8 mg Vitamin C; 3 mg Cholesterol

Lunches and Light Meals

These meals are equally good for lunch or dinner, but they represent a little lighter fare than some of the ones in following chapters. Most are around our 400-calorie target for a meal, but there are a few that are quite a bit lower than that. There are lots of meal salads here, full of vegetables that help to fill you, combined with lean meat or grains to make them even more substantial. There also are sandwiches and wraps and a few meal in a bowl kind of things. We particularly like these kinds of meals in warm weather, when you tend to want something cooler and lighter, but there are things here that are good year round.

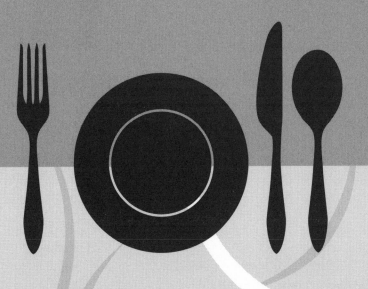

Antipasto Supper Salad

We usually have a salad dinner at least once a week, especially during the summer when fresh, locally grown vegetables are available. This meal on a plate antipasto salad has a great assortment of vegetables, with a tomato-based sauce that eliminates the need for any additional salad dressing.

½ cup (120 ml) white vinegar

2 tablespoons (28 ml) olive oil

3 ounces (85 g) no-salt-added tomato paste

4 ounces (115 g) pimento

10 ounces (280 g) frozen green beans, cooked and cooled

1 cup (122 g) carrot, sliced

¼ cup (25 g) green olives, sliced

8 ounces (225 g) mushrooms, sliced

1 cup (160 g) red onion, sliced

24 cherry tomatoes

1½ cups (180 g) zucchini, sliced

2 cups (480 g) garbanzo beans

8 ounces (225 g) roasted red pepper

9 cups (423 g) romaine lettuce, torn into bite-sized pieces

4 ounces (115 g) salami

12 ounces (340 g) tuna, water packed

6 tablespoons (30 g) Parmesan cheese, grated

Combine vinegar, olive oil, and tomato paste in a saucepan and heat over medium heat until hot and well combined. Remove and let cool. Cut vegetables into bite-sized pieces and add to the cooled mixture. Add garbanzo beans and stir to combine. Divide lettuce among serving plates and top with vegetable mixture, meat, and fish. Sprinkle with the Parmesan cheese.

6 SERVINGS

Each with: 393 Calories (31% from Fat, 28% from Protein, 41% from Carb); 29 g Protein; 14 g Total Fat; 3 g Saturated Fat; 7 g Monounsaturated Fat; 3 g Polyunsaturated Fat; 43 g Carb; 12 g Fiber; 10 g Sugar; 374 mg Phosphorus; 119 mg Calcium; 738 mg Sodium; 1436 mg Potassium; 10 218 IU Vitamin A; 4 mg ATE Vitamin E; 144 mg Vitamin C; 42 mg Cholesterol

Asian Beef and Barley Salad to Keep You from Being Hungry in an Hour

We made this hearty salad using some leftover beef brisket that we had grilled. Although it doesn't actually contain any soy sauce, the flavor is definitely Asian. The barley adds bulk and nutrition to make this a complete meal.

Marinade/Dressing

¼ cup (60 ml) balsamic vinegar

2 tablespoons (28 ml) sesame oil

½ teaspoon ground ginger

1 tablespoon sugar

1 clove garlic, minced

1 ounce (28 g) sesame seeds

Salad

8 ounces (225 g) leftover roast beef

½ pound (225 g) lettuce, shredded

8 ounces (225 g) snow peas

1 cup (122 g) carrot, sliced

1 cup (70 g) cabbage, shredded

8 ounces (225 g) mushrooms, sliced

1 cup (150 g) red bell pepper, sliced

4 ounces (115 g) mung bean sprouts

2 cups (314 g) cooked barley

Combine marinade ingredients. Slice beef and place in a plastic baggie with marinade for 1 to 2 hours. Drain, reserving liquid. Toss salad ingredients and top with beef slices. Spoon remaining dressing over top.

4 SERVINGS

Each with: 406 Calories (35% from Fat, 25% from Protein, 41% from Carb); 26 g Protein; 16 g Total Fat; 3 g Saturated Fat; 6 g Monounsaturated Fat; 5 g Polyunsaturated Fat; 43 g Carb; 10 g Fiber; 12 g Sugar; 359 mg Phosphorus; 151 mg Calcium; 75 mg Sodium; 987 mg Potassium; 5889 IU Vitamin A; 0 mg ATE Vitamin E; 122 mg Vitamin C; 48 mg Cholesterol

Asian Chicken Pasta Salad

This Asian-style salad of chicken, pasta, and fresh vegetables goes together quickly, tastes great, and leaves you feeling filled. We like to have a salad meal like this about once a week because it offers so many things to like.

8 ounces (225 g) whole wheat orzo, or other small pasta

3 tablespoons (45 ml) red wine vinegar

1½ tablespoons (30 g) chili sauce

1 tablespoon (15 ml) low sodium soy sauce

1 tablespoon (15 ml) sesame oil

1 tablespoon (6 g) ginger root, peeled and grated

2 teaspoons low sodium teriyaki sauce

2 cups (280 g) cooked chicken breast, cubed

4 ounces (115 g) fresh spinach, sliced into strips

½ cup (52 g) bean sprouts

8 ounces (225 g) mushrooms, sliced

½ cup (75 g) red bell pepper, cut into strips

¼ cup (25 g) green onion, sliced

2 tablespoons (14 g) slivered almonds, toasted

Prepare pasta according to package directions; drain and transfer to bowl. Meanwhile, in small bowl, mix together vinegar, chili sauce, soy sauce, oil, ginger, and teriyaki sauce; whisk well. To pasta in bowl add chicken, spinach, sprouts, mushrooms, red bell pepper, and green onion; toss to combine. Toss dressing with pasta mixture; refrigerate for 2 hours or until ready to serve. Sprinkle with almonds.

4 SERVINGS

Each with: 421 Calories (21% from Fat, 32% from Protein, 48% from Carb); 34 g Protein; 10 g Total Fat; 2 g Saturated Fat; 4 g Monounsaturated Fat; 3 g Polyunsaturated Fat; 50 g Carb; 4 g Fiber; 4 g Sugar; 346 mg Phosphorus; 88 mg Calcium; 307 mg Sodium; 642 mg Potassium; 4174 IU Vitamin A; 4 mg ATE Vitamin E; 40 mg Vitamin C; 60 mg Cholesterol

Chicken Chef's Salad

This is a quick, light main dish salad. It's good with just about any dressing from chapter 2, but I particularly like it with *A Peppercorn Ranch Dressing That You Can Actually Eat.*

4 cups (228 g) mixed salad greens

¼ cup (28 g) carrot, sliced

1 cup (180 g) tomato, cut in wedges

¼ cup (38 g) red bell pepper, sliced

4 ounces (115 g) mushrooms, sliced

4 ounces (115 g) chicken breast, cooked and sliced

2 ounces (55 g) Swiss cheese, cut in strips

2 eggs, hard boiled and sliced

¼ cup (55 g) peppercorn ranch dressing, see recipe in chapter 2

Layer the veggies and other ingredients in the above order. Apply dressing and eat.

2 SERVINGS

Each with: 390 Calories (38% from Fat, 38% from Protein, 24% from Carb); 37 g Protein; 17 g Total Fat; 8 g Saturated Fat; 5 g Monounsaturated Fat; 2 g Polyunsaturated Fat; 23 g Carb; 5 g Fiber; 9 g Sugar; 549 mg Phosphorus; 373 mg Calcium; 507 mg Sodium; 1007 mg Potassium; 10 162 IU Vitamin A; 144 mg ATE Vitamin E; 74 mg Vitamin C; 320 mg Cholesterol

Citrus and Avocado Chicken Salad

This is a great salad. I like to make a double batch of the dressing and use half to marinate boneless chicken breasts to grill for other meals.

1½ pounds (680 g) spinach, torn into bite-sized pieces

3 red grapefruits

3 oranges

2 avocados

3 cups (420 g) cooked chicken breast, sliced into strips

¼ cup (60 ml) orange juice

2 tablespoons (28 ml) lemon juice

1 teaspoon sugar

2 tablespoons (28 ml) white wine vinegar

¼ cup (60 ml) olive oil

Remove stems from spinach. Wash spinach thoroughly and dry. Tear leaves into bite-size pieces. Wrap gently in paper towels and refrigerate in plastic bags until ready to toss salad. Peel and section grapefruit and oranges. Slice avocados into quarters and then cut each slice into 2-inch (5 cm) chunks. Combine remaining ingredients for dressing. At serving time, toss spinach with dressing. Add grapefruit, orange, avocados, and chicken and gently toss again.

6 SERVINGS

Each with: 407 Calories (44% from Fat, 26% from Protein, 30% from Carb); 28 g Protein; 21 g Total Fat; 3 g Saturated Fat; 13 g Monounsaturated Fat; 3 g Polyunsaturated Fat; 32 g Carb; 10 g Fiber; 10 g Sugar; 272 mg Phosphorus; 187 mg Calcium; 146 mg Sodium; 1458 mg Potassium; 11 267 IU Vitamin A; 4 mg ATE Vitamin E; 137 mg Vitamin C; 60 mg Cholesterol

Colorful Chickpea, Chicken, and Rice Salad

I really like the flavor of this salad, but perhaps that's because I enjoy the taste of cumin, which is the main spice in the dressing. I also like the color (not to mention the nutrition) of the multicolor peppers.

2 cups (480 g) chickpeas, cooked

2 cups (380 g) brown rice, cooked

2 cups (280 g) cooked chicken breast, diced

½ cup (75 g) red bell pepper, diced

½ cup (75 g) green bell pepper, diced

½ cup (75 g) yellow bell pepper, diced

¼ cup (25 g) green onion, sliced

1 teaspoon sesame oil

½ teaspoon ground cumin

2 tablespoons (28 ml) lemon juice

1 tablespoon (15 ml) olive oil

2 teaspoons sesame seeds, toasted

Toss together chickpeas, rice, chicken, red, green, and yellow bell pepper, and green onion in a large bowl. Whisk together the sesame oil, cumin, lemon juice, and olive oil. Toss with salad. Sprinkle toasted sesame seeds on top.

4 SERVINGS

Each with: 427 Calories (22% from Fat, 30% from Protein, 48% from Carb); 32 g Protein; 10 g Total Fat; 2 g Saturated Fat; 5 g Monounsaturated Fat; 3 g Polyunsaturated Fat; 51 g Carb; 8 g Fiber; 6 g Sugar; 365 mg Phosphorus; 89 mg Calcium; 62 mg Sodium; 654 mg Potassium; 848 IU Vitamin A; 4 mg ATE Vitamin E; 141 mg Vitamin C; 60 mg Cholesterol

Cool and Curried Rice Salad

This rice salad actually makes a great lunch or light dinner. You could also reduce the serving size and use it as a side dish. I prefer it with the *Reduced Fat Italian Dressing* from chapter 2, but feel free to try the others.

6 cups (1.2 kg) brown rice, cooked, cold

1 cup (164 g) frozen corn, cooked and cooled

1 cup (100 g) celery, thinly sliced

1 cup (150 g) green bell pepper, chopped

¼ cup (25 g) olives, sliced

1 cup (180 g) plum tomato, chopped

½ cup (90 g) red onion, minced

¼ cup (60 g) dill pickles, chopped

½ teaspoon black pepper, or to taste

¼ teaspoon curry powder

2 tablespoons (32 g) chutney

⅓ cup (85 g) dressing of your choice, see recipes in chapter 2

6 cups (432 g) iceberg lettuce, torn into bite-sized pieces

3 eggs, hard boiled

Combine first 9 ingredients. Stir curry powder and chutney into dressing; pour over salad. Toss lightly and chill until serving time. To serve, mound on lettuce. Garnish with slices of hard-boiled eggs.

6 SERVINGS

Each with: 391 Calories (27% from Fat, 10% from Protein, 63% from Carb); 10 g Protein; 12 g Total Fat; 2 g Saturated Fat; 3 g Monounsaturated Fat; 4 g Polyunsaturated Fat; 62 g Carb; 6 g Fiber; 7 g Sugar; 264 mg Phosphorus; 72 mg Calcium; 312 mg Sodium; 545 mg Potassium; 853 IU Vitamin A; 40 mg ATE Vitamin E; 29 mg Vitamin C; 123 mg Cholesterol

Fiesta Salad

Here's a simple but flavorful main dish salad. It's good for warmer evenings or for lunch.

2 tablespoons (28 ml) olive oil
¼ cup (60 ml) lime juice
2 tablespoons (28 ml) lemon juice
1 teaspoon garlic, minced
1 teaspoon ground cumin
½ teaspoon dried oregano
2 boneless skinless chicken breast
8 cups (376 g) romaine lettuce,
   torn into bite-sized pieces
16 cherry tomatoes, halved
2 avocados, peeled and sliced
¼ cup (28 g) Swiss cheese,
   shredded
1 cup (63 g) tortilla chips, crumbled
¼ cup (60 g) fat-free sour cream
½ cup (130 g) salsa

Combine first 6 ingredients in a plastic zipper bag. Add chicken breast and marinate at least two hours, turning occasionally. Grill or sauté chicken breast until no longer pink. Cut into ½-inch (1.3 cm) thick slices. Divide lettuce between plates. Top with tomatoes, avocado, and chicken. Sprinkle with cheese and tortilla chips. Combine sour cream and salsa and pour over top.

4 SERVINGS

Each with: 403 Calories (55% from Fat, 16% from Protein, 30% from Carb); 17 g Protein; 26 g Total Fat; 5 g Saturated Fat; 15 g Monounsaturated Fat; 4 g Polyunsaturated Fat; 31 g Carb; 11 g Fiber; 4 g Sugar; 278 mg Phosphorus; 195 mg Calcium; 366 mg Sodium; 1137 mg Potassium; 7384 IU Vitamin A; 20 mg ATE Vitamin E; 61 mg Vitamin C; 30 mg Cholesterol

French Style Bean Salad

This makes a great luncheon salad. It can also be a main dish and will provide plenty of nutrition and bulk to get you through the night. If you can't find cannellini beans, use great northern or navy beans.

2 cups (512 g) cannellini beans,
   drained and rinsed
13 ounces (365 g) tuna, drained
1 cup (180 g) tomato, seeded and
   diced
½ cup (80 g) red onion, chopped
2 tablespoons (28 ml) lemon juice
1 tablespoon (11 g) Dijon mustard
¼ cup (60 ml) olive oil
¼ cup (10 g) fresh basil, chopped
6 cups (432 g) iceberg lettuce,
   torn into bite-sized pieces

Combine beans, tuna, tomato, and onion in large bowl. Combine lemon juice and mustard in small bowl. Gradually whisk in olive oil. Add to salad. Mix in basil. Serve over lettuce.

4 SERVINGS

Each with: 375 Calories (40% from Fat, 32% from Protein, 27% from Carb); 31 g Protein; 17 g Total Fat; 3 g Saturated Fat; 11 g Monounsaturated Fat; 3 g Polyunsaturated Fat; 26 g Carb; 9 g Fiber; 4 g Sugar; 393 mg Phosphorus; 146 mg Calcium; 312 mg Sodium; 894 mg Potassium; 798 IU Vitamin A; 6 mg ATE Vitamin E; 15 mg Vitamin C; 39 mg Cholesterol

He Went to Paris (for This Nicoise Salad)

OK, so maybe the name of the recipe was influenced by just seeing Jimmy Buffett in concert last week. (*He Went to Paris* is one of his songs for anyone that doesn't recognize the reference.) The ingredients in this salad are typical of the type of salad served in Nice, France.

1 ounce (28 g) anchovies, minced

2 teaspoons Dijon mustard

3 tablespoons (45 ml) red wine vinegar

2 tablespoons (28 ml) olive oil

4 cups (228 g) butter lettuce

1 can (5 ounces, or 140 g) tuna, drained

2 eggs, hard boiled, halved

1 large tomato, cut into wedges

2 medium potatoes, peeled, cooked, and sliced

½ cup (50 g) green beans, cooked, drained, and cooled

½ cup (75 g) green bell pepper, sliced and slivered

½ cup (80 g) red onion, cut in rounds

½ cup (85 g) black olives, drained

½ cup (35 g) mushrooms, thinly sliced

14 ounces (390 g) artichoke hearts, drained

½ cup (17 g) alfalfa sprouts

Combine first 4 ingredients to make dressing. Line a platter with butter lettuce. Place tuna in center. Arrange rest of ingredients in groups around tuna. Allow guest to choose their own ingredients for their salad or divide among 4 plates.

4 SERVINGS

Each with: 397 Calories (32% from Fat, 24% from Protein, 44% from Carb); 24 g Protein; 14 g Total Fat; 3 g Saturated Fat; 8 g Monounsaturated Fat; 2 g Polyunsaturated Fat; 45 g Carb; 10 g Fiber; 5 g Sugar; 385 mg Phosphorus; 126 mg Calcium; 567 mg Sodium; 1538 mg Potassium; 2391 IU Vitamin A; 44 mg ATE Vitamin E; 63 mg Vitamin C; 147 mg Cholesterol

Italian Dinner Salad

This is a meal on a plate. This may be only a salad, but I guarantee you won't walk away from the table hungry.

Salad

4 cups (188 g) romaine lettuce, finely chopped

2 cups (180 g) cabbage, finely chopped

1 cup (150 g) green bell pepper, chopped

1 cup (150 g) red bell pepper, chopped

4 ounces (115 g) black olives

½ cup (50 g) celery, thinly sliced

2 cups (480 g) garbanzo beans, drained

4 ounces (115 g) dry salami, cut up

4 ounces (115 g) Swiss cheese, cut up

6 ounces (170 g) boneless chicken breast, cooked and chopped

Dressing

¼ cup (60 ml) olive oil

2 tablespoons (28 ml) red wine vinegar

1 teaspoon balsamic vinegar

½ teaspoon garlic, minced

1 teaspoon lemon juice

1 tablespoon (11 g) Dijon mustard

1 teaspoon sugar

2 tablespoons (12 g) Italian seasoning

⅛ teaspoon black pepper, fresh ground

Divide lettuce between 6 plates. Arrange other vegetables, meats, and cheese over lettuce. Shake dressing ingredients together and drizzle over salads.

6 SERVINGS

Each with: 403 Calories (51% from Fat, 22% from Protein, 27% from Carb); 23 g Protein; 23 g Total Fat; 7 g Saturated Fat; 13 g Monounsaturated Fat; 2 g Polyunsaturated Fat; 28 g Carb; 7 g Fiber; 5 g Sugar; 313 mg Phosphorus; 282 mg Calcium; 846 mg Sodium; 611 mg Potassium; 3468 IU Vitamin A; 42 mg ATE Vitamin E; 91 mg Vitamin C; 52 mg Cholesterol

Italian Salad Meal

Sort of like an antipasto tray, this salad is sure to be a hit. For best presentation and eating, chop all the salad pieces the same size.

Dressing

½ cup (120 ml) red wine vinegar

2 tablespoons (28 ml) lemon juice, freshly squeezed

1 tablespoon (11 g) Dijon mustard

1 teaspoon garlic, minced

2 teaspoons dried oregano

1 teaspoon black pepper, freshly ground

½ teaspoon sugar

¼ cup (60 ml) olive oil

Salad

9 cups (423 g) romaine lettuce, finely chopped

1½ cups (270 g) plum tomatoes, finely chopped

1 cup (150 g) green bell pepper, seeded and diced

4 ounces (115 g) salami, diced

4 ounces (115 g) fresh mozzarella, diced

1 cup (140 g) smoked turkey breast, diced

1½ cups (360 g) garbanzo beans, drained

½ cup (50 g) scallions, thinly sliced

To make the dressing, place the vinegar, lemon juice, mustard, garlic, oregano, black pepper, and sugar in a blender or food processor and blend for 30 seconds. Slowly drizzle in the oil, blending until emulsified. Combine the salad ingredients in a large bowl and toss to mix. Pour the dressing over and toss again to distribute evenly. Serve immediately.

6 SERVINGS

Each with: 366 Calories (53% from Fat, 23% from Protein, 25% from Carb); 21 g Protein; 22 g Total Fat; 6 g Saturated Fat; 12 g Monounsaturated Fat; 3 g Polyunsaturated Fat; 23 g Carb; 6 g Fiber; 4 g Sugar; 272 mg Phosphorus; 223 mg Calcium; 897 mg Sodium; 652 mg Potassium; 5421 IU Vitamin A; 24 mg ATE Vitamin E; 56 mg Vitamin C; 48 mg Cholesterol

Meal on a Plate Chicken Caesar Salad

This is a pretty traditional chicken Caesar salad, except for the mushrooms, which I happened to like even before I found out they added bulk with almost no calories. This is a great quick meal when you don't feel like spending a long time cooking.

Dressing

¼ cup (60 ml) olive oil

1 clove garlic, minced

1 tablespoon (15 ml) lemon juice

2 tablespoons (28 ml) red wine vinegar

½ teaspoon Worcestershire sauce

Salad

1 pound (455 g) boneless chicken breasts

1 pound (455 g) romaine lettuce

8 ounces (225 g) mushrooms, sliced

1 cup (30 g) croutons

¼ cup (25 g) Parmesan cheese, grated

¼ teaspoon black pepper, fresh ground

Mix together dressing ingredients. Shake well in a jar with a tight fitting lid. Place ½ of dressing in a zipper baggie with chicken breasts and marinate several hours. Remove and discard dressing. Grill chicken until done. Slice into strips. Place lettuce on plates. Place mushrooms and chicken on top. Add croutons and sprinkle with cheese and black pepper. Serve with remaining dressing.

4 SERVINGS

Each with: 399 Calories (46% from Fat, 42% from Protein, 12% from Carb); 42 g Protein; 20 g Total Fat; 4 g Saturated Fat; 12 g Monounsaturated Fat; 3 g Polyunsaturated Fat; 12 g Carb; 3 g Fiber; 3 g Sugar; 397 mg Phosphorus; 133 mg Calcium; 250 mg Sodium; 785 mg Potassium; 6637 IU Vitamin A; 14 mg ATE Vitamin E; 31 mg Vitamin C; 102 mg Cholesterol

Mediterranean Chicken Rice Salad

This is one of those salads that I'm always glad makes a lot so I have some
left over for lunch the next day.

Salad

2½ cups (488 g) brown rice,
cooked and cooled

1 cup (100 g) celery, chopped

1 cup (150 g) green bell pepper,
chopped

¼ cup (48 g) pimento, chopped

¼ cup (25 g) green onion,
chopped

3 boneless skinless chicken
breast, cooked and cut into
strips

Dressing

6 ounces (170 g) artichoke hearts,
undrained, chopped

1 cup (225 g) low fat mayonnaise

1 teaspoon dried oregano

Mix salad ingredients well. Combine dressing ingredients.
Pour over salad mixture and stir to blend.

6 SERVINGS

Each with: 396 Calories (10% from Fat, 17% from Protein, 74% from Carb);
16 g Protein; 4 g Total Fat; 1 g Saturated Fat; 1 g Monounsaturated Fat; 1 g
Polyunsaturated Fat; 70 g Carb; 6 g Fiber; 5 g Sugar; 368 mg Phosphorus; 47 mg
Calcium; 382 mg Sodium; 481 mg Potassium; 543 IU Vitamin A; 2 mg ATE Vitamin E;
30 mg Vitamin C; 25 mg Cholesterol

Mega Waldorf Salad with Chicken and Blue Cheese Dressing

The trouble with Waldorf salad is that it usually has more calories than you want in a side salad, but it isn't enough for a meal. We decided to attack the second part of the problem, adding more veggies and chicken breast to make it into a complete meal. Then to add a little more interest, we topped it with a tangy blue cheese dressing. Now it not only fills you like a full meal, but it has the taste that will keep you coming back.

¼ cup (60 ml) lime juice

¼ cup (60 g) low fat mayonnaise

2 ounces (55 g) blue cheese, crumbled

¼ cup (60 g) fat-free sour cream

4 boneless skinless chicken breast, cooked and cut into bite-sized pieces

4 granny smith apples, cored and chopped into bite-sized pieces

1 cup (122 g) carrot, sliced

1 cup (71 g) broccoli florets

1 cup (100 g) celery, sliced

½ cup (75 g) raisins

6 cups (342 g) lettuce, preferably red

2 ounces (55 g) walnuts, chopped and toasted

Squeeze juice from lime into medium bowl; add mayonnaise, cheese, and sour cream. Whisk until well blended (or blend in food processor or blender). Add remaining ingredients except lettuce and walnuts, stirring until coated with dressing. Divide lettuce among 4 plates, mound a quarter of the chicken mixture in middle of each plate, and top with a quarter of the walnuts.

4 SERVINGS

Each with: 414 Calories (34% from Fat, 24% from Protein, 42% from Carb); 26 g Protein; 16 g Total Fat; 5 g Saturated Fat; 4 g Monounsaturated Fat; 6 g Polyunsaturated Fat; 46 g Carb; 7 g Fiber; 31 g Sugar; 372 mg Phosphorus; 175 mg Calcium; 434 mg Sodium; 981 mg Potassium; 4654 IU Vitamin A; 47 mg ATE Vitamin E; 37 mg Vitamin C; 59 mg Cholesterol

Not 400-Calorie Strawberry Spinach Salad

This recipe is an old family favorite, and it seemed like an ideal 400-calorie meal. Only problem is, no matter how much I add to the quantities, it isn't even close to 400 calories. But I can tell you that it has plenty to fill you up and keep you full. I know that from personal experience.
So here it is, a genuine 281-calorie mega meal.

Salad

2 pounds (910 g) spinach, torn into bite-sized pieces

3 cups (510 g) strawberries, hulled and halved

1 cup (160 g) red onion, sliced

2 cups (238 g) cucumber, sliced

1 cup (71 g) broccoli florets

8 ounces (225 g) mushrooms, sliced

⅓ cup (31 g) sliced almonds

Dressing

2 lemons, zested and squeezed

4 tablespoons (60 ml) white wine vinegar

2 tablespoons (28 ml) olive oil

½ cup (12 g) sugar substitute, such as Splenda

Chicken

6 boneless skinless chicken breast

¼ cup (60 g) strawberry syrup

Prepare fruit and veggies for salad. Zest lemons. Squeeze juice into bowl. Mix with other dressing ingredients. Reserve half of dressing. Combine remaining dressing with strawberry syrup and marinate chicken in this mixture for 2 hours. Remove chicken and grill or pan-fry until done. Slice into strips. Toss chicken, salad ingredients, and reserved dressing just before serving.

6 SERVINGS

Each with: 281 Calories (31% from Fat, 31% from Protein, 38% from Carb); 23 g Protein; 10 g Total Fat; 1 g Saturated Fat; 6 g Monounsaturated Fat; 2 g Polyunsaturated Fat; 28 g Carb; 6 g Fiber; 17 g Sugar; 300 mg Phosphorus; 151 mg Calcium; 130 mg Sodium; 1145 mg Potassium; 8862 IU Vitamin A; 4 mg ATE Vitamin E; 98 mg Vitamin C; 41 mg Cholesterol

Pasta, White Bean, and Tuna Salad

This is a tasty main dish salad with two-thirds of your daily fiber requirements in one helping. Not to mention that is has all kinds of other good things.

Vinaigrette

2 tablespoons (28 ml) olive oil

½ cup (120 ml) fresh lemon juice

½ teaspoon garlic, peeled and minced

1 teaspoon dried basil

½ teaspoon black pepper

Vegetables

1 can (6 ounces, or 170 g) artichoke hearts

6 ounces (170 g) green beans, blanched and drained

½ pound (225 g) beets, cooked or canned, drained and sliced

1½ cups (270 g) tomatoes, sliced in wedges

Pasta mixture

8 ounces (225 g) whole wheat pasta, cooked, rinsed and drained

2 cups (524 g) white beans, drained

1 can (5 ounces, or 140 g) tuna, drained

Whisk all vinaigrette ingredients together. Using half the vinaigrette mixture, marinate the vegetables for at least 1 hour before serving. Stir together drained pasta, beans, and tuna and mix. Immediately before serving, toss vegetables and pasta mixture with the remaining vinaigrette.

5 SERVINGS

Each with: 416 Calories (16% from Fat, 22% from Protein, 62% from Carb); 24 g Protein; 8 g Total Fat; 1 g Saturated Fat; 4 g Monounsaturated Fat; 2 g Polyunsaturated Fat; 68 g Carb; 13 g Fiber; 4 g Sugar; 370 mg Phosphorus; 112 mg Calcium; 142 mg Sodium; 850 mg Potassium; 629 IU Vitamin A; 2 mg ATE Vitamin E; 34 mg Vitamin C; 14 mg Cholesterol

Tuna and Pasta Salad

This is a great main dish salad for those hot summer days when you don't feel like cooking.

8 ounces (225 g) whole wheat
  pasta
½ pound (225 g) pea pods
1 can (5 ounces, or 140 g) tuna
6 ounces (170 g) artichoke hearts
½ cup (50 g) green olives, sliced
½ pound (225 g) fresh
  mushrooms
½ cup (120 ml) *Reduced Fat
  Italian Dressing*, see recipe in
  chapter 2
½ teaspoon lemon pepper
4 cups (288 g) iceberg lettuce,
  torn into bite-sized pieces

¼ cup (25 g) Parmesan cheese

Cook pasta according to package directions. Drain and let cool. Cook pea pods one minute in boiling water. Remove and let cool. Put pasta and pea pods into a bowl. Drain water from tuna and add to above. Add artichokes and artichoke liquid, sliced olives, and sliced mushrooms. Pour dressing over it all. Add lemon pepper and mix well. Serve over lettuce, sprinkled with Parmesan cheese.

4 SERVINGS

Each with: 383 Calories (18% from Fat, 26% from Protein, 56% from Carb); 26 g Protein; 8 g Total Fat; 2 g Saturated Fat; 3 g Monounsaturated Fat; 2 g Polyunsaturated Fat; 57 g Carb; 10 g Fiber; 6 g Sugar; 406 mg Phosphorus; 163 mg Calcium; 710 mg Sodium; 749 mg Potassium; 971 IU Vitamin A; 10 mg ATE Vitamin E; 40 mg Vitamin C; 25 mg Cholesterol

More than the Usual Shrimp Remoulade

Shrimp remoulade is a dish of French origin that is often found on luncheon menus and typically consists of just lettuce, shrimp, and the remoulade sauce. Here we add more vegetables to make it a more complete meal. It's perfect for lunch or a summer evening dinner.

¼ cup (44 g) mustard, Creole or Dijon

2 tablespoons (14 g) paprika

1 teaspoon cayenne pepper

½ cup (120 ml) tarragon vinegar

⅓ cup (60 ml) olive oil

1½ cups (150 g) scallions, coarsely chopped

½ cup (50 g) celery, finely chopped

½ cup (30 g) fresh parsley, coarsely chopped

3 pounds (1⅓ kg) shrimp

1 large iceberg lettuce, trimmed and cut into ¼-inch (6 mm) wide shred

8 ounces (225 g) mushrooms, sliced

1 cup (110 g) carrot, shredded

1 cup (120 g) zucchini, shredded

1 cup (150 g) red bell pepper, finely chopped

To prepare the remoulade sauce, combine the mustard, paprika, and cayenne pepper in a deep bowl and stir with a wire whisk until all the ingredients are thoroughly combined. Beat in the vinegar. Then, whisking constantly, pour in the oil in a slow, thin stream and continue to beat until the sauce is smooth and thick. Add the scallions, celery, and parsley and mix well. Cover the bowl tightly with plastic wrap and let the sauce rest at room temperature for at least 4 hours before serving. Meanwhile, shell the shrimp. Bring 2 quarts (1.9 L) of water to a simmer, drop in the shrimp and cook, uncovered, for 3 to 5 minutes, until the shrimp are pink and firm. With a slotted spoon, transfer the shrimp to a plate to cool. Then chill them until ready to serve. Just before serving, mound the shredded lettuce on 8 chilled individual serving plates, add the mushrooms, carrot, zucchini, and red bell pepper, and arrange the shrimp on top. Spoon the remoulade sauce over the shrimp and serve at once.

8 SERVINGS

Each with: 312 Calories (37% from Fat, 48% from Protein, 15% from Carb); 38 g Protein; 13 g Total Fat; 2 g Unsaturated Fat; 7 g Monounsaturated Fat; 2 g Polyunsaturated Fat; 12 g Carb; 4 g Fiber; 6 g Sugar; 429 mg Phosphorus; 148 mg Calcium; 287 mg Sodium; 844 mg Potassium; 4694 IU Vitamin A; 92 mg ATE Vitamin E; 57 mg Vitamin C; 259 mg Cholesterol

Ziti Salmon Salad

Pasta salad can be high in carbohydrates, but this one holds the line by being more vegetables than pasta. Canned salmon makes the recipe easy to fix as well as full of enough nutrition to make it a meal all by itself.

8 ounces (225 g) whole wheat pasta, such as ziti

16 ounces (455 g) salmon, drained, skin and bone removed

6 ounces (170 g) snow pea pods, thawed

1 cup (150 g) red bell pepper, chopped

1 cup (150 g) yellow bell pepper, chopped

½ cup (50 g) green onion, sliced

1 cup (110 g) carrot, shredded

10 cherry tomatoes, halved

1 cup (119 g) cucumber, sliced

½ cup (120 ml) *Reduced Fat Italian Dressing*, see recipe in chapter 2

6 cups (180 g) spinach, torn into bite-sized pieces

Prepare pasta as package directs; drain. In large bowl, combine pasta and remaining ingredients except spinach. Mix well. Cover; chill thoroughly. Stir and serve over spinach.

5 SERVINGS

Each with: 378 Calories (18% from Fat, 30% from Protein, 52% from Carb); 30 g Protein; 8 g Total Fat; 2 g Saturated Fat; 2 g Monounsaturated Fat; 2 g Polyunsaturated Fat; 51 g Carb; 8 g Fiber; 6 g Sugar; 520 mg Phosphorus; 327 mg Calcium; 451 mg Sodium; 1095 mg Potassium; 8300 IU Vitamin A; 16 mg ATE Vitamin E; 234 mg Vitamin C; 37 mg Cholesterol

Black Bean Taco Salad

Black beans take the place of meat in this taco salad, providing a low calorie,
high fiber alternative that tastes really good.

4½ cups (212 g) romaine lettuce,
shredded

1 cup (180 g) tomatoes, diced

1 cup (150 g) green bell pepper,
diced

1½ cups (258 g) black beans,
rinsed and drained

½ cup (130 g) salsa

2 ounces (55 g) tortilla chips,
crushed

2 ounces (55 g) low fat cheddar
cheese, shredded

Divide lettuce between two plates. Toss tomatoes, green bell
pepper, and black beans with salsa. Place on lettuce. Top with
chips and cheese.

2 SERVINGS

Each with: 435 Calories (18% from Fat, 20% from Protein, 61% from Carb);
23 g Protein; 9 g Total Fat; 2 g Unsaturated Fat; 3 g Monounsaturated Fat; 3 g
Polyunsaturated Fat; 69 g Carb; 15 g Fiber; 15 g Sugar; 607 mg Phosphorus; 294 mg
Calcium; 2134 mg Sodium; 1695 mg Potassium; 8595 IU Vitamin A; 17 mg ATE
Vitamin E; 122 mg Vitamin C; 7 mg Cholesterol

Hot Chinese Chicken Salad

In some ways, this is more like fried rice than a salad. But we've come to really like the addition of wilted lettuce to Chinese dishes. And this one gives you lots of things to like, from crispy chicken to vegetables, all for fewer than 350 calories.

6 boneless skinless chicken breasts, cut up

3 tablespoons (24 g) cornstarch

3 tablespoons (45 ml) canola oil

⅛ teaspoon garlic powder

8 ounces (225 g) sliced mushrooms

1 cup (100 g) celery, sliced diagonally

1 cup (160 g) onion, chopped

1 cup (110 g) carrot, shredded

1 cup (180 g) fresh tomato, cut in chunks

1 cup (124 g) water chestnuts, sliced

¼ cup (60 ml) low sodium soy sauce

3 cups (216 g) iceberg lettuce, shredded

3 cups (576 g) brown rice, cooked

Roll or shake chicken in cornstarch. Heat oil in large fry pan or wok at medium-high. Cook chicken 15 to 20 minutes in oil. Sprinkle with garlic powder while cooking. Add all vegetables. Stir. Stir in soy sauce. Cover and reduce heat. Simmer 5 minutes. Add lettuce. Remove from heat, toss, and serve at once with rice.

6 SERVINGS

Each with: 327 Calories (24% from Fat, 26% from Protein, 49% from Carb); 22 g Protein; 9 g Total Fat; 1 g Unsaturated Fat; 5 g Monounsaturated Fat; 3 g Polyunsaturated Fat; 41 g Carb; 5 g Fiber; 6 g Sugar; 303 mg Phosphorus; 52 mg Calcium; 441 mg Sodium; 777 mg Potassium; 2968 IU Vitamin A; 4 mg ATE Vitamin E; 10 mg Vitamin C; 41 mg Cholesterol

Mediterranean Roast Beef Salad

Goat cheese and Balsamic vinegar give this salad its Mediterranean flavor. Lots of vegetables add nutrition, and lean roast beef from the deli or a leftover roast provides protein. The result is a healthy, filling taste treat.

2 heads Bibb lettuce, torn into pieces

12 ounces (340 g) sliced roast beef

1 large tomato, cut into wedges

½ cup (80 g) red onion, sliced

4 ounces (115 g) goat cheese, crumbled

¼ cup (60 ml) olive oil

2 tablespoons (28 ml) balsamic vinegar

2 teaspoons (22 g) Dijon mustard

¼ teaspoon black pepper

Divide the lettuce, roast beef, tomato, onion, and goat cheese among bowls. In a small bowl, whisk together the oil, vinegar, mustard, and black pepper. Drizzle over the salad.

4 SERVINGS

Each with: 393 Calories (63% from Fat, 30% from Protein, 6% from Carb); 30 g Protein; 28 g Total Fat; 9 g Unsaturated Fat; 15 g Monounsaturated Fat; 2 g Polyunsaturated Fat; 6 g Carb; 2 g Fiber; 3 g Sugar; 255 mg Phosphorus; 85 mg Calcium; 170 mg Sodium; 515 mg Potassium; 3307 IU Vitamin A; 80 mg ATE Vitamin E; 9 mg Vitamin C; 102 mg Cholesterol

Sweet Treat Chinese Chicken Salad

This is a great dinner salad and a good use for leftover chicken (or turkey breast).
The dressing is very flavorful with the sesame oil and seeds, and to me,
the mandarin oranges really push it over the top.

Dressing

¼ cup (60 ml) rice vinegar

¼ cup (60 ml) sesame oil

¼ cup (60 ml) low sodium soy
sauce

¼ cup (36 g) sesame seeds

Salad

2 cups (280 g) cooked chicken,
diced

8 cups (576 g) iceberg lettuce,
torn into bite-sized pieces

¼ cup (25 g) green onion, sliced

½ cup (8 g) cilantro, chopped

½ cup (30 g) fresh parsley,
chopped

½ cup (50 g) celery, sliced

½ cup (61 g) carrot, sliced

1 cup (71 g) broccoli florets

1 cup (150 g) red bell pepper,
sliced

½ cup (55 g) slivered almonds

1 cup (189 g) mandarin oranges

For dressing, combine vinegar, oil, soy sauce, and sesame seeds. Marinate the chopped chicken in the dressing for a few hours or overnight. Chop lettuce, onion, cilantro, parsley, celery, carrot, broccoli, and red bell pepper and toss all together. Just before serving, add almonds, oranges, and chicken with dressing to salad. Toss well.

4 SERVINGS

Each with: 380 Calories (56% from Fat, 24% from Protein, 19% from Carb); 24 g Protein; 25 g Total Fat; 4 g Saturated Fat; 11 g Monounsaturated Fat; 8 g Polyunsaturated Fat; 19 g Carb; 5 g Fiber; 12 g Sugar; 280 mg Phosphorus; 111 mg Calcium; 634 mg Sodium; 855 mg Potassium; 5652 IU Vitamin A; 9 mg ATE Vitamin E; 127 mg Vitamin C; 53 mg Cholesterol

Chicken Kabobs with Chickpea Salad

It's kind of hard to say where this dish gets its flavor from (maybe I just need to travel more). But to me it seems Middle Eastern or possibly Indian. Chicken breasts kabobs are marinated in a yogurt sauce similar to tandoori chicken and then grilled and served over a salad featuring chickpeas and onion for a delightful taste sensation as well as great fiber and nutrient content.

1 cup (230 g) plain yogurt

½ teaspoon garlic, finely chopped

½ teaspoon ground cumin

½ teaspoon black pepper, divided

1 pound (455 g) boneless skinless chicken breast, cut in 1-inch (2.5 cm) cubes

2 cups (480 g) chickpeas, rinsed and drained

½ cup (90 g) red onion, thinly sliced

¼ cup (25 g) celery, sliced

1 cup (60 g) fresh parsley

2 tablespoons (28 ml) olive oil

2 teaspoons red wine vinegar

Heat grill to medium-high. In a shallow baking dish, combine the yogurt, garlic, cumin, and ¼ teaspoon black pepper. Thread the chicken onto 8 skewers and set them in the yogurt marinade, turning to coat. Refrigerate at least 10 minutes or as much as overnight. Meanwhile, in a large bowl, combine the chickpeas, onion, celery, parsley, oil, vinegar, and ¼ teaspoon black pepper. Remove the chicken from the marinade and cook on a well-oiled grill, turning occasionally, until cooked through, about 10 minutes. Divide the chickpea salad among plates and serve with the chicken.

4 SERVINGS

Each with: 397 Calories (25% from Fat, 37% from Protein, 38% from Carb); 37 g Protein; 11 g Total Fat; 2 g Unsaturated Fat; 6 g Monounsaturated Fat; 2 g Polyunsaturated Fat; 38 g Carb; 7 g Fiber; 17 g Sugar; 445 mg Phosphorus; 170 mg Calcium; 128 mg Sodium; 779 mg Potassium; 1371 IU Vitamin A; 14 mg ATE Vitamin E; 24 mg Vitamin C; 69 mg Cholesterol

Chicken Zucchini Pie

This is an easy and tasty one dish meal. It's based on the concept of the Bisquick impossible pies, which make their own crust and are full of veggies and chicken for low calorie nutrition.

2 cups (280 g) cooked chicken breast, cubed

2 cups (240 g) zucchini, cubed

1 cup (180 g) tomatoes, chopped

1 cup (160 g) onion, chopped

¼ cup (25 g) Parmesan cheese

1 cup (235 ml) skim milk

½ cup (80 g) whole wheat pastry flour

½ cup (120 ml) egg substitute

¼ teaspoon black pepper

¾ teaspoon baking powder

½ cup (58 g) low fat cheddar cheese

Preheat oven to 400°F (200°C, or gas mark 6) and spray 9-inch (23 cm) pie plate with nonstick vegetable oil spray. Mix chicken, veggies, and cheese and spoon evenly into pie plate. Beat remaining ingredients in the blender or with wire whisk until smooth. Pour evenly over chicken mixture. Bake about 35 minutes or until knife inserted in center comes out clean. Let stand 5 minutes before cutting.

4 SERVINGS

Each with: 309 Calories (21% from Fat, 49% from Protein, 30% from Carb); 38 g Protein; 7 g Total Fat; 3 g Saturated Fat; 2 g Monounsaturated Fat; 1 g Polyunsaturated Fat; 23 g Carb; 4 g Fiber; 3 g Sugar; 506 mg Phosphorus; 329 mg Calcium; 443 mg Sodium; 779 mg Potassium; 672 IU Vitamin A; 59 mg ATE Vitamin E; 23 mg Vitamin C; 70 mg Cholesterol

Tomatoes Stuffed with Goodness

This is a good meal for the hot weather and a great use of fresh tomatoes. The pasta will help to fill you up and the wide assortment of veggies will keep you full and handle the nutrition side. This is another of those meals that has everything you need to keep you going all afternoon or evening that still doesn't make it all the way to 400 calories. But I think with a whole large tomato and almost a cup and a half of vegetables, not to mention the tuna and pasta, you will be quite full.

1 can (5 ounces, or 140 g) tuna, water packed

1½ cups (210 g) whole wheat pasta, cooked, drained, and cooled

1 cup (120 g) zucchini, chopped

¾ cup (75 g) celery, chopped

¾ cup (83 g) carrot, shredded

½ cup (75 g) green bell pepper, chopped

1 cup (119 g) cucumber, chopped

10 ounces (280 g) frozen corn, cooked and cooled

¼ cup (60 g) low fat mayonnaise

½ cup (115 g) fat-free sour cream

½ teaspoon celery seed

½ teaspoon onion powder

4 large tomatoes

4 cups (228 g) mixed greens

Mix together tuna, pasta, veggies, mayonnaise, sour cream, and spices. Remove stems and hard centers from tomatoes. Cut almost through in both directions, leaving 4 wedges. Place tomatoes on lettuce on 4 plates, spreading them out. Pile the salad in the middle.

4 SERVINGS

Each with: 305 Calories (21% from Fat, 24% from Protein, 54% from Carb); 19 g Protein; 8 g Total Fat; 3 g Saturated Fat; 2 g Monounsaturated Fat; 2 g Polyunsaturated Fat; 43 g Carb; 8 g Fiber; 13 g Sugar; 328 mg Phosphorus; 120 mg Calcium; 234 mg Sodium; 1306 mg Potassium; 9303 IU Vitamin A; 35 mg ATE Vitamin E; 67 mg Vitamin C; 45 mg Cholesterol

Chicken in a Pot

This is a healthier variation on chicken pot pie. Reduced-fat biscuits replace the buttery crust covering a steaming pot of chicken and vegetables.

2 teaspoons olive oil

2 cups (140 g) mushrooms, sliced

½ teaspoon garlic, minced

4 cups (950 ml) low sodium chicken broth

1 medium potato, diced

1½ cups (183 g) carrot, sliced

1 cup (150 g) green bell pepper, chopped

¾ cup (75 g) celery, sliced

¼ cup (31 g) all purpose flour

¼ cup (60 ml) water

3 cups (420 g) cooked chicken breast

½ teaspoon black pepper

1 cup (125 g) reduced-fat biscuit baking mix, see recipe in chapter 2

⅓ cup (60 ml) skim milk

Preheat the oven to 400°F (200°C, or gas mark 6). Heat the olive oil in a large heavy saucepan over medium heat. Add the mushrooms and garlic; sauté 5 minutes. Add chicken broth, potato, carrot, green bell pepper, and celery; bring to a boil. Cover, reduce heat, and simmer 10 minutes or until vegetables are just tender. In a cup, stir together the flour and water until smooth; stir into broth mixture. Add the chicken and black pepper; bring to a boil, stirring constantly. Pour into a 2-quart (1.9 L) baking dish coated with nonstick vegetable oil spray. Stir together the baking mix and skim milk to make a soft dough. Drop by tablespoonfuls onto the chicken mixture. Bake 20 to 25 minutes or until topping is golden.

5 SERVINGS

Each with: 397 Calories (23% from Fat, 36% from Protein, 41% from Carb); 36 g Protein; 10 g Total Fat; 2 g Unsaturated Fat; 5 g Monounsaturated Fat; 2 g Polyunsaturated Fat; 41 g Carb; 4 g Fiber; 7 g Sugar; 499 mg Phosphorus; 116 mg Calcium; 468 mg Sodium; 1093 mg Potassium; 4871 IU Vitamin A; 16 mg ATE Vitamin E; 35 mg Vitamin C; 72 mg Cholesterol

Italian Veggie Noodles

This is kind of a poor man's lasagna. It's quick to throw together for lunch or dinner but full of veggies and nutrition.

8 ounces (225 g) whole wheat noodles, uncooked

1½ cups (375 g) low fat ricotta cheese

2 cups (240 g) zucchini, chopped

1 cup (150 g) red bell pepper, diced

2 cups (140 g) mushrooms chopped

½ cup (20 g) fresh herbs, chives, basil, and parsley

Cook noodles. Drain and return to pot. Add other ingredients and cook for 5 to 7 minutes until warmed.

4 SERVINGS

Each with: 357 Calories (20% from Fat, 23% from Protein, 57% from Carb); 21 g Protein; 9 g Total Fat; 5 g Unsaturated Fat; 2 g Monounsaturated Fat; 1 g Polyunsaturated Fat; 54 g Carb; 3 g Fiber; 4 g Sugar; 383 mg Phosphorus; 306 mg Calcium; 129 mg Sodium; 617 mg Potassium; 1873 IU Vitamin A; 97 mg ATE Vitamin E; 90 mg Vitamin C; 29 mg Cholesterol

Thai Noodle Bowl

This is a healthy version of the noodle bowls that have become so popular. Flavored with peanut butter, lime juice, and garlic, it will satisfy the taste buds without excess calories.

4 ounces (115 g) whole wheat spaghetti

2 tablespoons (32 g) peanut butter

3 tablespoons (45 ml) lime juice

1 teaspoon garlic, minced

1 teaspoon fresh ginger, peeled and grated

½ cup (75 g) edamame

10 ounces (280 g) frozen stir-fry vegetables

2 tablespoons (18 g) chopped peanuts

¼ cup (25 g) scallions, sliced

Cook pasta according to directions. In a skillet, sauté peanut butter, lime juice, garlic, and ginger for 1 minute. Add edamame and vegetables and cook for 12 minutes until vegetables are tender; pour over pasta. Top with peanuts and scallions.

2 SERVINGS

Each with: 411 Calories (21% from Fat, 16% from Protein, 63% from Carb); 18 g Protein; 11 g Total Fat; 2 g Unsaturated Fat; 4 g Monounsaturated Fat; 3 g Polyunsaturated Fat; 70 g Carb; 12 g Fiber; 2 g Sugar; 299 mg Phosphorus; 82 mg Calcium; 106 mg Sodium; 627 mg Potassium; 7336 IU Vitamin A; 0 mg ATE Vitamin E; 24 mg Vitamin C; 0 mg Cholesterol

Better BLT

Make your BLT healthier by stacking the tomato thickly and serving with fruit on the side for extra nutrition.

8 slices low sodium bacon

2 tablespoons (28 g) low fat mayonnaise

4 slices whole wheat bread, toasted

4 leaves romaine lettuce

1 large tomato, sliced

1 pear

Cook bacon. Spread mayonnaise on toast and top with bacon, lettuce, and tomato. Serve pear on the side.

2 SERVINGS

Each with: 412 Calories (35% from Fat, 18% from Protein, 47% from Carb); 18 g Protein; 16 g Total Fat; 5 g Unsaturated Fat; 7 g Monounsaturated Fat; 2 g Polyunsaturated Fat; 49 g Carb; 8 g Fiber; 18 g Sugar; 304 mg Phosphorus; 88 mg Calcium; 726 mg Sodium; 817 mg Potassium; 2454 IU Vitamin A; 4 mg ATE Vitamin E; 28 mg Vitamin C; 37 mg Cholesterol

Turkey and Avocado Wrap

This recipe features low calorie turkey, healthy avocado, high nutrient density spinach, and fresh fruit. How could you ask for a better low calorie lunch?

5 ounces (140 g) turkey breast, sliced

1 avocado, chopped

2 cups (60 g) spinach

2 whole wheat tortillas, 8-inch (20 cm)

2 nectarines or peaches

Wrap turkey, avocado, and spinach in tortilla. Serve nectarines or peaches on the side.

2 SERVINGS

Each with: 397 Calories (38% from Fat, 23% from Protein, 40% from Carb); 23 g Protein; 17 g Total Fat; 3 g Unsaturated Fat; 10 g Monounsaturated Fat; 3 g Polyunsaturated Fat; 41 g Carb; 10 g Fiber; 11 g Sugar; 281 mg Phosphorus; 70 mg Calcium; 228 mg Sodium; 1137 mg Potassium; 3392 IU Vitamin A; 0 mg ATE Vitamin E; 23 mg Vitamin C; 43 mg Cholesterol

Tuna Garden Wrap

A tasty tuna salad with lots of vegetables makes this wrap filling as well as delicious.
An apple adds extra nutrition as well as appeal.

3 tablespoons (45 ml) *Reduced Fat Italian Dressing*, see recipe in chapter 2

7 ounces (200 g) tuna, packed in water

1 cup (110 g) carrot, shredded

1 cucumber, sliced

2 whole wheat tortillas, 8-inch (20 cm)

2 apples

Mix dressing with tuna. Wrap tuna and veggies in tortilla. Serve with apples on the side.

2 SERVINGS

Each with: 358 Calories (18% from Fat, 31% from Protein, 51% from Carb); 28 g Protein; 7 g Total Fat; 2 g Unsaturated Fat; 2 g Monounsaturated Fat; 2 g Polyunsaturated Fat; 47 g Carb; 5 g Fiber; 19 g Sugar; 330 mg Phosphorus; 80 mg Calcium; 557 mg Sodium; 837 mg Potassium; 7931 IU Vitamin A; 6 mg ATE Vitamin E; 13 mg Vitamin C; 43 mg Cholesterol

Tasty Tuna Wrap

A tuna salad with lots of veggies and topped with spinach provides a nutrient rich lunch
or light dinner without adding calories.

6 ounces (170 g) tuna, in water

¼ cup (15 g) fresh parsley, chopped

2 tablespoons (28 ml) lemon juice

1 tablespoon (15 ml) olive oil

½ cup (60 g) cucumber, diced

½ cup (60 g) zucchini, diced

½ cup (75 g) red bell pepper, diced

1 cup (180 g) tomatoes, diced

⅛ teaspoon black pepper

2 whole wheat tortillas, 8-inch (20 cm)

1 cup (30 g) baby spinach

Combine tuna with parsley, lemon, oil, black pepper, and all vegetables except spinach. Place in tortillas and top with spinach. Roll up.

2 SERVINGS

Each with: 361 Calories (32% from Fat, 29% from Protein, 39% from Carb); 26 g Protein; 13 g Total Fat; 2 g Unsaturated Fat; 7 g Monounsaturated Fat; 2 g Polyunsaturated Fat; 35 g Carb; 4 g Fiber; 3 g Sugar; 300 mg Phosphorus; 111 mg Calcium; 288 mg Sodium; 771 mg Potassium; 3778 IU Vitamin A; 5 mg ATE Vitamin E; 117 mg Vitamin C; 36 mg Cholesterol

Hail Caesar Turkey Wrap

Low in calories, but big on nutrition, this Caesar salad flavored wrap in a big hit for lunches around our house.

2 whole wheat tortillas, 8-inch (20 cm)

6 ounces (170 g) turkey breast, sliced

1 cup (47 g) romaine lettuce, shredded

1 cup (180 g) tomatoes, diced

2 tablespoons (28 g) Caesar salad dressing, low fat

2 apples

Fill tortilla with turkey, lettuce, tomatoes, and dressing. Serve with apple.

2 SERVINGS

Each with: 344 Calories (15% from Fat, 29% from Protein, 56% from Carb); 25 g Protein; 6 g Total Fat; 1 g Unsaturated Fat; 2 g Monounsaturated Fat; 1 g Polyunsaturated Fat; 49 g Carb; 5 g Fiber; 16 g Sugar; 273 mg Phosphorus; 90 mg Calcium; 442 mg Sodium; 673 mg Potassium; 2139 IU Vitamin A; 0 mg ATE Vitamin E; 31 mg Vitamin C; 51 mg Cholesterol

Dinners: Chicken and Turkey

C hicken and turkey are naturals for our 400-calorie meals. They are naturally low in fat and calories. There are a couple of things to remember to help you make the best choices when having chicken or turkey. First is that much of the fat is in the skin, so you should avoid eating that. The second is that white meat is leaner than dark meat. In keeping with both of these suggestions, you'll find that many of these recipes call for boneless, skinless chicken breasts. These have the additional advantage that they can be used in a wide variety of recipes. This can easily be seen in this chapter as we have not only traditional food from the United States, but around the world, with recipes that came from Italy, Spain, Mexico, Greece, France, and a variety of Asian recipes. And that's just the beginning.

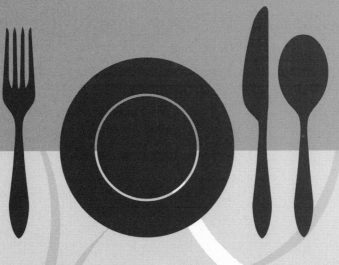

Honey Fried Chicken Dinner

Here's a complete fried chicken dinner for less than 400 calories. To make this possible, we oven fry lean chicken breasts, drizzled with a honey glaze, and then serve it with red potatoes and broccoli.

1 pound (455 g) boneless skinless chicken breast

2 tablespoons (22 g) Dijon mustard

4 tablespoons (28 g) dry bread crumbs

4 small red potatoes, quartered

2 teaspoons olive oil

4 cups (284 g) fresh broccoli florets

¼ cup (85 g) honey

2 tablespoons (28 ml) low sodium chicken broth, or water

Preheat oven to 450°F (230°C, or gas mark 8). Coat a large baking sheet with nonstick vegetable oil spray. Butterfly chicken by cutting each piece in half horizontally, almost through to the other side, but not completely. Open chicken breast half to make one thin piece. Brush Dijon mustard over both sides. Place seasoned bread crumbs in a shallow dish; add chicken breasts and turn to coat each side. Transfer chicken to prepared baking sheet and spray the chicken breasts with nonstick vegetable oil spray. Bake 8 to 10 minutes until chicken is cooked through. Meanwhile, place red potatoes in a microwave-safe container with a lid, add olive oil, and toss to coat potatoes. Cover and microwave on high for 5 minutes until potatoes are tender. Place broccoli in a microwave-safe container with a lid, cover, and microwave on high for 3 minutes until broccoli is crisp-tender. In a small bowl, whisk together honey and chicken broth. Transfer chicken to individual plates and drizzle honey mixture over top. Serve red potatoes and broccoli on the side.

4 SERVINGS

Each with: 395 Calories (11% from Fat, 33% from Protein, 56% from Carb); 33 g Protein; 5 g Total Fat; 1 g Unsaturated Fat; 2 g Monounsaturated Fat; 1 g Polyunsaturated Fat; 56 g Carb; 4 g Fiber; 20 g Sugar; 403 mg Phosphorus; 85 mg Calcium; 244 mg Sodium; 1402 mg Potassium; 2176 IU Vitamin A; 7 mg ATE Vitamin E; 104 mg Vitamin C; 66 mg Cholesterol

Creamy Pasta with Chicken and Vegetables

This is a good way to use up a few fresh vegetables. And it is
a healthy way to eat Italian.

10 ounces (280 g) whole wheat
linguine, or spaghetti

2 tablespoons (28 ml) olive oil

2 cups (240 g) zucchini, cut in
strips

12 ounces (340 g) mushrooms,
sliced

2 cups (71 g) broccoli florets

1 cup (160 g) onion, chopped

½ teaspoon garlic, minced

½ teaspoon dried basil

1 cup (235 ml) skim milk

2 cups (280 g) chicken breast,
cooked and cubed

⅛ teaspoon black pepper

1 cup (180 g) roma tomatoes,
sliced

¼ cup (25 g) Parmesan cheese

Cook linguini or spaghetti according to package directions. In a
skillet, heat oil. Add zucchini, mushrooms, broccoli, onion,
garlic, and basil. Cook and stir until zucchini is crisp-tender,
about 2 to 3 minutes. Drain pasta and return to saucepan. Stir
in skim milk, chicken, zucchini mixture, and black pepper and
heat through. Add tomatoes and cheese. Toss and serve.

6 SERVINGS

Each with: 377 Calories (23% from Fat, 29% from Protein, 47% from Carb);
28 g Protein; 10 g Total Fat; 2 g Saturated Fat; 5 g Monounsaturated Fat; 2 g
Polyunsaturated Fat; 45 g Carb; 4 g Fiber; 5 g Sugar; 381 mg Phosphorus; 158 mg
Calcium; 151 mg Sodium; 790 mg Potassium; 630 IU Vitamin A; 41 mg ATE Vitamin
E; 40 mg Vitamin C; 89 mg Cholesterol

Pasta with Chicken and Broccoli

This is another meal in a pan. If you've longed for the days of Hamburger Helper, now is the time to cheer. This recipe is just as easy and a boxed meal never tasted this good or had this kind of nutrition.

¼ cup (60 ml) olive oil

2 garlic cloves, minced

½ pound (225 g) boneless skinless chicken breasts, cut in ½-inch strips

1½ cups (107 g) broccoli florets

1 teaspoon dried basil

black pepper to taste

¼ cup (60 ml) white wine

¾ cup (175 ml) low sodium chicken broth

½ pound (225 g) whole wheat bow tie pasta, cooked

Parmesan cheese (optional)

In a large skillet, heat oil over medium heat. Sauté garlic for about one minute, stirring constantly. Add the chicken and cook until well done. Add the broccoli and cook until crisp-tender. Add basil, black pepper to taste; wine, and chicken broth. Cook for about 5 minutes. Add the cooked and drained pasta to the skillet and toss to combine. Heat for 1 to 2 minutes. Serve. Top with grated Parmesan cheese if desired.

4 SERVINGS

Each with: 417 Calories (34% from Fat, 22% from Protein, 44% from Carb); 22 g Protein; 15 g Total Fat; 2 g Saturated Fat; 10 g Monounsaturated Fat; 2 g Polyunsaturated Fat; 45 g Carb; 1 g Fiber; 1 g Sugar; 230 mg Phosphorus; 36 mg Calcium; 63 mg Sodium; 380 mg Potassium; 826 IU Vitamin A; 3 mg ATE Vitamin E; 26 mg Vitamin C; 33 mg Cholesterol

Really Low in Calories Chicken Shepherd's Pie

Shepherd's pie can be a high calorie, low nutrient dish, with its ground beef, buttery mashed potatoes, and cheese. So I went to work making a lower fat and calorie version for this book using chicken. And the problem I had was it was too LOW in calories. No matter how many veggies I added and how big the serving got, it just wasn't 400 calories. So you'll just have to content yourself with a 350-calorie mega meal.

2 tablespoons (16 g) cornstarch

1 cup (235 ml) low sodium chicken broth

3 cups (420 g) cooked chicken breast, diced

1 cup (150 g) red bell pepper, chopped

1 cup (160 g) red onion, chopped

20 ounces (570 g) frozen mixed vegetables

20 ounces (570 g) frozen broccoli

3 cups (610 g) mashed potatoes, prepared according to package directions

½ cup (58 g) low fat cheddar cheese, shredded

Mix cornstarch with broth. Heat until thickened and bubbly. Stir in chicken. Place in the bottom of a 9 × 9-inch (23 × 23 cm) baking dish. Cook vegetables until almost tender. Spread over chicken mixture. Cover with prepared mashed potatoes. Top with cheddar cheese. Heat under broiler until potatoes start to brown and cheese melts.

6 SERVINGS

Each with: 350 Calories (11% from Fat, 39% from Protein, 50% from Carb); 33 g Protein; 4 g Total Fat; 2 g Saturated Fat; 1 g Monounsaturated Fat; 1 g Polyunsaturated Fat; 43 g Carb; 9 g Fiber; 8 g Sugar; 377 mg Phosphorus; 145 mg Calcium; 809 mg Sodium; 916 mg Potassium; 5932 IU Vitamin A; 15 mg ATE Vitamin E; 96 mg Vitamin C; 64 mg Cholesterol

Chicken and Stuffing Bake

Creamed chicken and stuffing is served with broccoli for an every night Thanksgiving dinner. The use of chicken breasts and low fat soup holds down the fat content and the calories, providing a filling meal with fewer than 400 calories total.

6 ounces (170 g) stuffing mix

1½ pounds (680 g) boneless skinless chicken breast, cut in bite-sized pieces

1 can (10¾ ounces, or 305 g) low sodium cream of chicken soup

¼ cup (60 g) fat-free sour cream

16 ounces (455 g) frozen mixed vegetables, thawed

½ teaspoon black pepper

½ teaspoon garlic powder

½ teaspoon onion powder

4½ cup (320 g) broccoli florets, steamed until crisp-tender

Preheat oven to 400°F (200°C, or gas mark 6). Prepare stuffing according to package directions. Mix chicken, soup, sour cream, and vegetables. Place in a 13 × 9-inch (33 × 23 cm) baking pan and sprinkle with black pepper, onion powder, and garlic powder. Cover the chicken mixture with the stuffing. Bake 30 to 40 minutes or until chicken is done. Serve with broccoli.

6 SERVINGS

Each with: 361 Calories (17% from Fat, 39% from Protein, 44% from Carb); 35 g Protein; 7 g Total Fat; 2 g Unsaturated Fat; 2 g Monounsaturated Fat; 1 g Polyunsaturated Fat; 39 g Carb; 4 g Fiber; 5 g Sugar; 363 mg Phosphorus; 110 mg Calcium; 969 mg Sodium; 715 mg Potassium; 4985 IU Vitamin A; 38 mg ATE Vitamin E; 54 mg Vitamin C; 74 mg Cholesterol

Fit for Chicken à la King

Loaded with vegetables, this easy version of chicken à la king will satisfy your appetite and your taste buds.

8 ounces (225 g) whole wheat pasta

4 boneless skinless chicken breasts

2 cups (200 g) celery, chopped

1 cup (160 g) onion, chopped

2 cups (260 g) peas

1 cup (150 g) green bell pepper, chopped

2 cups (142 g) broccoli florets

1 can (10¾ ounces, or 305 g) low sodium cream of mushroom soup

Cook pasta according to package directions. Cut chicken breasts into small cubes and brown in a nonstick pan and set aside. Chop vegetables and sauté until they just start to turn soft. Add the mushroom soup and one can of water to the vegetables. Add the chicken and cook until chicken is done. Add the pasta and heat through.

4 SERVINGS

Each with: 356 Calories (9% from Fat, 30% from Protein, 61% from Carb); 27 g Protein; 4 g Total Fat; 1 g Unsaturated Fat; 1 g Monounsaturated Fat; 1 g Polyunsaturated Fat; 55 g Carb; 10 g Fiber; 8 g Sugar; 381 mg Phosphorus; 128 mg Calcium; 1116 mg Sodium; 1465 mg Potassium; 1281 IU Vitamin A; 12 mg ATE Vitamin E; 92 mg Vitamin C; 46 mg Cholesterol

Barbecue Chicken Dinner

Barbecued chicken is teamed with a rice pilaf full of vegetables for this quick and easy dinner.

4 boneless skinless chicken
  breasts
¼ cup (65 g) barbecue sauce
1 tablespoon (15 ml) olive oil
20 ounces (570 g) frozen mixed
  vegetables
2 cups (390 g) brown rice, cooked
4 tablespoons (28 g) sliced
  almonds

Grill chicken breast until chicken is done, about 8 minutes, brushing with barbecue sauce while cooking. Sauté vegetables in olive oil until tender, about 8 minutes. Add rice and heat until warm through. Top with almonds.

4 SERVINGS

Each with: 393 Calories (23% from Fat, 25% from Protein, 52% from Carb); 25 g Protein; 10 g Total Fat; 1 g Unsaturated Fat; 6 g Monounsaturated Fat; 2 g Polyunsaturated Fat; 51 g Carb; 9 g Fiber; 11 g Sugar; 330 mg Phosphorus; 73 mg Calcium; 250 mg Sodium; 560 mg Potassium; 6077 IU Vitamin A; 4 mg ATE Vitamin E; 5 mg Vitamin C; 41 mg Cholesterol

Stuffed Zucchini

This is for perfect those times when you don't get back to check the garden as often as you should and find a couple of zucchini that would make great softball bats. Discard the seeds and any center part of the squash that has gotten hard or stringy and put the rest of what you scoop out into the filling.

3 large zucchini
1¼ pounds (570 g) ground turkey
1 cup (160 g) onion, chopped
1 teaspoon garlic, crushed
2 cups (360 g) no-salt-added
  tomatoes
1½ cups (293 g) brown rice,
  cooked or (236 g) small whole
  wheat pasta
1 teaspoon dried basil
3 ounces (85 g) Swiss cheese,
  shredded

Cut the zucchini is half lengthwise. Scrape out the center, leaving a thickness of about a half inch (1.3 cm). Discard the seeds and chop the remainder. Cook the ground turkey, onion, and garlic in a large skillet until meat is done. Stir in tomatoes, rice or pasta, and basil. Cook the zucchini in boiling water until it begins to soften. Drain and place in baking pan. Divide the filling between the zucchini. Place a ½ ounce (15 g) of cheese on top of each. Place under broiler until cheese is melted and bubbly.

6 SERVINGS

Each with: 349 Calories (34% from Fat, 45% from Protein, 22% from Carb); 39 g Protein; 13 g Total Fat; 7 g Saturated Fat; 3 g Monounsaturated Fat; 2 g Polyunsaturated Fat; 19 g Carb; 2 g Fiber; 4 g Sugar; 329 mg Phosphorus; 332 mg Calcium; 148 mg Sodium; 732 mg Potassium; 824 IU Vitamin A; 17 mg Vitamin C; 98 mg Cholesterol

To Die for Chicken with Avocado and Tomato

When we first tried this recipe, I couldn't believe how much I liked it. The chicken is incredibly tender and flavorful. And the combination of avocados and tomatoes cooked with the chicken in a cheesy sauce is a real winner, not only from the standpoint of taste, but looks and nutrition too.

4 boneless skinless chicken
  breasts
2 tablespoons (28 ml) olive oil,
  melted
2 avocados
1 cup (160 g) tomatoes, chopped
½ cup (115 g) fat-free sour cream
½ cup (58 g) low fat Monterey
  Jack cheese, shredded
1 cup (71 g) broccoli florets,
  steamed until crisp-tender
1 cup (100 g) cauliflower florets,
  steamed until crisp-tender
½ cup (61 g) carrot, sliced and
  steamed

Slice chicken ½-inch (1.3 cm) thick. In large skillet, heat oil on medium-high. Add chicken slices and sauté 3 to 5 minutes until they start to turn brown. Preheat oven to 350°F (180°C, or gas mark 4). Peel, pit, and thinly slice avocado. Cut tomatoes into thin wedges. In medium casserole, layer chicken, avocado, and tomato. Top with sour cream. Sprinkle with cheese. Bake 30 minutes. Serve with steamed vegetables.

4 SERVINGS

Each with: 381 Calories (60% from Fat, 25% from Protein, 15% from Carb); 25 g Protein; 26 g Total Fat; 6 g Saturated Fat; 15 g Monounsaturated Fat; 3 g Polyunsaturated Fat; 15 g Carb; 8 g Fiber; 2 g Sugar; 333 mg Phosphorus; 142 mg Calcium; 193 mg Sodium; 917 mg Potassium; 2595 IU Vitamin A; 44 mg ATE Vitamin E; 53 mg Vitamin C; 56 mg Cholesterol

Crispy Chicken and Garlicky Collards

There's a lot to like about this meal. Low calorie, low fat chicken breasts are given both a crisp coating and a huge fiber boost with a mustard and bran flakes coating. Then they are teamed with collards, which are the number one item at the top of the ANDI nutrient density charts. And with all that, you still have calories left for a helping of good old fashioned mashed potatoes.

4 boneless skinless chicken breasts

2 tablespoons (22 g) Dijon mustard

2 cups (80 g) bran flakes cereal, crushed

2 tablespoons (28 ml) olive oil

½ teaspoon black pepper, divided

1 pound (455 g) collard greens, thick stems removed and leaves cut into bite-sized pieces

½ teaspoon garlic, thinly sliced

1 lemon, cut into wedges

3 cups (630 g) mashed potatoes, prepared according to package directions

Preheat oven to 400°F (200°C, or gas mark 6). In a large bowl, toss the chicken in mustard to coat. In a separate bowl, mix the cereal, 1 tablespoon (15 ml) of the oil, and ¼ teaspoon black pepper. Coat the chicken with the cereal mixture and bake on a baking sheet until golden and cooked through, 45 to 50 minutes. Meanwhile, cook the collards in a large pot of boiling salted water until tender, about 10 minutes. Drain, rinse, and squeeze out the excess water. Heat the remaining oil in a skillet over medium heat. Add the garlic, collards, and ¼ teaspoon black pepper. Cook for 2 to 3 minutes. Serve with the chicken and lemon and mashed potatoes.

4 SERVINGS

Each with: 392 Calories (21% from Fat, 25% from Protein, 54% from Carb); 26 g Protein; 10 g Total Fat; 2 g Unsaturated Fat; 6 g Monounsaturated Fat; 1 g Polyunsaturated Fat; 56 g Carb; 11 g Fiber; 3 g Sugar; 370 mg Phosphorus; 230 mg Calcium; 861 mg Sodium; 1019 mg Potassium; 8699 IU Vitamin A; 11 mg ATE Vitamin E; 72 mg Vitamin C; 44 mg Cholesterol

Kickin' Chicken Stew

Beans, tomatoes, and salsa add flavor and nutrition to this southwestern stew. Cream cheese gives it a delightful creamy texture that is sure to please.

5 boneless skinless chicken breasts

16 ounces (455 g) salsa

4 cups (688 g) black beans, cooked

10 ounces (280 g) frozen corn

2 cups (360 g) no-salt-added tomatoes, diced

1 teaspoon ground cumin

3 ounces (85 g) fat-free cream cheese

Place chicken breasts in bottom of slow cooker. Add remaining ingredients except cream cheese. Cover and cook on low for 8–10 hours. Add cream cheese, cook on low setting for 30 minutes, and then stir.

5 SERVINGS

Each with: 408 Calories (15% from Fat, 31% from Protein, 54% from Carb); 32 g Protein; 7 g Total Fat; 3 g Unsaturated Fat; 2 g Monounsaturated Fat; 2 g Polyunsaturated Fat; 56 g Carb; 12 g Fiber; 17 g Sugar; 570 mg Phosphorus; 150 mg Calcium; 1976 mg Sodium; 1692 mg Potassium; 1011 IU Vitamin A; 35 mg ATE Vitamin E; 34 mg Vitamin C; 51 mg Cholesterol

Easy Fix Chicken and Bean Skillet

This is a great, quick dinner for those nights when you don't have something planned and everyone is hungry. It's simple and fast but loaded with flavor and nutrition.

1 cup (160 g) onion, chopped

⅓ cup (50 g) red bell pepper, chopped

¾ teaspoon garlic, crushed

2 teaspoons olive oil

½ pound (225 g) boneless chicken breast, cut in 1-inch (2.5 cm) cubes

¾ teaspoon ground cumin

½ teaspoon cinnamon

10 ounces (280 g) navy beans, drained

10 ounces (280 g) kidney beans, drained

2 cups (510 g) no-salt-added stewed tomatoes, undrained

black pepper to taste

½ cup (88 g) whole wheat couscous

Sauté onion, red bell pepper, and garlic in oil in medium saucepan 2 to 3 minutes. Add chicken, cumin, and cinnamon; cook over medium-high heat until chicken is lightly browned, about 3 to 4 minutes. Add beans and tomatoes; heat to boiling. Reduce heat and simmer, uncovered, until slightly thickened, about 5 to 8 minutes. Season to taste with black pepper. Cook couscous according to package directions. Serve chicken and bean mixture over couscous.

4 SERVINGS

Each with: 408 Calories (9% from Fat, 29% from Protein, 62% from Carb); 30 g Protein; 4 g Total Fat; 1 g Saturated Fat; 2 g Monounsaturated Fat; 1 g Polyunsaturated Fat; 65 g Carb; 14 g Fiber; 8 g Sugar; 399 mg Phosphorus; 169 mg Calcium; 327 mg Sodium; 1096 mg Potassium; 632 IU Vitamin A; 3 mg ATE Vitamin E; 39 mg Vitamin C; 33 mg Cholesterol

French Country Chicken Cassoulet

A traditional French country dish, cassoulet sometimes contains sausage as well as chicken. We've omitted that because it adds fat and calories and added extra vegetable for increased nutrition.

2 cups (524 g) navy beans, dried

4 cups (950 ml) water

8 boneless skinless chicken breast, cut up

2 tablespoons (28 ml) olive oil

1 cup (130 g) carrot, finely chopped

1 cup (100 g) celery, chopped

1 cup (160 g) onion, chopped

1½ cups (355 ml) low sodium tomato juice

1 tablespoon (15 ml) Worcestershire sauce

½ teaspoon dried basil

½ teaspoon dried oregano

½ teaspoon paprika

 Tip: You can also cook this in a covered casserole dish in the oven at 325°F (170°C, or gas mark 3) for 1½ hours.

In large sauce pan, bring beans and 4 cups (950 ml) water to boiling. Reduce heat and simmer, covered, for 1½ hours. Pour beans and liquid into bowl. Brown chicken in the oil. In slow cooker, place chicken, carrot, celery, and onion. Drain beans; mix with remaining ingredients. Pour over meat mixture. Cover; cook on low-heat setting for 8 hours. Mash bean mixture slightly, if desired.

6 SERVINGS

Each with: 412 Calories (15% from Fat, 37% from Protein, 49% from Carb); 38 g Protein; 7 g Total Fat; 1 g Saturated Fat; 4 g Monounsaturated Fat; 1 g Polyunsaturated Fat; 51 g Carb; 19 g Fiber; 6 g Sugar; 527 mg Phosphorus; 148 mg Calcium; 134 mg Sodium; 1358 mg Potassium; 3065 IU Vitamin A; 6 mg ATE Vitamin E; 23 mg Vitamin C; 55 mg Cholesterol

Healthy French Chicken Stew

This recipe comes from the Normandy region of France, where apples and apple brandy are grown and produced. Calvados is a dry apple brandy from that region. If you can't find it, you can substitute any apple brandy. The recipe was made healthier than the original by reducing the amount of butter, using fat-free evaporated milk instead of cream, and using chicken breasts rather than a whole chicken.

4 boneless skinless chicken breast, quartered

2 tablespoons (28 g) unsalted butter

1 tablespoon (15 ml) olive oil

1 cup (130 g) carrot, peeled and diced

¼ cup (40 g) shallot, sliced

1 cup (160 g) onion

1 cup (235 ml) dry white wine

1 cup (235 ml) water

1 clove garlic, minced

1 teaspoon dried thyme

2 bay leaves

black pepper, to taste

1½ cups (188 g) apples (pippin), peeled and chopped

1 pound (455 g) mushrooms, washed and minced

1 cup (235 ml) nonfat evaporated milk

1 ounce (28 ml) Calvados

¼ cup (60 ml) egg substitute

2 cups (320 g) egg noodles, cooked

In a cast iron casserole or heavy Dutch oven, lightly brown the chicken in half the butter and half the oil. When all the pieces are golden, add the carrot, shallots, and the sliced onion and cook for a few minutes. Pour the white wine and 1 cup (235 ml) of water over the chicken and then add the garlic. Add some thyme leaves and bay leaves and season with black pepper. Cover and simmer over low heat for 40 minutes. Remove the chicken from the heat, arrange the pieces of chicken in an ovenproof serving dish, and keep warm. Pass the cooking liquid through a sieve. Set the vegetables aside and keep warm. Meanwhile, melt the remaining butter in a skillet with the oil, add the apples, and cook until just lightly brown on all sides. Remove the apples from the skillet and arrange them around the chicken. Keep the dish warm in the oven. Sauté the mushrooms until they have lost all their juices. Set aside to add to the sauce. To make the sauce: Pour the strained cooking liquid into a saucepan and set over medium heat. With a whisk, beat in the evaporated milk, the Calvados, and the egg substitute in that order. Simmer until it has thickened to a light cream. Stir in the mushrooms and the vegetables. Adjust seasoning. Remove the dish from the oven, spoon some of the sauce over the chicken, and pour the remaining sauce into a sauce boat. Serve with noodles.

4 SERVINGS

Each with: 420 Calories (29% from Fat, 32% from Protein, 40% from Carb); 30 g Protein; 12 g Total Fat; 5 g Unsaturated Fat; 5 g Monounsaturated Fat; 1 g Polyunsaturated Fat; 37 g Carb; 5 g Fiber; 18 g Sugar; 451 mg Phosphorus; 248 mg Calcium; 184 mg Sodium; 1107 mg Potassium; 4515 IU Vitamin A; 130 mg ATE Vitamin E; 12 mg Vitamin C; 72 mg Cholesterol

Go to Italy Tonight with Chicken Breast Cacciatore

This made a great tasting sauce with no extra work. And it's always nice to come home to a meal that's done and has filled the house with such an aroma. Paired with a broccoli and cauliflower combination, it also provides great nutrition.

1 cup (160 g) onion, sliced
6 boneless chicken breast
12 ounces (340 g) no-salt-added tomato paste
¼ teaspoon black pepper
½ teaspoon garlic powder
1 teaspoon dried oregano
1 teaspoon dried basil
¼ cup (60 ml) dry white wine
¼ cup (60 ml) water
4½ cups (320 g) broccoli florets, steamed until crisp-tender
4½ cups (450 g) cauliflower florets, steamed until crisp-tender
12 ounces (340 g) whole wheat pasta

Place onion in bottom of slow cooker. Place chicken on top. Combine remaining ingredients and pour over top. Cook on low for 8 to 10 hours. Serve with steamed broccoli and cauliflower and pasta cooked according to package directions.

6 SERVINGS

Each with: 385 Calories (6% from Fat, 31% from Protein, 64% from Carb); 31 g Protein; 3 g Total Fat; 1 g Saturated Fat; 0 g Monounsaturated Fat; 1 g Polyunsaturated Fat; 65 g Carb; 12 g Fiber; 10 g Sugar; 416 mg Phosphorus; 109 mg Calcium; 144 mg Sodium; 1275 mg Potassium; 1349 IU Vitamin A; 4 mg ATE Vitamin E; 115 mg Vitamin C; 42 mg Cholesterol

Pesto Chicken and Pasta

Pine nuts and fresh basil provide a pesto flavor to this flavorful dish, without the fat and sodium that canned pesto usually contains. The result is a healthier meal that's low in calories.

8 ounces (225 g) whole wheat pasta
1 teaspoon garlic, minced
30 cherry tomatoes, halved
2 cups (280 g) cooked chicken breast
1 tablespoon (15 ml) olive oil
½ cup (68 g) pine nuts
1 cup (40 g) chopped basil

Boil pasta according to directions. Sauté garlic, tomatoes, and chicken in olive oil for 3 to 5 minutes until warm. Add cooked pasta, pine nuts, and basil. Stir to combine and continue cooking for a few minutes longer until basil is limp.

4 SERVINGS

Each with: 378 Calories (42% from Fat, 30% from Protein, 29% from Carb); 29 g Protein; 18 g Total Fat; 2 g Unsaturated Fat; 7 g Monounsaturated Fat; 7 g Polyunsaturated Fat; 28 g Carb; 7 g Fiber; 1 g Sugar; 349 mg Phosphorus; 207 mg Calcium; 57 mg Sodium; 879 mg Potassium; 1602 IU Vitamin A; 4 mg ATE Vitamin E; 30 mg Vitamin C; 60 mg Cholesterol

Home-Style Italian Chicken Spaghetti Pie

Adding lots of chicken breast and vegetables and reducing the amount of pasta makes this one dish meal both satisfying and tasty.

8 ounces (225 g) whole wheat spaghetti, cooked

½ cup (120 ml) egg substitute

1 cup (225 g) fat-free cottage cheese

½ cup (80 g) onion, chopped

½ cup (75 g) green bell pepper, chopped

16 ounces (455 g) frozen Italian vegetable mix

2 cups (360 g) no-salt-added tomatoes, drained

1 teaspoon dried oregano

½ teaspoon garlic powder

3 cups (420 g) cooked chicken, cubed

¾ cup (83 g) part skim mozzarella, shredded

Cook spaghetti according to package directions. Drain. Mix in egg substitute. Form into a crust in a greased 10-inch (25 cm) pie pan. Top with cottage cheese. In a large skillet, cook onion and green bell pepper until tender. Add remaining ingredients except cheese and heat through. Spread over noodles and cottage cheese. Bake in 350°F (180°C, or gas mark 4) oven for 20 minutes. Sprinkle with mozzarella cheese about 5 minutes before the end of baking.

6 SERVINGS

Each with: 397 Calories (18% from Fat, 37% from Protein, 44% from Carb); 38 g Protein; 8 g Total Fat; 3 g Saturated Fat; 3 g Monounsaturated Fat; 2 g Polyunsaturated Fat; 45 g Carb; 7 g Fiber; 4 g Sugar; 446 mg Phosphorus; 244 mg Calcium; 232 mg Sodium; 724 mg Potassium; 4148 IU Vitamin A; 20 mg ATE Vitamin E; 30 mg Vitamin C; 62 mg Cholesterol

Mexican Chicken and Black Beans Skillet Meal

This is a quick one pan meal. If you have a little leftover rice, you can have this meal on the table in less than a half hour. The flavor is excellent and the nutrition is way beyond the old meal in a box days.

4 boneless skinless chicken breast, cut in 1-inch (2.5 cm) cubes

½ cup (80 g) onion, chopped

1 teaspoon garlic, crushed

2 cups (344 g) black beans, rinsed, drained

1 cup (180 g) tomatoes, chopped

¼ cup (65 g) salsa, mild or hot

½ cup (115 g) fat-free sour cream

2 cups (390 g) cooked brown rice

1 avocado, sliced

Spray large skillet with nonstick vegetable oil spray; heat over medium heat until hot. Sauté chicken, onion, and garlic until chicken is cooked, 5 to 8 minutes. Stir in beans, tomato, salsa, and sour cream. Cook until hot, 1 to 2 minutes. Serve over rice, garnished with avocado.

4 SERVINGS

Each with: 436 Calories (26% from Fat, 26% from Protein, 48% from Carb); 29 g Protein; 13 g Total Fat; 4 g Saturated Fat; 6 g Monounsaturated Fat; 2 g Polyunsaturated Fat; 53 g Carb; 13 g Fiber; 2 g Sugar; 406 mg Phosphorus; 90 mg Calcium; 138 mg Sodium; 970 mg Potassium; 536 IU Vitamin A; 35 mg ATE Vitamin E; 18 mg Vitamin C; 53 mg Cholesterol

Mole Tostadas

Low fat chicken and black beans, simmered in a chocolate chili mole sauce, combine for the stuffing for these tostadas. Lettuce and fresh tomato add additional bulk and nutrition.

8 corn tortillas

1 teaspoon canola oil

1 cup (160 g) onion, chopped

½ teaspoon garlic, minced

1 tablespoon (6 g) cocoa powder

1 teaspoon chili powder

1 teaspoon ground cumin

½ teaspoon cinnamon

½ teaspoon sugar

½ teaspoon dried oregano

2 cups (360 g) no-salt-added tomatoes, drained

2 cups (344 g) black beans, rinsed and drained

2 cups (280 g) cooked chicken breast, shredded

2 cups (94 g) romaine lettuce, shredded

2 cups (360 g) tomato, chopped

Preheat oven to 425°F (220°C, or gas mark 7). Lightly spray large baking sheet with nonstick vegetable oil spray. Arrange tortillas in single layer on baking sheet and lightly spray them with nonstick vegetable oil spray. Bake until crisp, 6 to 8 minutes. Transfer tortillas to wire rack to cool. Meanwhile, heat oil in large nonstick skillet over medium heat. Add onion and garlic; cook, stirring frequently, until golden, about 7 minutes. Add cocoa, chili, cumin, cinnamon, sugar, and oregano; cook, stirring constantly, until fragrant, about 1 minute. Add tomatoes, beans, and chicken; bring to boil. Reduce heat and simmer, stirring occasionally, until thickened, 10 to 12 minutes. Spoon about ⅓ cup (85 g) of chili onto each tortilla. Top evenly with lettuce and tomato.

4 SERVINGS

Each with: 399 Calories (15% from Fat, 32% from Protein, 53% from Carb); 33 g Protein; 7 g Total Fat; 1 g Unsaturated Fat; 2 g Monounsaturated Fat; 2 g Polyunsaturated Fat; 54 g Carb; 11 g Fiber; 14 g Sugar; 546 mg Phosphorus; 190 mg Calcium; 1055 mg Sodium; 1428 mg Potassium; 2636 IU Vitamin A; 4 mg ATE Vitamin E; 39 mg Vitamin C; 60 mg Cholesterol

Lower Calorie Chicken Fajitas

Fajitas are often a high calorie item. Here we reduce the number of calories by using low fat chicken and a minimum amount of oil. Most large groceries now carry whole grain, lower carb tortillas, which also reduce the overall calorie count while increasing the nutrition level.

2 teaspoons olive oil, divided

2 cups (320 g) onion, sliced

1 cup (150 g) yellow bell pepper, cut into strips

1 cup (150 g) red bell pepper, cut into strips

1 cup (150) green bell pepper, cut into strips

¼ cup (23 g) jalapeño pepper (about 2 peppers), thinly sliced seeded

⅓ cup (5 g) fresh cilantro, chopped

⅛ teaspoon black pepper

12 ounces (340 g) boneless chicken breast, cut into 2 × ¼-inch (5 × 0.6 cm) strips

4 whole wheat tortillas, 8-inch (20 cm)

2 tablespoons (30 g) fat-free cream cheese

2 cups (476 g) refried beans, see recipe in chapter 14

Heat 1 teaspoon oil in a large nonstick skillet over medium-high heat. Add the onion, yellow, red, and green bell pepper, and jalapeno pepper; stir-fry until crisp-tender. Remove pepper mixture from skillet; stir in cilantro and black pepper. Heat 1 teaspoon oil in skillet over medium-high heat. Add chicken; sauté 3 minutes or until done. Return pepper mixture to skillet; cook 1 minute or until thoroughly heated. Heat tortillas according to package directions. Spread 1½ teaspoons of cream cheese over each tortilla. Divide chicken mixture evenly among tortillas; roll up. Heat beans and serve with fajitas.

4 SERVINGS

Each with: 401 Calories (19% from Fat, 30% from Protein, 51% from Carb); 32 g Protein; 9 g Total Fat; 3 g Unsaturated Fat; 4 g Monounsaturated Fat; 1 g Polyunsaturated Fat; 53 g Carb; 11 g Fiber; 6 g Sugar; 380 mg Phosphorus; 107 mg Calcium; 268 mg Sodium; 998 mg Potassium; 1747 IU Vitamin A; 19 mg ATE Vitamin E; 204 mg Vitamin C; 64 mg Cholesterol

Enchiladas Verde Casserole

Here's a great tasty chicken enchilada dish with a creamy green chili sauce. It tastes rich and full of calories, but is just full of nutrition.

3 boneless skinless chicken breasts
1 cup (160 g) onion, chopped
1 teaspoon garlic, minced
8 ounces (225 g) fat-free sour cream
⅓ cup (5 g) fresh cilantro
1 teaspoon ground cumin
1 teaspoon black pepper
2 tablespoons (28 ml) lime juice
1 cup (115 g) low fat Monterey Jack cheese, shredded, divided
2 cups (354) great northern beans
8 corn tortillas
16 ounces (455 g) salsa verde

Cut up chicken and cook in skillet sprayed with nonstick vegetable oil spray until lightly brown. Remove from skillet. In same skillet, sauté chopped onion and chopped garlic. In large bowl, mix sour cream, chopped cilantro, cumin, black pepper, lime juice, ½ cup (58 g) cheese, beans, cooked onion, and garlic mixture. Shred chicken and add to bowl. Mix well. Spread half of mixture in 9 × 13-inch (23 × 33 cm) baking dish. Quarter all tortillas. Spread half of tortillas over mixture. Spread half of salsa verde over tortillas. Repeat layers. Top with remaining cheese. Bake at 350°F (180°C, or gas mark 4) for 20 minutes.

4 SERVINGS

Each with: 429 Calories (20% from Fat, 31% from Protein, 49% from Carb); 34 g Protein; 10 g Total Fat; 5 g Unsaturated Fat; 3 g Monounsaturated Fat; 1 g Polyunsaturated Fat; 53 g Carb; 9 g Fiber; 2 g Sugar; 617 mg Phosphorus; 342 mg Calcium; 324 mg Sodium; 833 mg Potassium; 487 IU Vitamin A; 66 mg ATE Vitamin E; 9 mg Vitamin C; 54 mg Cholesterol

Old Mexico Chicken and Rice Meal

This Mexican skillet meal may remind you of some of the popular boxed meal mixes. But the flavor is superior, and the nutrition is much better.

1 tablespoon (15 ml) olive oil

1 pound (455 g) boneless skinless chicken breast, cubed

1 cup (160 g) onion, chopped

¾ cup (113 g) green bell pepper, chopped

10 ounces (280 g) frozen corn, thawed

1 cup (235 ml) low sodium chicken broth

1 cup (260 g) mild salsa

1½ cups (143) instant brown rice, uncooked

½ cup (58 g) low fat cheddar cheese, shredded

Heat oil in large skillet on medium-high heat. Add chicken, onion, and green bell pepper; cook and stir until chicken is cooked through. Add corn, broth, and salsa; bring to boil. Stir in rice; cover. Remove from heat. Let stand 5 minutes. Fluff with fork. Sprinkle with cheese; cover. Let stand 2 minutes or until cheese melts.

4 SERVINGS

Each with: 371 Calories (18% from Fat, 39% from Protein, 43% from Carb); 37 g Protein; 8 g Total Fat; 2 g Saturated Fat; 4 g Monounsaturated Fat; 1 g Polyunsaturated Fat; 40 g Carb; 4 g Fiber; 7 g Sugar; 442 mg Phosphorus; 122 mg Calcium; 660 mg Sodium; 808 mg Potassium; 596 IU Vitamin A; 17 mg ATE Vitamin E; 40 mg Vitamin C; 69 mg Cholesterol

Spanish Chicken

This is a Spanish-style dish full of chicken, rice, and vegetables. The slow cooker makes preparation easy, and both the flavor and nutrition are great.

4 boneless skinless chicken breast, diced

2 cups (260 g) carrot, diced

1 cup (160 g) onion, diced

2 cups (248 g) frozen green beans

1 pound (455 g) mushrooms, sliced

2 bay leaves

½ teaspoon dried tarragon

½ teaspoon savory

¼ teaspoon garlic powder

¼ teaspoon black pepper, coarsely ground

2 cups (360 g) no-salt-added tomatoes, chopped

3 cups (585 g) brown rice, cooked

½ cup (120 ml) water

½ cup (70 g) green olives, sliced

Place chicken, carrot, onion, green beans, mushrooms, bay leaves, tarragon, savory, garlic powder, black pepper, and tomatoes in slow cooker. Cover and cook on low 4 to 5 hours; stir in rice and water. Finish cooking for a total of 8 to 9 hours. Stir in olives during last half hour of cooking. Remove bay leaves before serving.

4 SERVINGS

Each with: 369 Calories (11% from Fat, 28% from Protein, 61% from Carb); 27 g Protein; 5 g Total Fat; 1 g Unsaturated Fat; 2 g Monounsaturated Fat; 1 g Polyunsaturated Fat; 58 g Carb; 10 g Fiber; 12 g Sugar; 436 mg Phosphorus; 129 mg Calcium; 266 mg Sodium; 1257 mg Potassium; 8326 IU Vitamin A; 4 mg ATE Vitamin E; 36 mg Vitamin C; 41 mg Cholesterol

Classic Spanish Arroz Con Pollo, and Then Some

In this recipe, we've taken the classic Spanish chicken and rice dish and reduced the fat by using boneless skinless chicken breast and then added mushrooms and more vegetables than usual to make it even more filling without adding to the calories. Finally, we made it an easy to fix slow cooker recipe. If you prefer, you can still make it in a large covered skillet, following the same preparation steps, but simmer it in the skillet until the rice is tender, about 45 minutes, adding the peas and green bell pepper for the final 10 minutes.

1 tablespoon (15 ml) olive oil

2½ pounds (1.1 kg) boneless skinless chicken breast

1 cup (160 g) onion, finely chopped

6 ounces (170 g) mushrooms, sliced

1 teaspoon garlic, minced

¼ teaspoon black pepper

1½ cups (285 g) brown rice

¼ teaspoon saffron, or 1 teaspoon turmeric

2 cups (360 g) no-salt-added tomatoes

1½ cups (355 ml) low sodium chicken broth

½ cup (120 ml) white wine

¾ cups (113 g) green bell pepper, finely chopped

2 cups (260 g) frozen peas

In a nonstick skillet, heat oil over medium-high heat. Add chicken, in batches, and brown lightly on all sides. Transfer to slow cooker. Reduce heat to medium. Add onion and mushrooms and cook, stirring, until softened. Add garlic and black pepper and cook, stirring, for 1 minute. Add rice and stir until grains are well coated with mixture. Stir in saffron or turmeric, tomatoes, chicken broth, and white wine. Transfer to slow cooker and stir to combine with chicken. Cover and cook on low for 6 to 8 hours or on high for 3 to 4 hours until chicken is cooked through and rice is tender. Stir in green bell pepper and peas, cover, and cook on high for 20 minutes until vegetables are heated through.

6 SERVINGS

Each with: 384 Calories (14% from Fat, 55% from Protein, 30% from Carb); 51 g Protein; 6 g Total Fat; 1 g Saturated Fat; 3 g Monounsaturated Fat; 1 g Polyunsaturated Fat; 28 g Carb; 6 g Fiber; 7 g Sugar; 524 mg Phosphorus; 77 mg Calcium; 193 mg Sodium; 974 mg Potassium; 1332 IU Vitamin A; 11 mg ATE Vitamin E; 36 mg Vitamin C; 110 mg Cholesterol

Full of Flavor Greek Salad

Chicken turns this Greek-inspired salad into a substantial main course. Loaded with vegetables and full of flavor, it will become a favorite.

⅓ cup (80 ml) red wine vinegar

2 tablespoons (28 ml) olive oil

1 tablespoon (4 g) fresh oregano, chopped or 1 teaspoon dried

1 teaspoon garlic powder

¼ teaspoon black pepper, freshly ground

6 cups (282 g) romaine lettuce, chopped

2½ cups (350 g) cooked chicken breast, chopped

2 cups (360 g) tomatoes, chopped

1 medium cucumber, peeled, seeded and chopped

½ cup (80 g) red onion, finely chopped

½ cup (75 g) ripe olives, sliced

½ cup (75 g) feta cheese, crumbled

2 whole wheat pita breads, 6-inch (15 cm)

 Tip: Feel free to substitute other chopped fresh vegetables, such as broccoli florets or bell peppers, for the tomatoes or cucumber.

Whisk vinegar, oil, oregano, garlic powder, and black pepper in a large bowl. Add lettuce, chicken, tomatoes, cucumber, onion, olives, and feta; toss to coat. Toast pita bread and serve with salad.

4 SERVINGS

Each with: 413 Calories (36% from Fat, 34% from Protein, 30% from Carb); 35 g Protein; 17 g Total Fat; 5 g Unsaturated Fat; 8 g Monounsaturated Fat; 2 g Polyunsaturated Fat; 32 g Carb; 5 g Fiber; 6 g Sugar; 365 mg Phosphorus; 208 mg Calcium; 598 mg Sodium; 827 mg Potassium; 5638 IU Vitamin A; 29 mg ATE Vitamin E; 44 mg Vitamin C; 91 mg Cholesterol

Greek Mousaka

This variation of the typical Greek dish uses ground turkey rather than the more common lamb to hold down the fat. But the taste is still traditional, and it will definitely fill you up.

3 cups (700 ml) water

1½ pounds (680 g) eggplant, peeled and sliced

½ pound (225 g) ground turkey

1 cup (160 g) onion, chopped

2 teaspoons garlic, minced

½ teaspoon cinnamon

½ teaspoon dried oregano

1 cup (235 ml) low sodium chicken broth

⅔ cup (127 g) brown rice

8 ounces (225 g) no-salt-added tomato sauce

2 tablespoons unsalted butter

¼ cup (30 g) whole wheat pastry flour

1½ cups (355 ml) skim milk

½ cup (120 ml) egg substitute

¼ teaspoon nutmeg

Lightly grease a shallow 2-quart (1.9 L) baking dish. Bring 3 cups (700 ml) water to boil in a large nonstick skillet. Add eggplant, cover, reduce heat, and simmer 10 minutes or until tender. Remove to paper towels to drain. Wipe skillet. Add turkey, onion, and garlic. Cook until no longer pink. Stir in cinnamon and oregano, then broth and rice. Cover and simmer 10 minutes, stirring 2 or 3 times. Stir in tomato sauce. Remove from heat. Melt butter in a 2-quart (1.9 L) saucepan. Whisk in flour and cook, stirring 1 to 2 minutes, without letting mixture brown. Gradually whisk in skim milk. Cook, whisking constantly, 4 to 5 minutes until thickened and smooth. Whisk about ⅓ the hot mixture into beaten egg substitute and then whisk egg mixture into remaining sauce. Remove from heat; stir in nutmeg. Preheat oven to 350°F (180°C, or gas mark 4). To assemble, cover bottom of prepared baking dish with half the eggplant slices. Spoon on all the filling and then cover with remaining eggplant. Pour on topping. Bake 20 to 25 minutes or until hot and bubbly and top is lightly golden.

4 SERVINGS

Each with: 388 Calories (22% from Fat, 23% from Protein, 56% from Carb); 22 g Protein; 10 g Total Fat; 5 g Saturated Fat; 2 g Monounsaturated Fat; 2 g Polyunsaturated Fat; 55 g Carb; 9 g Fiber; 9 g Sugar; 355 mg Phosphorus; 220 mg Calcium; 451 mg Sodium; 1116 mg Potassium; 732 IU Vitamin A; 104 mg ATE Vitamin E; 12 mg Vitamin C; 37 mg Cholesterol

Cajun Chicken and Sausage Jambalaya

I love a good Jambalaya, but it is often not the best thing when you are trying to watch your calories. This one uses chicken and turkey sausage to hold down the fat level and includes more than the usual vegetables to add to the nutrition and that feeling of fullness.

1 pound (455 g) boneless chicken breast

4 cups (950 ml) water

2 cups (320 g) onion, chopped

1 cup (10 g) celery, sliced

1 tablespoon (10 g) garlic, minced

1 tablespoon (15 ml) olive oil

½ pound (225 g) turkey sausage

3 tablespoons (28 g) green bell pepper, chopped

¼ cup (25 g) green onion

2 cups (360 g) no-salt-added tomatoes

2 tablespoons (28 ml) Worcestershire sauce

¼ teaspoon dried thyme

¼ teaspoon cayenne pepper

1½ cups (285 g) brown rice

In a large saucepan, combine the chicken breasts, water, half the chopped onion, half the chopped celery, and one third of the garlic. Bring to a simmer over medium-high heat. Reduce the heat to medium-low and cook, partially covered, until the chicken juices run clear when pierced with a fork, 20 to 25 minutes. Remove the chicken breasts from the cooking liquid. In a sieve set over a large bowl, drain and reserve the cooking liquid. You should have about 4 cups (950 ml) of liquid; add water, if necessary. Chop the chicken breast meat coarsely and set it aside. Heat the oil in a 5-quart (4.7 L) Dutch oven. Add the sausage and cook over medium heat, stirring often, until lightly browned, about 5 minutes. Then stir in the remaining ingredients, breaking up the tomatoes with a spoon. Cook over medium-low heat, tightly covered, until the rice has absorbed all the liquid, about 45 minutes. Remove the Dutch oven from the heat, stir in the reserved chicken, cover, and let stand for 5 minutes.

6 SERVINGS

Each with: 416 Calories (25% from Fat, 28% from Protein, 47% from Carb); 29 g Protein; 12 g Total Fat; 4 g Saturated Fat; 4 g Monounsaturated Fat; 2 g Polyunsaturated Fat; 49 g Carb; 4 g Fiber; 6 g Sugar; 421 mg Phosphorus; 87 mg Calcium; 353 mg Sodium; 783 mg Potassium; 382 IU Vitamin A; 5 mg ATE Vitamin E; 58 mg Vitamin C; 67 mg Cholesterol

Cajun Chicken and Rice

Cajun seasoning flavors grilled chicken breasts and a sort of quick jambalaya is made with brown rice and the holy trinity of Cajun cooking, onion, bell pepper, and celery. The result is a high flavor, low calorie meal that can be prepared quickly.

1 teaspoon Cajun seasoning

4 boneless skinless chicken breasts

2 teaspoons olive oil

½ teaspoon garlic, minced

1 cup (160 g) chopped onion

1 cup (150 g) green bell pepper, diced

1 cup (100 g) celery, sliced

2 tablespoons (32 g) no-salt-added tomato paste

A few dashes Tabasco sauce, to taste

4 cups (780 g) brown rice, cooked

Sprinkle Cajun seasoning on chicken and bake or grill. Add oil to skillet; sauté garlic, onion, green bell pepper, celery, tomato paste, and Tabasco sauce for 2 to 3 minutes. Add precooked rice and sauté for 5 more minutes. Serve chicken on rice.

4 SERVINGS

Each with: 352 Calories (13% from Fat, 25% from Protein, 62% from Carb); 22 g Protein; 5 g Total Fat; 1 g Unsaturated Fat; 2 g Monounsaturated Fat; 1 g Polyunsaturated Fat; 54 g Carb; 6 g Fiber; 4 g Sugar; 322 mg Phosphorus; 55 mg Calcium; 83 mg Sodium; 620 mg Potassium; 412 IU Vitamin A; 4 mg ATE Vitamin E; 36 mg Vitamin C; 41 mg Cholesterol

Cantonese Chicken Stir-Fry

This recipe has a very nice light sauce, without the usual soy sauce. It's loaded with vegetables and will fill you up and keep you that way.

2 tablespoons (28 ml) oil

1 cup (122 g) carrot, sliced

2 cups (142 g) broccoli florets

1 cup (160 g) onion, chopped

8 ounces (225 g) mushrooms, sliced

1 cup (70 g) bok choy, chopped

¼ teaspoon ground ginger

¼ teaspoon garlic powder

¼ teaspoon black pepper

3 boneless skinless chicken breast, sliced thinly

1 tablespoon (15 ml) sherry

1 tablespoon (20 g) no-salt-added chili sauce

1 cup (235 ml) low sodium chicken broth

1 tablespoon (8 g) cornstarch

1 cup (195 g) brown rice

In a wok, heat half the oil. Add the carrot, broccoli , onion, and half the spices and stir-fry for 2 minutes. Add the mushrooms and bok choy and stir-fry 1 additional minute. Remove vegetables. Add the remaining oil and heat. Add chicken and remaining spices and stir-fry until chicken is no longer pink. Return the vegetables to the wok. Stir together the sherry, chili sauce, broth, and cornstarch. Add to wok and heat until mixture thickens and begins to bubble. Serve over brown rice cooked according to package directions.

4 SERVINGS

Each with: 375 Calories (22% from Fat, 22% from Protein, 56% from Carb); 21 g Protein; 9 g Total Fat; 1 g Saturated Fat; 2 g Monounsaturated Fat; 5 g Polyunsaturated Fat; 53 g Carb; 5 g Fiber; 6 g Sugar; 374 mg Phosphorus; 72 mg Calcium; 242 mg Sodium; 797 mg Potassium; 4183 IU Vitamin A; 3 mg ATE Vitamin E; 48 mg Vitamin C; 31 mg Cholesterol

Chicken with Snow Peas and Broccoli

The stir-frying and ingredients give this an Asian feel, although it doesn't use the typical seasonings. Whatever you call it, it tastes great and is full of nutrient dense ingredients.

2 tablespoons (28 ml) olive oil, divided

1 pound (455 g) boneless chicken breasts, sliced

¼ cup (60 ml) egg substitute

¼ cup (32 g) cornstarch

1½ cups (240 g) onion, sliced

1 cup (150 g) green bell pepper, sliced

12 ounces (340 g) snow peas

1½ cups (107 g) broccoli florets

2 tablespoons (40 g) honey

½ cup (120 ml) low sodium chicken broth

1 tablespoon (8 g) cornstarch

2 tablespoons (8 g) almonds, slivered

Heat 1 tablespoon (15 ml) of the oil in a wok. Dip half the chicken in the egg substitute and dust with cornstarch. Stir-fry until just cooked, about 4 to 5 minutes. Remove and repeat with remaining chicken. Remove and add the rest of the oil to the wok. Stir-fry the onion until it begins to soften. Add the green bell pepper, snow peas, and broccoli and stir-fry until crisp cooked, about 4 minutes. Stir together honey, broth, and cornstarch. Add to the vegetables and cook until slightly thickened. Add the chicken and toss until coated and heated through. Sprinkle the almonds over the top.

4 SERVINGS

Each with: 379 Calories (27% from Fat, 35% from Protein, 37% from Carb); 34 g Protein; 12 g Total Fat; 2 g Saturated Fat; 7 g Monounsaturated Fat; 2 g Polyunsaturated Fat; 36 g Carb; 5 g Fiber; 16 g Sugar; 364 mg Phosphorus; 102 mg Calcium; 130 mg Sodium; 830 mg Potassium; 1361 IU Vitamin A; 7 mg ATE Vitamin E; 116 mg Vitamin C; 66 mg Cholesterol

Sure You Can Have Fried Rice

You can have fried rice! The trick is to make the stir-fried rice part of a bigger production that includes lots of meat and vegetables. And that is what this does, starting with low fat, low calorie chicken breasts and then adding lots of vegetables to give you a meal that you can eat.

2 tablespoons (28 ml) olive oil

4 boneless skinless chicken breast, sliced into strips

1 cup (150 g) red bell pepper, chopped

1 cup (124 g) water chestnuts, sliced

2 cups (142 g) broccoli florets

½ cup (50 g) green onion, chopped

3 cups (585 g) cooked brown rice

1 tablespoon (15 ml) rice wine vinegar

¼ cup (60 ml) low sodium soy sauce

1 cup (130 g) frozen peas, thawed

Heat large nonstick skillet over medium heat. Add 1 tablespoon (15 ml) oil. Add chicken, red bell pepper, water chestnuts, broccoli, and green onion. Cook 5 minutes until chicken is cooked through. Remove to a plate. Heat remaining tablespoon (15 ml) of oil in skillet. Add rice and cook 1 minute. Stir in soy sauce, vinegar, and peas; cook 1 minute. Stir in chicken and vegetable mixture.

4 SERVINGS

Each with: 395 Calories (21% from Fat, 25% from Protein, 54% from Carb); 25 g Protein; 9 g Total Fat; 1 g Saturated Fat; 6 g Monounsaturated Fat; 2 g Polyunsaturated Fat; 54 g Carb; 7 g Fiber; 4 g Sugar; 363 mg Phosphorus; 67 mg Calcium; 725 mg Sodium; 806 mg Potassium; 2637 IU Vitamin A; 4 mg ATE Vitamin E; 112 mg Vitamin C; 41 mg Cholesterol

Sweet and Sour Chicken

This is a simple, quick to prepare version that has a very nice sauce. Because the chicken is stir-fried instead of battered and deep fried, you can actually eat this version and still stay on your diet.

8½ ounces (240 g) pineapple chunks

½ cup (120 g) duck sauce, divided

2 tablespoons (2 g) brown sugar substitute, such as Splenda

¼ cup (60 ml) rice vinegar

1 teaspoon low sodium soy sauce

¼ cup (60 ml) orange juice

1 pound (455 g) boneless skinless chicken breast, cut in ½-inch (1.3 cm) pieces

1 pound (455 g) Asian vegetable mix, frozen

¼ teaspoon ground ginger

1 tablespoon (15 ml) water

2 teaspoons cornstarch

½ cup (80 g) long grain brown rice, cooked according to package directions

Mix juice from pineapple with duck sauce, brown sugar, vinegar, soy sauce, and orange juice. Set aside. In a large skillet with a tight fitting lid, place chicken and sauté until no longer pink on the outside, about 5 minutes. Add ¼ cup (60 ml) of sauce, pineapple chunks, vegetables, and ginger. Cover and simmer until chicken is done and vegetables are crisp-tender. Stir together water and cornstarch. Add to pan with remaining sauce. Cook until mixture is thickened and bubbly. Serve over rice.

4 SERVINGS

Each with: 387 Calories (5% from Fat, 33% from Protein, 61% from Carb); 32 g Protein; 2 g Total Fat; 1 g Saturated Fat; 1 g Monounsaturated Fat; 1 g Polyunsaturated Fat; 59 g Carb; 6 g Fiber; 9 g Sugar; 322 mg Phosphorus; 64 mg Calcium; 365 mg Sodium; 731 mg Potassium; 4924 IU Vitamin A; 7 mg ATE Vitamin E; 15 mg Vitamin C; 66 mg Cholesterol

Chicken in Orange Sauce

This is not exactly a traditional Chinese flavor combination, but it's one that works well. It's kind of similar to sweet and sour (or maybe I just think so because of the pineapple) and full of things that are good for you.

4 boneless skinless chicken breasts

1 tablespoon (10 g) tapioca

¾ cup (175 ml) low sodium chicken broth

¼ cup (60 ml) orange juice

¼ cup (60 ml) teriyaki sauce

1 teaspoon mustard seed

1 cup (165 g) pineapple chunks

1 pound (455 g) broccoli, chopped into florets

4 cups (760 g) brown rice, uncooked

Place chicken on the bottom of slow cooker. In a bowl, mix together tapioca, broth, orange juice, teriyaki sauce, mustard seed, and pineapple. Pour over chicken. Cover and cook on low for 7 to 8 hours. Add broccoli for last 20 minutes of cooking so it remains crisp. Cook rice according to package directions and serve chicken mixture over rice.

4 SERVINGS

Each with: 410 Calories (9% from Fat, 26% from Protein, 64% from Carb); 27 g Protein; 4 g Total Fat; 1 g Unsaturated Fat; 1 g Monounsaturated Fat; 1 g Polyunsaturated Fat; 67 g Carb; 7 g Fiber; 9 g Sugar; 408 mg Phosphorus; 101 mg Calcium; 540 mg Sodium; 896 mg Potassium; 799 IU Vitamin A; 4 mg ATE Vitamin E; 112 mg Vitamin C; 42 mg Cholesterol

Easy Baked Chicken Egg Foo Young

Rather than fried, this egg foo young dish is baked in the oven and saves the fat from the oil. It produces a filling dish full of eggs, chicken, and vegetables at just a little over 300 calories.

Casserole

2 cups (475 ml) egg substitute

1½ cups (150 g) celery, sliced

3 cups (420 g) cooked chicken breast

1½ cups (225 g) red bell pepper, chopped

16 ounces (455 g) bean sprouts, drained

½ cup (64 g) nonfat dry milk powder

2 tablespoons (20 g) onion, chopped

1 tablespoon (4 g) fresh parsley, chopped

⅛ teaspoon black pepper

Mushroom Sauce

2½ tablespoons (20 g) cornstarch

1½ cups (355 ml) low sodium chicken broth, divided

1 tablespoon (15 ml) low sodium soy sauce

4 ounces (115 g) mushrooms, sliced

2 tablespoons (13 g) green onion, sliced

Stir together all casserole ingredients; pour into greased 12 × 8 × 2-inch (30 × 20 × 5 cm) baking dish. Bake at 350°F (180°C, or gas mark 4) for 30 to 35 minutes or until knife inserted in center comes out clean. To make the sauce, combine cornstarch with ¼ cup (60 ml) broth. Heat remaining broth to boiling in a saucepan; gradually whisk in cornstarch, broth mixture, and soy sauce. Cook, stirring until thickened and smooth; add mushrooms and green onion. To serve, cut casserole into squares and top with mushroom sauce.

6 SERVINGS

Each with: 322 Calories (21% from Fat, 58% from Protein, 22% from Carb); 40 g Protein; 6 g Total Fat; 1 g Unsaturated Fat; 2 g Monounsaturated Fat; 2 g Polyunsaturated Fat; 15 g Carb; 2 g Fiber; 6 g Sugar; 401 mg Phosphorus; 159 mg Calcium; 369 mg Sodium; 980 mg Potassium; 1825 IU Vitamin A; 44 mg ATE Vitamin E; 103 mg Vitamin C; 61 mg Cholesterol

(Just Like at the Mall) Bourbon Chicken

This is a lower sodium, lower fat, lower calorie taste-alike for the kind of chicken they are always giving out samples of at the mall food court. Chicken breasts replace the more common and fattier thighs and sugar substitute sweetens it.

Marinade

3 tablespoons (45 ml) low sodium soy sauce

½ cup (8 g) brown sugar substitute, such as Splenda

½ teaspoon garlic powder

1 teaspoon ground ginger

2 tablespoons (10 g) dried minced onion

½ cup (120 ml) bourbon

Chicken

1 pound (455 g) boneless skinless chicken breast, cut in bite-sized pieces

Side Dishes

1½ cups (293 g) brown rice, cooked

1½ cups (107 g) broccoli florets, steamed until crisp-tender

 Tip: We like it the way it's shown here, with brown rice and steamed broccoli, but you could substitute other vegetables.

Mix all the marinade ingredients and pour over chicken pieces in a bowl. Cover and refrigerate for several hours or overnight. Bake chicken at 350°F (180°C, or gas mark 4) for one hour in a single layer, basting occasionally. Serve with rice and broccoli.

3 SERVINGS

Each with: 411 Calories (8% from Fat, 51% from Protein, 41% from Carb); 40 g Protein; 3 g Total Fat; 1 g Unsaturated Fat; 1 g Monounsaturated Fat; 1 g Polyunsaturated Fat; 32 g Carb; 3 g Fiber; 3 g Sugar; 438 mg Phosphorus; 68 mg Calcium; 648 mg Sodium; 688 mg Potassium; 322 IU Vitamin A; 9 mg ATE Vitamin E; 42 mg Vitamin C; 88 mg Cholesterol

You Can Have (and Love) Chicken Lo Mein

This classic Chinese dish is made more healthy and lower in calories than usual by adding lots more vegetables and using whole wheat pasta. I find that I prefer this to plain white noodles.

8 ounces (225 g) whole wheat spaghetti

4 boneless skinless chicken breasts

6 ounces (170 g) fresh mushrooms, sliced

½ cup (50 g) green onion, sliced

3 tablespoons (42 g) unsalted butter

2 cups (475 ml) low sodium chicken broth

2 teaspoons cornstarch

6 ounces (170 g) snow pea pods

4 ounces (115 g) water chestnuts, sliced

1 pound (455 g) broccoli

2 tablespoons (24 g) pimento, chopped

2 tablespoons (28 ml) low sodium soy sauce

½ teaspoon ground ginger

Prepare spaghetti according to package directions. Drain. In large skillet or Dutch oven, cook chicken, mushrooms, and onion in butter until chicken is tender and liquid is absorbed. Meanwhile, stir together broth and cornstarch. Add to chicken mixture along with cooked spaghetti and remaining ingredients; mix well. Heat through and serve.

4 SERVINGS

Each with: 353 Calories (27% from Fat, 31% from Protein, 42% from Carb); 29 g Protein; 11 g Total Fat; 6 g Unsaturated Fat; 3 g Monounsaturated Fat; 1 g Polyunsaturated Fat; 39 g Carb; 8 g Fiber; 7 g Sugar; 394 mg Phosphorus; 111 mg Calcium; 398 mg Sodium; 1116 mg Potassium; 1777 IU Vitamin A; 76 mg ATE Vitamin E; 137 mg Vitamin C; 64 mg Cholesterol

Traditional Sweet and Sour Chicken

This is just like at the restaurant or in one of the boxed mixes. Except that this version is much lower in calories. We accomplish that by stir-frying rather than deep frying the chicken while adding vegetables and being careful about the amount of rice. But I can guarantee you won't go away hungry.

1 pound (455 g) boneless skinless chicken breasts, cut in strips

16 ounces (455 g) frozen Asian vegetable mix

⅔ cup (160 ml) pineapple juice

¼ cup (60 ml) rice vinegar

4 teaspoons (11 g) cornstarch

1 tablespoon (15 ml) low sodium soy sauce

2 cups (330 g) pineapple chunks, in juice

2 cups (390 g) brown rice, cooked

Spray 10-inch (25 cm) skillet with nonstick vegetable oil spray and stir-fry chicken until done. Meanwhile, cook vegetables according to package directions. In small bowl, combine pineapple juice, rice vinegar, cornstarch, and soy sauce. Add pineapple chunks to cooked chicken and then add cooked vegetables. Pour in sauce mixture. Cook over medium heat until thick and bubbly. Serve over rice.

4 SERVINGS

Each with: 385 Calories (6% from Fat, 34% from Protein, 60% from Carb); 33 g Protein; 3 g Total Fat; 1 g Unsaturated Fat; 1 g Monounsaturated Fat; 1 g Polyunsaturated Fat; 57 g Carb; 8 g Fiber; 19 g Sugar; 370 mg Phosphorus; 78 mg Calcium; 249 mg Sodium; 792 mg Potassium; 4922 IU Vitamin A; 7 mg ATE Vitamin E; 19 mg Vitamin C; 66 mg Cholesterol

Chinese Chicken Pasta Stir-Fry

This is an Asian flavored use for leftover chicken that's quick and easy to make. This recipe uses whole wheat pasta rather than the higher calorie rice that is more common for Chinese dishes.

2 tablespoons (28 ml) oil

1½ cups (240 g) onion, coarsely chopped

1 cup (150 g) bell pepper, coarsely chopped

2 cups (200 g) cauliflower florets

2 cups (142 g) broccoli florets

1 cup (145 g) snow pea pods

1 cup (140 g) cooked chicken, cubed

8 ounces (225 g) whole wheat pasta, cooked

1 teaspoon garlic, minced

¼ cup (60 ml) soy sauce

3 tablespoons (45 ml) rice wine

1½ tablespoons sugar

1½ tablespoons (23 ml) Worcestershire sauce

½ teaspoon ground ginger

Heat oil in wok or skillet. Sauté vegetables in hot oil until just tender. Stir in chicken and pasta. Mix together remaining ingredients and stir in until meat, pasta, and vegetables are well coated.

4 SERVINGS

Each with: 377 Calories (19% from Fat, 13% from Protein, 68% from Carb); 13 g Protein; 8 g Total Fat; 1 g Saturated Fat; 2 g Monounsaturated Fat; 5 g Polyunsaturated Fat; 66 g Carb; 9 g Fiber; 11 g Sugar; 254 mg Phosphorus; 81 mg Calcium; 994 mg Sodium; 629 mg Potassium; 2513 IU Vitamin A; 0 mg ATE Vitamin E; 160 mg Vitamin C; 0 mg Cholesterol

Cook All Day, Fill You All Night Chicken Curry

I'm fond of curries. They make a particularly nice slow cooker meal because they fill the house with such a great aroma for you to come home to. This one calls for a number of spices that are typical of curry powder. If you have a favorite curry powder on the shelf, you could substitute a couple of tablespoons (13 g) of that for the other spices.

4 medium potatoes, diced

1 cup (150 g) green bell pepper, coarsely chopped

1 cup (160 g) onion, coarsely chopped

1½ cups (180 g) zucchini, sliced

1½ cups (150 g) cauliflower florets

1 pound (455 g) boneless skinless chicken breast, cubed

2 cups (360 g) no-salt-added tomatoes

1 tablespoon (6 g) coriander

1½ tablespoons (11 g) paprika

1 tablespoon (6 g) ground ginger

¼ teaspoon cayenne pepper

½ teaspoon turmeric

¼ teaspoon cinnamon

⅛ teaspoon ground cloves

1 cup (235 ml) low sodium chicken broth

4 tablespoons (32 g) cornstarch

2 tablespoons (28 ml) cold water

Place vegetables in slow cooker. Place chicken on top. Mix together tomatoes, spices, and chicken broth. Pour over chicken. Cook on low for 8 to 10 hours or on high for 5 to 6 hours. Remove meat and vegetables. Turn heat to high. Stir cornstarch into water. Add to cooker. Cook until sauce is slightly thickened, about 15 to 20 minutes.

5 SERVINGS

Each with: 406 Calories (6% from Fat, 30% from Protein, 65% from Carb); 30 g Protein; 3 g Total Fat; 1 g Saturated Fat; 0 g Monounsaturated Fat; 1 g Polyunsaturated Fat; 67 g Carb; 9 g Fiber; 10 g Sugar; 434 mg Phosphorus; 95 mg Calcium; 116 mg Sodium; 2121 mg Potassium; 1508 IU Vitamin A; 5 mg ATE Vitamin E; 97 mg Vitamin C; 53 mg Cholesterol

Easy Slow Cooker Curry

There's a lot to like about this recipe. You could start with the taste, which is mildly spicy and well developed from the long cooking. Or perhaps you want to start with the generous portion of creamy chicken and vegetables; or the low fat, high protein, and fiber nutrient content; or don't choose at all and just enjoy.

4 boneless skinless chicken breast, diced

1 can (10¾ ounces, or 305 g) low sodium cream of chicken soup

¼ cup (60 ml) sherry

½ cup (50 g) green onion, finely chopped

1 teaspoon curry powder

⅛ teaspoon black pepper

2 cups (200 g) cauliflower florets

1 cup (160 g) onion, coarsely chopped

1 cup (150 g) green bell pepper, cut in cubes

2 cups (240 g) zucchini, sliced

3 cups (585 g) brown rice, cooked

Cut chicken into small pieces and place in slow cooker. Add all remaining ingredients except rice. Cover and cook on low setting 6 to 8 hours. Serve over hot rice, cooked according to package directions.

4 SERVINGS

Each with: 349 Calories (16% from Fat, 29% from Protein, 56% from Carb); 24 g Protein; 6 g Total Fat; 2 g Unsaturated Fat; 2 g Monounsaturated Fat; 1 g Polyunsaturated Fat; 46 g Carb; 6 g Fiber; 6 g Sugar; 240 mg Phosphorus; 74 mg Calcium; 631 mg Sodium; 674 mg Potassium; 543 IU Vitamin A; 33 mg ATE Vitamin E; 74 mg Vitamin C; 47 mg Cholesterol

Chicken and Chickpea Curry

Low fat chicken and chickpeas give this a super boost of protein and other vegetables provide additional nutrients. And the combination provides plenty of volume without the need for rice or other filler.

1 tablespoon (15 ml) canola oil
½ cup (80 g) onion, chopped
1 tablespoon (1 g) fresh coriander, chopped
½ cup (75 g) green bell pepper, chopped
½ teaspoon garlic, chopped
1 cup (240 g) chickpeas
1 tablespoon (6 g) curry powder
1 tablespoon (7 g) turmeric
12 ounces (340 g) boneless skinless chicken breast, chopped
1 tablespoon (15 ml) lemon juice
1 cup (230 g) plain low fat yogurt

Heat the canola oil in a large pan and add the onion, coriander, green bell pepper, garlic, and chickpeas. Fry lightly. Add the curry powder and turmeric to the onion mix. Add a little bit of water if fluid is needed. Remove from pan. Put chicken in pan and fry until cooked through. Sprinkle with lemon juice. Add onion and curry mix to chicken and simmer for about 20 minutes. Add yogurt, heat through, and remove from stove.

3 SERVINGS

Each with: 341 Calories (24% from Fat, 43% from Protein, 33% from Carb); 36 g Protein; 9 g Total Fat; 2 g Unsaturated Fat; 4 g Monounsaturated Fat; 2 g Polyunsaturated Fat; 28 g Carb; 6 g Fiber; 10 g Sugar; 461 mg Phosphorus; 220 mg Calcium; 140 mg Sodium; 846 mg Potassium; 228 IU Vitamin A; 18 mg ATE Vitamin E; 31 mg Vitamin C; 71 mg Cholesterol

Low Calorie Turkey Meat Loaf Meal

Low fat turkey adds a generous helping of protein to this tasty meat loaf while keeping the calorie count down. Serve with buttermilk mashed potatoes and carrots for a complete meal.

Meat Loaf

1½ pounds (680 g) ground turkey

1 cup (160 g) onion, chopped

8 ounces (225 g) spinach, thick stems removed and leaves chopped

1 cup (30 g) fresh parsley, chopped

½ cup (60 g) bread crumbs

2 tablespoons (22 g) Dijon mustard

2 tablespoons (28 ml) egg substitute

½ teaspoon black pepper

¼ cup (60 ml) low sodium catsup

Potatoes

2 pounds (900 g) red potatoes, quartered

1 cup (235 ml) low fat buttermilk

1 tablespoon (15 ml) olive oil

3 cups (366 g) carrot, sliced

¼ cup (63 g) low sodium spaghetti sauce

Preheat oven to 400°F (200°C, or gas mark 6). In a bowl, combine the ground turkey, onion, spinach, parsley, bread crumbs, mustard, egg substitute, and black pepper. Transfer the mixture to a baking sheet and form it into a 10-inch (25 cm) loaf. Spread with the ketchup. Bake until cooked through, 45 to 50 minutes. Meanwhile, place the potatoes in a large pot of enough water to cover and bring to a boil. Reduce heat and simmer until tender, 15 to 18 minutes. Drain the potatoes and return them to the pot. Mash with the low fat buttermilk, oil, and ¼ teaspoon black pepper. Cook carrots in boiling water until tender. Serve the meat loaf with the potatoes and carrots and pass the spaghetti sauce.

6 SERVINGS

Each with: 385 Calories (14% from Fat, 37% from Protein, 49% from Carb); 36 g Protein; 6 g Total Fat; 1 g Unsaturated Fat; 2 g Monounsaturated Fat; 1 g Polyunsaturated Fat; 48 g Carb; 7 g Fiber; 11 g Sugar; 448 mg Phosphorus; 183 mg Calcium; 386 mg Sodium; 1738 mg Potassium; 12 284 IU Vitamin A; 3 mg ATE Vitamin E; 62 mg Vitamin C; 70 mg Cholesterol

Turkey and Barley Stuffed Green Peppers

Stuffed peppers can turn out to be diet nightmare. Here we've avoided that by using turkey instead of beef and limiting the cheese and making it low fat. But the flavor is still rich and the added volume of the mushrooms and onions will help to fill you up.

1 tablespoon (15 ml) olive oil

1 pound (455 g) ground turkey

2 cups (140 g) mushrooms, chopped

1 cup (160 g) onion, chopped

1 cup (157 g) cooked pearl barley

2 tablespoons (8 g) fresh parsley, chopped

¼ teaspoon dried thyme

¼ teaspoon black pepper

½ cup (58 g) low fat Monterey Jack cheese, shredded

4 green bell peppers

1 cup (245 g) no-salt-added tomato sauce

Preheat oven to 350°F (180°C, or gas mark 4) degrees. Heat the oil in a large skillet. Add turkey, mushrooms, and onion and cook, stirring until the onions are browned and turkey is no longer pink. Stir in the barley, parsley, thyme, and black pepper. Stir in the cheese; set aside. Cut off the tops of the peppers; remove and discard the seeds. Spoon ¼ of the mixture into each pepper. Stand the peppers upright in a baking dish just large enough to accommodate them. Pour the sauce over the peppers. Bake 30 minutes or until the peppers are tender.

4 SERVINGS

Each with: 400 Calories (17% from Fat, 39% from Protein, 44% from Carb); 39 g Protein; 8 g Total Fat; 2 g Saturated Fat; 3 g Monounsaturated Fat; 1 g Polyunsaturated Fat; 44 g Carb; 10 g Fiber; 5 g Sugar; 494 mg Phosphorus; 120 mg Calcium; 188 mg Sodium; 971 mg Potassium; 417 IU Vitamin A; 10 mg ATE Vitamin E; 14 mg Vitamin C; 72 mg Cholesterol

Fill Yourself Up on Thai Turkey

If you like the flavor of Thai food, you will like this. Loaded with extra vegetables, it provides a filling and flavorful meal. And it's a great use for leftover turkey.

3 cups (420 g) cooked turkey, cut into ¾-inch (1.9 cm) pieces

1 cup (150 g) red bell pepper, cut into short, thin strips

1 cup (160 g) onion, chopped

4 ounces (115 g) mushrooms, sliced

2 cups (142 g) broccoli florets

1¼ cups (285 ml) low sodium chicken broth

¼ cup (60 ml) low sodium soy sauce

¾ teaspoon garlic, minced

½ teaspoon red pepper flakes

2 tablespoons (16 g) cornstarch

¼ cup (25 g) green onion, cut in ½-inch (1.3 cm) pieces

⅓ cup (87 g) peanut butter

1½ cups (293 g) brown rice, prepared according to package directions

½ cup (8 g) fresh cilantro, chopped

Place turkey, red bell pepper, onion, mushrooms, broccoli, 1 cup (235 ml) broth, soy sauce, garlic, and red pepper flakes in large sauce pan. Cover and simmer until vegetables are crisp-tender, about 10 minutes. Mix cornstarch with remaining ¼ cup (60 ml) of broth in small bowl until smooth. Stir green onion, peanut butter, and cornstarch mixture into turkey. Cook and stir until sauce is thickened. Serve over rice and garnish with cilantro.

6 SERVINGS

Each with: 429 Calories (26% from Fat, 29% from Protein, 46% from Carb); 31 g Protein; 12 g Total Fat; 3 g Saturated Fat; 5 g Monounsaturated Fat; 4 g Polyunsaturated Fat; 49 g Carb; 4 g Fiber; 4 g Sugar; 426 mg Phosphorus; 64 mg Calcium; 438 mg Sodium; 746 mg Potassium; 1826 IU Vitamin A; 0 mg ATE Vitamin E; 74 mg Vitamin C; 54 mg Cholesterol

Black Eyed Peas and Rice Salad

This is a nice dinner salad of rice and black eyed peas with cooked turkey. It will definitely fill you up as well as satisfy the taste buds.

---

3 cup (585 g) brown rice, cooked

1½ cups (257 g) black eyed peas, cooked

1 tablespoon (11 g) Dijon mustard

½ teaspoon black pepper, fresh ground

¼ cup (60 ml) red wine vinegar

¼ cup (60 ml) olive oil

2 cups (280 g) cooked turkey

½ cup (80 g) red onion, sliced

½ teaspoon garlic, minced

½ cup (55 g) carrot, grated

4 cups (120 g) spinach, torn into bite-sized pieces

Cook the rice and the peas in advance. Whisk the mustard, black pepper, and vinegar until dissolved. Drizzle in the oil while whisking. Toss the black-eyed peas, rice, and turkey with the vinaigrette. Mix in the onion, garlic, carrot, and parsley. Serve over spinach.

8 SERVINGS

Each with: 425 Calories (21% from Fat, 18% from Protein, 60% from Carb); 19 g Protein; 10 g Total Fat; 2 g Saturated Fat; 6 g Monounsaturated Fat; 2 g Polyunsaturated Fat; 64 g Carb; 5 g Fiber; 3 g Sugar; 359 mg Phosphorus; 54 mg Calcium; 72 mg Sodium; 508 mg Potassium; 2878 IU Vitamin A; 0 mg ATE Vitamin E; 7 mg Vitamin C; 34 mg Cholesterol

Dinners: Beef

Unlike the chicken and turkey of the previous chapter, beef has a reputation of being bad for you. It tends to be high in saturated fat and that is doubly bad, because it not only adds calories, but it is a contributor to heart problems. However, this doesn't have to be the case if you are careful about the cuts of beef you use. Many of the recipes in this chapter call for low fat cuts of beef like round steak. If they are cooked properly, they can be just as good as the fatter cuts (which also are usually more expensive, so that's another advantage). The recipes using ground beef call for extra lean. I usually buy either the 93% lean or for an even leaner and cheaper alternative buy cuts like top round steak, often called London broil, and grind it myself. We do still try to limit the number of meals we have with beef, but it has a place in our meal plan.

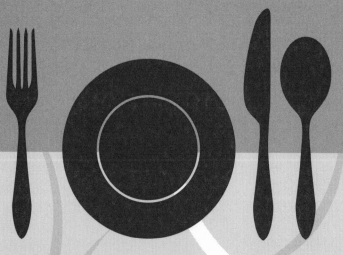

Easy Creamy Beef and Vegetables

This hearty casserole is perfect for a winter meal. Extra lean ground beef
helps to hold down the fat content, and canned soup gives it a creamy texture.
It's a true comfort food.

---

2 pounds (900 g) extra lean
  ground beef
2 cups (320 g) onion, sliced
2 cups (244 g) carrot, thinly
  sliced
⅛ teaspoon black pepper
1 can (10¾ ounces, or 305 g) low
  sodium cream of mushroom
  soup
¼ cup (60 ml) skim milk
3 medium potatoes, thinly sliced

Layer the following in a greased slow cooker: ground beef,
onion, carrot, and black pepper. Combine soup and skim milk.
Toss with potatoes. Arrange potatoes in slow cooker. Cover.
Cook on low for 7 to 9 hours.

8 SERVINGS

Each with: 417 Calories (44% from Fat, 24% from Protein, 31% from Carb);
25 g Protein; 20 g Total Fat; 8 g Unsaturated Fat; 9 g Monounsaturated Fat; 1 g
Polyunsaturated Fat; 32 g Carb; 4 g Fiber; 5 g Sugar; 293 mg Phosphorus; 57 mg
Calcium; 247 mg Sodium; 1258 mg Potassium; 3882 IU Vitamin A; 6 mg ATE Vitamin
E; 32 mg Vitamin C; 79 mg Cholesterol

Cheeseburger Pie

A beef and tomato filling with a cheesy topping makes this pie a real favorite with teenagers as well as adults. The lean ground beef and low fat cheese help to hold the calories to the level we are looking for.

Pie

1 pie shell

1 pound (455 g) extra lean ground beef

¼ cup (40 g) onion, chopped

¼ cup (38 g) green bell pepper, chopped

¼ cup (30 g) bread crumbs

½ teaspoon dried oregano

¼ teaspoon black pepper

8 ounces (225 g) no-salt-added tomato sauce

Cheese topping

8 ounces (225 g) low fat cheddar cheese, grated

½ teaspoon Worcestershire sauce

¼ cup (60 ml) egg substitute

¼ cup (60 ml) skim milk

½ teaspoon dry mustard

Bake pie shell at 425°F (220°C, or gas mark 7) until just set and partially baked. Set aside. Brown beef and drain. Mix beef with remaining ingredients and spoon into shell. Mix topping ingredients and spread over pie. Bake at 350°F (180°C, or gas mark 4) for approximately 25 minutes.

6 SERVINGS

Each with: 400 Calories (53% from Fat, 28% from Protein, 19% from Carb); 27 g Protein; 23 g Total Fat; 9 g Unsaturated Fat; 10 g Monounsaturated Fat; 2 g Polyunsaturated Fat; 19 g Carb; 1 g Fiber; 5 g Sugar; 350 mg Phosphorus; 204 mg Calcium; 483 mg Sodium; 493 mg Potassium; 473 IU Vitamin A; 29 mg ATE Vitamin E; 18 mg Vitamin C; 60 mg Cholesterol

Bar B Que Meat Loaf

The sauce makes this meat loaf especially good. The lean beef keeps the calories low enough for you to have the traditional (at least for us) mashed potatoes and carrots.

1½ pounds (680 g) extra lean ground beef

½ cup (60 g) bread crumbs

1 cup (160 g) onion, finely chopped

¼ cup (60 ml) egg substitute

¼ teaspoon black pepper

16 ounces (455 g) no-salt-added tomato sauce, divided

½ cup (120 ml) water

3 tablespoons (45 ml) cider vinegar

3 tablespoons (3 g) brown sugar substitute, such as Splenda

2 tablespoons (22 g) mustard

2 tablespoons (28 ml) Worcestershire sauce

4 cups (840 g) mashed potatoes, prepared according to package directions

4 cups (488 g) carrot, cut in 2-inch (5 cm) pieces and cooked

Mix together beef, bread crumbs, onion, beaten egg substitute, black pepper, and 4 ounces (115 g) tomato sauce. Form into loaf. Put in to a shallow pan about 7 inches (18 cm). Combine the rest of the sauce and all other ingredients. Pour over loaf. Bake in moderate oven, 350°F (180°C, or gas mark 4), for one hour and 15 minutes. Cook carrots and make mashed potatoes according to package directions. Serve with meat loaf.

8 SERVINGS

Each with: 382 Calories (38% from Fat, 23% from Protein, 39% from Carb); 22 g Protein; 16 g Total Fat; 6 g Unsaturated Fat; 7 g Monounsaturated Fat; 1 g Polyunsaturated Fat; 37 g Carb; 5 g Fiber; 9 g Sugar; 239 mg Phosphorus; 82 mg Calcium; 525 mg Sodium; 1078 mg Potassium; 7957 IU Vitamin A; 4 mg ATE Vitamin E; 26 mg Vitamin C; 61 mg Cholesterol

Sirloin Steak with Golden Fried Zucchini

Do you think that you can't have good steak while trying to lose weight? Think again. The trick to being able to eat steak like this sirloin is to limit the portion size and team it with other healthy filling foods like the zucchini and whole wheat couscous featured here.

2 tablespoons (28 ml) olive oil

1½ pound (680 g) sirloin steak

½ teaspoon black pepper

6 small zucchini, halved lengthwise

1 teaspoon lemon zest, grated

½ teaspoon garlic, finely chopped

3 tablespoons (20 g) fresh herbs, such as parsley, cilantro, or basil

2 tablespoons (14 g) bread crumbs

12 ounces (340 g) whole wheat couscous

Heat 1 tablespoon (15 ml) of the oil in a large skillet over medium-high heat. Season the steak with black pepper. Cook the steak to desired doneness, 4 to 5 minutes per side for medium-rare. Transfer to a cutting board. Let rest 10 minutes before slicing. Meanwhile, return the pan to medium heat and add 2 teaspoons of the oil. Cook the zucchini, cut-side down, covered, until browned and tender, about 6 minutes. Cut crosswise into ½-inch (1.3 cm) pieces and divide among plates. In a bowl, combine the lemon zest, garlic, herbs, bread crumbs, and remaining oil. Sprinkle the mixture over the zucchini. Serve the zucchini and couscous with the steak.

6 SERVINGS

Each with: 413 Calories (55% from Fat, 26% from Protein, 19% from Carb); 27 g Protein; 25 g Total Fat; 9 g Unsaturated Fat; 12 g Monounsaturated Fat; 1 g Polyunsaturated Fat; 19 g Carb; 3 g Fiber; 2 g Sugar; 266 mg Phosphorus; 62 mg Calcium; 89 mg Sodium; 717 mg Potassium; 306 IU Vitamin A; 0 mg ATE Vitamin E; 24 mg Vitamin C; 74 mg Cholesterol

Low Fat Smothered Steak with Noodles

The slow cooker can turn what is usually a tough cut of beef into something tender. This steak, covered in a mushroom and onion sauce, is an excellent example. And it's also an example of how a rich looking and tasting meal can be made healthier by carefully choosing the ingredients.

2 pound (900 g) beef round steak
1 package onion soup mix
¼ cup (60 ml) water
1 can (10¾ ounces, or 305 g) low sodium cream of mushroom soup
4 cups (640 g) egg noodles, cooked
3 cups (300 g) green beans

Cut steak into 6 serving size pieces. Place in slow cooker. Add dry onion soup mix, water, and soup. Cover and cook for 6 to 8 hours. Cook noodles according to package directions. Serve sauce and steak over noodles with green beans.

6 SERVINGS

Each with: 379 Calories (18% from Fat, 44% from Protein, 38% from Carb); 41 g Protein; 7 g Total Fat; 2 g Unsaturated Fat; 3 g Monounsaturated Fat; 1 g Polyunsaturated Fat; 35 g Carb; 3 g Fiber; 2 g Sugar; 450 mg Phosphorus; 46 mg Calcium; 372 mg Sodium; 901 mg Potassium; 406 IU Vitamin A; 7 mg ATE Vitamin E; 9 mg Vitamin C; 123 mg Cholesterol

Wine Sauced Steak

Kind of like a combination of beef Burgundy and Swiss steak, this dish is sure to please. And it's also low in calories while providing a filling meal.

2 pound (900 g) beef round steak

2 tablespoons (16 g) all purpose flour

½ teaspoon black pepper

2 tablespoons (28 ml) olive oil

1 cup (160 g) onion, chopped

½ cup (61 g) carrot, sliced

14 ounces (390 g) no-salt-added tomatoes

¾ cup (175 ml) dry red wine

½ teaspoon garlic, minced

¼ cup (60 ml) water

2 tablespoons (16 g) all purpose flour

3 cups (585 g) brown rice, cooked

Trim fat from steak; cut meat into 6 equal pieces. Coat with mixture of flour and black pepper. Pound steak to ½-inch (1.3 cm) thickness using a meat mallet. Brown meat in hot oil; drain. Place onion and carrot in slow cooker. Place meat atop. Combine undrained tomatoes, wine, and garlic. Pour over meat. Cover; cook on low heat setting for 8 to 10 hours. Transfer meat and vegetables to serving platter. Reserve 1½ cups (355 ml) of the cooking liquid for wine sauce. To make the wine sauce, pour reserved liquid into saucepan. Blend cold water slowly into flour; stir into liquid. Cook and stir until thickened and bubbly. Serve meat and vegetables over rice. Spoon some sauce over meat; pass remaining sauce.

6 SERVINGS

Each with: 410 Calories (25% from Fat, 40% from Protein, 36% from Carb); 38 g Protein; 10 g Total Fat; 3 g Unsaturated Fat; 6 g Monounsaturated Fat; 1 g Polyunsaturated Fat; 34 g Carb; 3 g Fiber; 4 g Sugar; 440 mg Phosphorus; 48 mg Calcium; 96 mg Sodium; 921 mg Potassium; 1372 IU Vitamin A; 0 mg ATE Vitamin E; 12 mg Vitamin C; 86 mg Cholesterol

Pure Comfort Beef and Barley Casserole

This quick casserole has a great flavor from a unique combination of ingredients. Use of extra lean ground beef helps to hold down the calories, while whole grain barley and vegetables pack in the nutrition.

⅓ cup (67 g) pearl barley

1 pound (455 g) extra lean ground beef, browned

1 cup (160 g) onion, cut up

1 cup (122 g) carrot, sliced

2 tablespoons (40 g) molasses

2 tablespoons (28 ml) low sodium soy sauce

In a 2-quart (1.9 L) casserole, mix barley, browned beef, onion, carrot, and molasses. Mix well. Add enough water to cover. Bake at 350°F (180°C, or gas mark 4) for 1 hour covered. Before serving, stir in soy sauce. Mix. You may have to add more water during baking.

4 SERVINGS

Each with: 384 Calories (47% from Fat, 25% from Protein, 28% from Carb); 24 g Protein; 20 g Total Fat; 8 g Unsaturated Fat; 8 g Monounsaturated Fat; 1 g Polyunsaturated Fat; 27 g Carb; 4 g Fiber; 9 g Sugar; 234 mg Phosphorus; 55 mg Calcium; 369 mg Sodium; 720 mg Potassium; 3856 IU Vitamin A; 0 mg ATE Vitamin E; 4 mg Vitamin C; 78 mg Cholesterol

Squash That Hamburger

OK, maybe I've been at this too long tonight, but Hamburger Zucchini Casserole sounded so mundane. And this tastes anything but mundane. It a warm, filling tasty treat full of good things like extra lean ground beef, squash, and cheese. So squash your resistance and give it a try.

6 cups (720 g) zucchini, diced

1 pound (455 g) extra lean ground beef

1 cup (160 g) onion, chopped

2 cups (390 g) brown rice, cooked

1 teaspoon dried oregano

1 teaspoon garlic powder

16 ounces (455 g) fat-free cottage cheese

1 can (10¾ ounces, or 305 g) low sodium cream of mushroom soup

1 cup (115 g) low fat Monterey Jack cheese, shredded

Cook squash and drain well. Sauté beef and onion. Add rice and seasoning to beef. Place half of squash in 2½-quart (2.4 L) casserole. Cover with beef mix and spoon over the cottage cheese. Add squash and spread on soup. Sprinkle with cheese. Bake at 350°F (180°C, or gas mark 4) for 35 to 45 minutes, uncovered.

4 SERVINGS

Each with: 445 Calories (42% from Fat, 27% from Protein, 31% from Carb); 35 g Protein; 24 g Total Fat; 10 g Unsaturated Fat; 10 g Monounsaturated Fat; 2 g Polyunsaturated Fat; 40 g Carb; 5 g Fiber; 7 g Sugar; 516 mg Phosphorus; 205 mg Calcium; 569 mg Sodium; 1243 mg Potassium; 464 IU Vitamin A; 21 mg ATE Vitamin E; 34 mg Vitamin C; 87 mg Cholesterol

Hamburger Vegetable Skillet

It doesn't get any easier or better than this. Mix it all up in a skillet and let it cook. Then eat a meal that is way better and way healthier than anything you can get out of a box.

1½ pounds (680 g) extra lean ground beef

8 ounces (235 ml) tomato juice, unsalted

1 medium potato, diced

1 cup (90 g) cabbage, chopped

10 ounces (280 g) frozen green beans

1 bay leaf

¼ teaspoon dried thyme

¼ tablespoons dill weed

6 cups (1.4 L) water

1 cup (160 g) onion, chopped

1 cup (180 g) no-salt-added tomatoes

½ teaspoon dried basil

¼ teaspoon black pepper

½ teaspoon garlic powder

1 cup (150 g) green bell pepper, diced

½ cup (61 g) carrot, sliced

10 ounces (280 g) frozen corn

Brown meat in large skillet. Pour off fat. Add remaining ingredients. Bring mixture to a boil. Reduce heat. Cover and simmer 1 hour or until vegetables are tender. Stir occasionally. Remove bay leaf before serving.

6 SERVINGS

Each with: 405 Calories (44% from Fat, 25% from Protein, 30% from Carb); 26 g Protein; 20 g Total Fat; 8 g Unsaturated Fat; 9 g Monounsaturated Fat; 1 g Polyunsaturated Fat; 31 g Carb; 6 g Fiber; 8 g Sugar; 292 mg Phosphorus; 75 mg Calcium; 113 mg Sodium; 1159 mg Potassium; 2072 IU Vitamin A; 0 mg ATE Vitamin E; 57 mg Vitamin C; 78 mg Cholesterol

Stuffed Red Peppers

Red peppers contain a lot more vitamin A than green ones, so why not use them for stuffed peppers. I like the flavor better too.

6 red bell peppers
½ cup (60 g) bread crumbs
1 cup (235 ml) nonfat evaporated milk
¾ cup (120 g) chopped onion
2 tablespoons (28 ml) olive oil
1½ pounds (680 g) extra lean ground beef
¼ cup (25 g) scallions
2 cups (475 g) water

Blanch red bell peppers, cut off tops, and finely chop as much of the tops as possible. Combine bread crumbs and evaporated milk and let soak. Cook onion in oil until tender. Combine all ingredients and stuff peppers. Place in a dish, add water, and cook at 375°F (190°C, or gas mark 5) for one hour.

6 SERVINGS

Each with: 377 Calories (58% from Fat, 27% from Protein, 14% from Carb); 26 g Protein; 24 g Total Fat; 8 g Saturated Fat; 12 g Monounsaturated Fat; 1 g Polyunsaturated Fat; 14 g Carb; 2 g Fiber; 9 g Sugar; 273 mg Phosphorus; 152 mg Calcium; 154 mg Sodium; 665 mg Potassium; 2543 IU Vitamin A; 51 mg ATE Vitamin E; 144 mg Vitamin C; 80 mg Cholesterol

Better for You Beef Stroganoff

In this recipe, we've limited the amount of beef (but only to what a serving is supposed to be) and added the nontraditional carrots for a nutritional boost. This makes a great comfort food meal for a chilly evening.

1¼ pound (570 g) beef round steak
2 tablespoons (28 ml) olive oil
1½ cups (105 g) mushrooms, sliced
1 cup (110 g) carrot, shredded
½ teaspoon sherry flavoring
¾ cup (125 ml) low sodium beef broth
½ cup (115 g) fat-free sour cream
3 cups (480 g) egg noodles

Cut meat into ¼-inch (6 mm) strips. Heat oil in skillet. Brown meat quickly, 2 to 4 minutes. Remove meat. Add mushrooms and carrot to skillet. Cook for 2 to 3 minutes. Remove mushrooms. Add sherry and broth to skillet and cook until liquid is reduced to about ⅓ cup (80 ml). Stir in sour cream. Stir in meat and mushrooms. Heat through without boiling.

6 SERVINGS

Each with: 376 Calories (32% from Fat, 43% from Protein, 25% from Carb); 40 g Protein; 13 g Total Fat; 4 g Unsaturated Fat; 6 g Monounsaturated Fat; 1 g Polyunsaturated Fat; 23 g Carb; 2 g Fiber; 2 g Sugar; 314 mg Phosphorus; 44 mg Calcium; 89 mg Sodium; 504 mg Potassium; 2660 IU Vitamin A; 25 mg ATE Vitamin E; 2 mg Vitamin C; 119 mg Cholesterol

Beef with Asparagus and Mushrooms

Sophisticated steak and vegetables with wood-scented rosemary results in deep full flavor. Lean London broil keeps the calories low in this tasty recipe.

1 pound (455 g) London broil, 1-inch (2.5 cm) thick

1 teaspoon garlic, minced

4 teaspoons (3 g) crushed rosemary

2 tablespoons (28 ml) olive oil

1 cup (160 g) onion, sliced

1 pound (455 g) asparagus, cut into 2-inch (2.5 cm) pieces

1 pound (455 g) mushrooms, sliced

⅛ teaspoon black pepper

1 tablespoon (6 g) lemon zest

Score both sides of the steak in diamond pattern by carefully making ⅛-inch (3 mm) deep diagonal cuts with a sharp knife at 1-inch (2.5 cm) intervals. Rub half of the garlic and 2 teaspoons of the rosemary into both sides of meat. Heat a tablespoon (15 ml) of the oil in a large nonstick skillet over medium heat. Add steak and cook, turning once, about 4 minutes per side for medium rare or until desired doneness. Transfer to a plate and loosely cover with foil to keep warm. Heat remaining oil in the same skillet. Add onion and cook stirring often, for 2 minutes. Add remaining garlic and cook, stirring constantly, until fragrant, about 30 seconds. Add asparagus and mushrooms and cook, stirring often, until asparagus is crisp and tender and almost all the liquid has evaporated, about 5 minutes. Stir in lemon zest, black pepper, and remaining rosemary. Cut steak into thin slices and serve with the vegetables.

4 SERVINGS

Each with: 364 Calories (35% from Fat, 51% from Protein, 14% from Carb); 47 g Protein; 15 g Total Fat; 4 g Unsaturated Fat; 8 g Monounsaturated Fat; 1 g Polyunsaturated Fat; 13 g Carb; 5 g Fiber; 6 g Sugar; 421 mg Phosphorus; 49 mg Calcium; 60 mg Sodium; 1027 mg Potassium; 876 IU Vitamin A; 0 mg ATE Vitamin E; 14 mg Vitamin C; 102 mg Cholesterol

Better Than Traditional Beef Stew

Here is the kind of meal you need as the weather starts to turn cooler. But this is comfort food made healthy, with lean meat and lots of vegetables. It has a wonderful aroma and flavor (thanks to a couple of unusual ingredients). And it can cook while you're away, so it's ready when you arrive home.

2 tablespoons (16 g) all purpose flour

1 pound (455 g) beef round steak, cubed

2 tablespoons (28 ml) olive oil

3 medium potatoes, cubed

1 cup (122 g) carrot, sliced

½ cup (80 g) onion, coarsely chopped

2 cups (240 g) zucchini, cubed

1 cup (235 ml) low sodium beef broth

2 cups (360 g) no-salt-added tomatoes

½ cup (120 ml) water

2 tablespoons (30 g) brown sugar

1 tablespoon (15 ml) Worcestershire sauce

1 tablespoon (15 ml) vinegar

1½ teaspoons instant coffee

1 teaspoon ground cumin

½ teaspoon ground ginger

¼ teaspoon allspice, ground

Place flour in plastic bag. Add beef and shake to coat. Brown on all sides in hot oil. Place potatoes, carrot, onion, and zucchini in a slow cooker. Top with meat. Mix together remaining ingredients. Pour over meat and vegetables. Cover and cook on low for 8 to 10 hours or on high for 4 to 5 hours.

6 SERVINGS

Each with: 393 Calories (21% from Fat, 34% from Protein, 46% from Carb); 33 g Protein; 9 g Total Fat; 2 g Unsaturated Fat; 5 g Monounsaturated Fat; 1 g Polyunsaturated Fat; 45 g Carb; 5 g Fiber; 11 g Sugar; 339 mg Phosphorus; 73 mg Calcium; 123 mg Sodium; 1542 mg Potassium; 2776 IU Vitamin A; 0 mg ATE Vitamin E; 61 mg Vitamin C; 68 mg Cholesterol

European Beef Stew

I don't know why I called this European, but it just seems to me like the kind of thing you'd find in Germany, Austria, or the Netherlands. At any rate, it's loaded with vegetables in richly flavored broth and is the kind of thing you want to come home to on a chilly evening.

4 teaspoons (20 ml) canola oil, divided

2 pound (900 g) beef round steak, trimmed of fat and cut into 1-inch (2.5 cm) cubes

¾ pound (340 g) mushrooms, sliced

3 tablespoons (24 g) all purpose flour

2 cups (475 ml) ale, or dark beer

1 cup (122 g) carrot, peeled and cut into 1-inch (2.5 cm) pieces

1 cup (160 g) onion, chopped

3 cups (450 g) turnip, cubed

1 medium potato, cubed

½ teaspoon garlic, minced

1½ tablespoons (17 g) Dijon mustard

1 teaspoon caraway seeds

½ teaspoon freshly ground black pepper

1 bay leaf

Heat 2 teaspoons oil in a large skillet over medium heat. Add half the beef and brown on all sides, turning frequently, about 5 minutes. Transfer to a 6-quart (5.7 L) slow cooker. Drain any fat from the pan. Add the remaining 2 teaspoons oil and brown the remaining beef. Transfer to the slow cooker. Return the skillet to medium heat, add mushrooms, and cook, stirring often, until they give off their liquid and it evaporates to a glaze, 5 to 7 minutes. Sprinkle flour over the mushrooms; cook undisturbed for 10 seconds and then stir and cook for 30 seconds more. Pour in ale or beer; bring to a boil, whisking constantly to reduce foaming, until thickened and bubbling, about 3 minutes. Transfer the mushroom mixture to the slow cooker. Add carrot, onion, turnips, potato, garlic, mustard, caraway seeds, black pepper, and bay leaf to the slow cooker. Stir to combine. Cover and cook on low until the beef is very tender, about 8 hours. Discard the bay leaf before serving.

6 SERVINGS

Each with: 376 Calories (23% from Fat, 47% from Protein, 30% from Carb); 40 g Protein; 9 g Total Fat; 2 g Unsaturated Fat; 4 g Monounsaturated Fat; 1 g Polyunsaturated Fat; 25 g Carb; 4 g Fiber; 7 g Sugar; 475 mg Phosphorus; 83 mg Calcium; 208 mg Sodium; 1277 mg Potassium; 2580 IU Vitamin A; 0 mg ATE Vitamin E; 25 mg Vitamin C; 70 mg Cholesterol

Beef Stew Hungarian Style

Similar to what is usually called beef paprikash, this stew has just the right amount of spice to satisfy and just few enough calories to be perfect for our plans.

2 tablespoons (28 ml) olive oil

1 cup (160 g) onion, chopped

1½ pound (680 g) beef round steak, cubed

½ teaspoon black pepper, coarsely ground

1 tablespoon (7 g) paprika

½ teaspoon dried marjoram, crumbled

½ teaspoon caraway seeds

1 cup (122 g) carrot, cut in 2-inch (5 cm) pieces

½ cup (50 g) celery, cut in 2-inch (5 cm) pieces

1 cup (150 g) green bell pepper, cut in 1-inch (2.5 cm) pieces

1 cup (160 g) tomatoes, cut up

8 ounces (225 g) mushrooms, sliced

¾ cup (180 g) fat-free sour cream

 Tip: If you can find it, use Hungarian sweet paprika.

Heat oil and sauté onion until soft and golden. Add beef, stir, and then add all the other ingredients except for sour cream. Cover, reduce heat, and simmer until tender, up to 2 hours. Stir occasionally and add water if needed. Serve with a dollop of sour cream.

4 SERVINGS

Each with: 394 Calories (42% from Fat, 43% from Protein, 14% from Carb); 42 g Protein; 19 g Total Fat; 6 g Unsaturated Fat; 9 g Monounsaturated Fat; 1 g Polyunsaturated Fat; 14 g Carb; 4 g Fiber; 5 g Sugar; 474 mg Phosphorus; 123 mg Calcium; 168 mg Sodium; 1089 mg Potassium; 5376 IU Vitamin A; 45 mg ATE Vitamin E; 46 mg Vitamin C; 96 mg Cholesterol

Flavorful Beef Stew with Root Vegetables

This flavorful stew cooks well in a cast iron Dutch oven, but any large heavy pan will do. The flavor of the dark beer and root vegetables combine for a real taste treat but not a high calorie one.

2 pound (900 g) beef round steak, cut into 1-inch (2.5 cm) pieces

2 teaspoons black pepper, freshly ground, divided

2 bay leaves

1 tablespoon (2 g) thyme

1 tablespoon (2 g) rosemary

2 tablespoons (28 ml) olive oil

2 tablespoons (28 g) unsalted butter

1 cup (160 g) onions, peeled and diced

¼ cup (31 g) all purpose flour

12 ounces (355 ml) dark beer

1 quart (950 ml) low sodium beef broth

½ cup (90 g) crushed tomatoes

1 cup (130 g) carrots, peeled and diced

½ cup (50 g) celery, diced

1 cup (150 g) rutabaga, peeled and diced

1 cup (133 g) parsnips, peeled and diced

Season the beef with 1 teaspoon black pepper. Tie the bay leaves, thyme, and rosemary into cheesecloth. In a large skillet, combine the oil and butter and heat until the butter bubbles. Add the beef in one flat and not-too-tightly-packed layer and brown the beef well on all sides. Remove the beef, set aside, and add the onions and cook to a golden-caramelized color. Sprinkle the onions with the flour and stir to combine well. Return the beef to the pan, add the beer, broth, herbs, crushed tomatoes, and remaining 1 teaspoon pepper. Bring to a boil and reduce the heat to a slow simmer. Cover and cook for ¾ hour. Add the carrots, celery, rutabaga, and parsnips and continue to cook for 1 additional hour.

6 SERVINGS

Each with: 375 Calories (37% from Fat, 44% from Protein, 19% from carb); 38 g Protein; 14 g Total Fat; 5 g Saturated Fat; 6 g Monounsaturated Fat; 1 g Polyunsaturated Fat; 17 g carb; 3 g fiber; 3 g Sugar; 413 mg phosphorus; 65 mg calcium; 257 mg sodium; 977 mg potassium; 784 IU vitamin A; 32 mg ATE vitamin E; 15 mg vitamin C; 96 mg cholesterol

Pot Roast New Orleans Style

A taste of old New Orleans, this beef is nicely spiced and cooked with the traditional onion, celery and green bell pepper. Those Cajuns must know something about healthy cooking.

6 cups (1.2 kg) brown rice, cooked
2½ pound (1.1 kg) beef round roast
¼ teaspoon cayenne pepper
½ teaspoon black pepper
2 teaspoons olive oil
1 cup (160 g) onion, chopped
1 cup (100 g) celery, chopped
1 cup (150 g) green bell pepper, chopped
2 tablespoons (16 g) all purpose flour
1 teaspoon garlic, minced
28 ounces (785 g) no-salt-added tomatoes
1 cup (235 ml) low sodium beef broth
½ teaspoon dried thyme
½ teaspoon basil
1 bay leaf

 Tip: Feel free to add more cayenne pepper if you like things spicier (or more like real Cajun food).

Prepare rice according to package directions. Rub meat all over with cayenne pepper and black pepper. In Dutch oven, heat oil and brown meat. Take out meat and sauté vegetables. Add flour to vegetables and cook 2 minutes, stirring constantly. Add garlic, tomatoes, broth, thyme, basil, and bay leaf. Stir until well blended. Place meat back in Dutch oven. Bring liquid to boil on high heat. Reduce heat to simmer, cover, and cook 2½ to 3 hours. Remove bay leaf. Slice meat and serve sauce and vegetables over both meat and rice.

8 SERVINGS

Each with: 399 Calories (18% from Fat, 37% from Protein, 45% from Carb); 37 g Protein; 8 g Total Fat; 2 g Unsaturated Fat; 4 g Monounsaturated Fat; 1 g Polyunsaturated Fat; 44 g Carb; 5 g Fiber; 4 g Sugar; 459 mg Phosphorus; 93 mg Calcium; 130 mg Sodium; 980 mg Potassium; 302 IU Vitamin A; 0 mg ATE Vitamin E; 31 mg Vitamin C; 71 mg Cholesterol

Beef and Cabbage Stew

The vinegar gives this a vaguely Germanic flavor, but whatever you call it, it's good and filling. This is the kind of recipe you can't wait to get home to on a cold day.

2 tablespoons (16 g) all purpose flour

¼ teaspoon black pepper

1½ pound (680 g) beef round steak

2 tablespoons (28 ml) oil

2 cups (320 g) onion, sliced

2½ cups (225 g) cabbage

2 cups (360 g) no-salt-added tomatoes

2 cups (300 g) turnips, peeled and cubed

2 cups (244 g) carrot, sliced

1 medium potato, peeled and cubed

1 cup (235 ml) low sodium beef broth

2 tablespoons (28 ml) vinegar

Combine flour and black pepper. Coat meat with mixture. Brown meat in oil on all sides. Place vegetables in slow cooker and top with meat. Add broth and vinegar to skillet. Stir, scraping up browned bits from bottom. Pour over beef and vegetables in cooker. Cover and cook on low for 8 hours.

5 SERVINGS

Each with: 378 Calories (25% from Fat, 38% from Protein, 37% from Carb); 36 g Protein; 11 g Total Fat; 2 g Saturated Fat; 3 g Monounsaturated Fat; 4 g Polyunsaturated Fat; 35 g Carb; 7 g Fiber; 11 g Sugar; 429 mg Phosphorus; 110 mg Calcium; 167 mg Sodium; 1551 mg Potassium; 6340 IU Vitamin A; 0 mg ATE Vitamin E; 53 mg Vitamin C; 78 mg Cholesterol

Mostly Eggplant Stew

This recipe is a nice variation on the beef stew theme, with different vegetables and spices.
The combination is part Mediterranean, but the cumin adds a bit of a Latin taste.
The generous amount of vegetables just soaks up the flavor,
making this a family favorite around our house.

2 pound (900 g) beef round steak, cubed

2 tablespoons (28 ml) olive oil

2 cups (360 g) no-salt-added tomatoes

1 cup (160 g) onion, chopped

2 tablespoons (32 g) no-salt-added tomato paste

½ teaspoon dried oregano

½ teaspoon dried basil

½ teaspoon ground cumin

¼ teaspoon red pepper

½ teaspoon garlic powder

1 cup (235 ml) water

1 medium potato, peeled and cubed

1 cup (235 ml) white wine

2 eggplants, peeled and cubed

2 cups (240 g) zucchini, sliced

8 ounces (225 g) mushrooms, sliced

In a Dutch oven, brown half the beef at a time in the oil. Drain and return all meat to the pan. Add tomatoes, onion, tomato paste, and spices. Stir in water. Bring to a boil. Reduce heat and simmer, covered, for 45 minutes. Add potato and wine. Cover and simmer 10 minutes more. Stir in eggplant, zucchini, and mushrooms. Cover and simmer until meat and vegetables are tender, 15 to 20 minutes.

6 SERVINGS

Each with: 386 Calories (25% from Fat, 43% from Protein, 32% from Carb); 40 g Protein; 10 g Total Fat; 2 g Saturated Fat; 5 g Monounsaturated Fat; 1 g Polyunsaturated Fat; 29 g Carb; 9 g Fiber; 10 g Sugar; 472 mg Phosphorus; 70 mg Calcium; 107 mg Sodium; 1637 mg Potassium; 331 IU Vitamin A; 0 mg ATE Vitamin E; 30 mg Vitamin C; 86 mg Cholesterol

Healthy, Hearty Roast Beef Hash

This could also be eaten for breakfast, but it's loaded with lots of vegetables and makes an easy dinner. You can use whatever leftover roast beef you have, trimmed of fat. We've also made it using part of a leftover smoked beef roast.

1 pound (455 g) roast beef, cooked and chopped

1 medium potato, peeled and diced

1 cup (160 g) onion, chopped

1 cup (150 g) green bell pepper, chopped

¼ cup (25 g) celery, chopped

1 tablespoon (9 g) dry mustard

1 tablespoon (9 g) garlic powder

¼ tablespoon dried thyme

¾ cup (175 ml) low sodium beef broth

Combine all ingredients and pack into a well greased baking pan. Cover with foil and bake at 375°F (190°C, or gas mark 5) for 45 minutes. Uncover, turn oven to broil, and brown the top.

3 SERVINGS

Each with: 439 Calories (31% from Fat, 41% from Protein, 28% from Carb); 45 g Protein; 15 g Total Fat; 5 g Unsaturated Fat; 6 g Monounsaturated Fat; 1 g Polyunsaturated Fat; 30 g Carb; 4 g Fiber; 5 g Sugar; 332 mg Phosphorus; 52 mg Calcium; 105 mg Sodium; 917 mg Potassium; 246 IU Vitamin A; 0 mg ATE Vitamin E; 52 mg Vitamin C; 159 mg Cholesterol

Oven Smoked Roast

Spices and liquid smoke give this roast its right-out-of-the-smoker flavor.

2½ pound (1.1 kg) beef round roast

2 cups (475 ml) low sodium beef broth

¼ cup (60 ml) low sodium soy sauce

¼ cup (60 ml) lemon juice

1 tablespoon (10 g) garlic, minced

1 tablespoon (15 ml) Liquid Smoke

8 ounces (225 g) egg noodles, cooked

6 cups (600 g) green beans, cooked

Place roast in roasting pan. Combine broth, soy sauce, lemon juice, garlic, and Liquid Smoke in bowl. Mix well. Pour over roast. Marinate in refrigerator overnight. Bake covered at 300°F (150°C, or gas mark 3) for 2½ hours. Bake uncovered for 30 minutes longer. Serve with noodles and green beans.

8 SERVINGS

Each with: 327 Calories (18% from Fat, 47% from Protein, 34% from Carb); 38 g Protein; 7 g Total Fat; 2 g Unsaturated Fat; 3 g Monounsaturated Fat; 1 g Polyunsaturated Fat; 28 g Carb; 4 g Fiber; 2 g Sugar; 418 mg Phosphorus; 76 mg Calcium; 400 mg Sodium; 811 mg Potassium; 588 IU Vitamin A; 5 mg ATE Vitamin E; 17 mg Vitamin C; 98 mg Cholesterol

Low Fat Italian Steak with Pasta

This is another easy to fix slow cooker recipe that makes the most of leaner beef, while providing great flavor and nutrition.

2 pound (900 g) beef round steak

¼ teaspoon black pepper

1½ cups (240 g) onion, sliced

1 cup (150 g) green bell pepper, cut in strips

28 ounces (785 g) low sodium spaghetti sauce

3 cups (360 g) zucchini, sliced

12 ounces (340 g) whole wheat pasta, cooked

 Tip: For a one dish meal, stir the cooked pasta into the cooker along with the zucchini.

Cut beef into serving sized pieces. Sprinkle with black pepper. Layer beef, onion, and green bell pepper in slow cooker. Pour sauce over. Cover and cook on low for 8 to 10 hours. Stir in zucchini, cover, turn heat to high, and cook for 15 to 20 minutes more until zucchini is tender. While zucchini is cooking, prepare pasta according to package directions. Serve beef and vegetable mixture over pasta.

6 SERVINGS

Each with: 373 Calories (20% from Fat, 44% from Protein, 36% from Carb); 41 g Protein; 8 g Total Fat; 2 g Unsaturated Fat; 3 g Monounsaturated Fat; 1 g Polyunsaturated Fat; 33 g Carb; 5 g Fiber; 11 g Sugar; 471 mg Phosphorus; 92 mg Calcium; 652 mg Sodium; 1244 mg Potassium; 1190 IU Vitamin A; 0 mg ATE Vitamin E; 44 mg Vitamin C; 70 mg Cholesterol

Layered Spaghetti Bake

Extra lean beef is cooked in a creamy tomato sauce and then layered with spaghetti and cheese in this pleasing dish.

1 pound (455 g) extra lean ground beef

½ cup (75 g) green bell pepper, chopped

½ cup (80 g) onion, chopped

½ cup (115 g) low fat mayonnaise

16 ounces (455 g) no-salt-added tomato sauce

¼ cup (25 g) Parmesan cheese, grated

8 ounces (225 g) mushrooms, chopped

1 teaspoon dried oregano

½ teaspoon black pepper

½ teaspoon garlic powder

7 ounces (200 g) whole wheat spaghetti, cooked and drained

1 cup (115 g) low fat cheddar cheese, shredded, divided

Preheat oven to 350°F (180°C, or gas mark 4). Brown meat with green bell pepper and onion; drain. Stir in mayonnaise, tomato sauce, Parmesan cheese, mushrooms, oregano, black pepper, and garlic powder. Cook 2 to 3 minutes over low heat or until thoroughly heated. Place ½ of the spaghetti in 2-quart (1.9 L) casserole. Top with ½ of the meat mixture and ½ cup (58 g) cheddar cheese. Repeat layers. Bake 30 minutes.

6 SERVINGS

Each with: 418 Calories (37% from Fat, 27% from Protein, 36% from Carb); 28 g Protein; 17 g Total Fat; 7 g Unsaturated Fat; 7 g Monounsaturated Fat; 1 g Polyunsaturated Fat; 37 g Carb; 5 g Fiber; 6 g Sugar; 399 mg Phosphorus; 177 mg Calcium; 422 mg Sodium; 764 mg Potassium; 406 IU Vitamin A; 18 mg ATE Vitamin E; 22 mg Vitamin C; 63 mg Cholesterol

Ultimate Pasta

This pasta sauce contains just a bit of everything. It isn't difficult to make, but it is long simmered so you need to plan ahead. It has plenty of vegetables to provide lots of nutrition while holding down the calories compared to typical pasta meals.

2 slices bacon, low sodium

½ pound (225 g) extra lean ground beef, ground

1 cup (150 g) green bell pepper, chopped

8 ounces (225 g) mushrooms, sliced

1 cup (160 g) onion, chopped

2 cups (360 g) no-salt-added tomatoes, undrained

1 bay leaf

1 teaspoon black pepper, or to taste

dash cinnamon

dash ground cloves

½ teaspoon dried basil

½ teaspoon dried oregano

1 teaspoon garlic, sliced

6 ounces (170 g) no-salt-added tomato paste

¼ cup (60 ml) red wine

6 ounces (170 g) whole wheat spaghetti, cooked according to package directions

Sauté bacon in heavy skillet. Crumble. Add beef, green bell pepper, mushrooms, and onion. Cook until meat is browned. Then add tomatoes (with juice), bay leaf, and seasonings. Simmer for 1 hour. Add tomato paste and wine and simmer for another 30 minutes. Remove bay leaf. Serve over pasta.

4 SERVINGS

Each with: 404 Calories (27% from Fat, 22% from Protein, 51% from Carb); 23 g Protein; 13 g Total Fat; 5 g Saturated Fat; 5 g Monounsaturated Fat; 1 g Polyunsaturated Fat; 53 g Carb; 8 g Fiber; 11 g Sugar; 316 mg Phosphorus; 95 mg Calcium; 192 mg Sodium; 1222 mg Potassium; 964 IU Vitamin A; 1 mg ATE Vitamin E; 60 mg Vitamin C; 44 mg Cholesterol

One Dish Lasagna Pie

This recipe is a variation of the Bisquick impossible pies that make their own crust as they bake. In this case, we've increased the vegetables and held down the fat to give you a meal that is filling, tasty, and nutritious.

1 pound (455 g) extra lean ground beef
1 cup (245 g) low sodium spaghetti sauce
⅓ cup (85 g) ricotta cheese
3 tablespoons (15 g) Parmesan cheese, grated
1 tablespoon (15 ml) skim milk
1 cup (120 g) zucchini, sliced
1 cup (150 g) red bell pepper, sliced
1 cup (160 g) onion, sliced
1 cup (150 g) fresh mozzarella, grated
½ cup (63 g) all purpose flour
¾ teaspoon baking powder
2 tablespoons (28 g) unsalted butter
1 cup (235 ml) skim milk
½ cup (120 ml) egg substitute

Preheat oven to 400°F (200°C, or gas mark 6). Grease a 9-inch (23 cm) pie plate. Cook beef in a 10-inch (25 cm) skillet over medium heat, stirring occasionally, until brown; drain. Stir in ½ cup (123 g) spaghetti sauce; heat until bubbly. Stir together ricotta cheese, Parmesan cheese, and 1 tablespoon (15 ml) skim milk. Spread half of the beef mixture in pie plate. Drop cheese mixture by spoonfuls onto the beef mixture. Top with vegetables. Sprinkle with ½ cup (75 g) of the mozzarella cheese. Top with remaining beef mixture. Stir together flour and baking powder. Cut in butter. Stir in skim milk and egg substitute until blended. Pour into pie plate. Bake 30 to 35 minutes or until knife inserted in center comes out clean. Sprinkle with remaining ½ cup (75 g) mozzarella cheese. Bake 2 to 3 minutes longer or until cheese is melted.

4 SERVINGS

Each with: 369 Calories (41% from Fat, 25% from Protein, 34% from Carb); 23 g Protein; 17 g Total Fat; 10 g Saturated Fat; 5 g Monounsaturated Fat; 2 g Polyunsaturated Fat; 32 g Carb; 3 g Fiber; 5 g Sugar; 494 mg Phosphorus; 535 mg Calcium; 485 mg Sodium; 855 mg Potassium; 2172 IU Vitamin A; 160 mg ATE Vitamin E; 85 mg Vitamin C; 45 mg Cholesterol

Southwestern Beef with Chili Dumplings

Here's a great southwestern meal in a pot. With the dumplings, nothing else is even needed. Well-trimmed round steak helps to hold down the fat and calories while beans give a nutrition boost.

1½ pounds (680 g) beef round steak
¼ cup (31 g) all purpose flour
1 teaspoon chili powder
½ teaspoon ground cumin
¼ teaspoon black pepper
2 tablespoons (28 ml) olive oil
1 cup (160 g) onion, chopped
2 cups (512 g) kidney beans, cooked
10 ounces (280 g) frozen corn
Dumplings
2 cups (250 g) all purpose flour
1 teaspoon chili powder
1 tablespoon (14 g) baking powder
3 tablespoons (42 g) unsalted butter
¾ cup (175 ml) skim milk

Trim fat from beef and cut into 1-inch (2.5 cm) cubes. Shake meat with flour, chili powder, cumin, and black pepper in a zipper baggie to coat well. Heat oil in a large Dutch oven. Add beef cubes to oil, a few at a time, and brown. Stir in onion and sauté until soft. Return beef to pot. Drain liquid from beans into a large measuring container and add water to make 3 cups (700 ml). Stir into beef mixture and cover. Heat to boiling. Lower heat and simmer for 2 hours or until beef is tender. Stir in corn and beans; heat to boiling again. In large bowl, combine flour, chili powder, and baking powder. Cut in butter until mixture resembles coarse crumbs. Add skim milk all at once and stir with a fork until evenly moist. Drop batter by tablespoon on top of boiling stew. Cook uncovered, 10 minutes. Cover. Cook 10 minutes longer or until dumplings are done.

8 SERVINGS

Each with: 412 Calories (25% from Fat, 29% from Protein, 46% from Carb); 30 g Protein; 12 g Total Fat; 4 g Unsaturated Fat; 5 g Monounsaturated Fat; 1 g Polyunsaturated Fat; 48 g Carb; 7 g Fiber; 2 g Sugar; 394 mg Phosphorus; 197 mg Calcium; 267 mg Sodium; 723 mg Potassium; 442 IU Vitamin A; 50 mg ATE Vitamin E; 5 mg Vitamin C; 51 mg Cholesterol

Southwestern Beef Stew

Salsa helps to give this stew its southwestern flavor. I particularly like this as a meal to serve when we have people over, not just because it taste great, but it makes a great presentation with all the fresh vegetables. And thanks to low fat round steak, it is still less than 400 calories per serving.

1½ pound (680 g) beef round steak
2 tablespoons (28 ml) olive oil
2 cups (320 g) onion, quartered
½ teaspoon garlic, minced
28 ounces (785 g) no-salt-added tomatoes
2 cups (475 ml) low sodium beef broth
1 cup (235 ml) water
¾ teaspoons dried thyme
¾ teaspoons marjoram
½ cup (30 g) fresh parsley, chopped
2 cups (200 g) celery, cut in 1-inch (2.5 cm) pieces
2 cups (244 g) carrot, sliced
1 cup (150 g) red bell pepper, diced
¼ cup (65 g) salsa
½ cup (53 g) whole wheat elbow macaroni
1 pound (455 g) frozen corn

Brown meat in oil in 5- or 6-quart (4.7 or 5.7 L) pot. Add onion and garlic; stir until limp. Add tomatoes and break up with spoon. Add liquids and spices. Bring to a boil. Cover and simmer until meat is very tender, approximately 2 hours. Stir in vegetables and continue to simmer for 15 minutes. Stir in salsa, macaroni, and corn. Cook until carrot and macaroni are tender, about 10 minutes.

6 SERVINGS

Each with: 372 Calories (24% from Fat, 35% from Protein, 42% from Carb); 34 g Protein; 10 g Total Fat; 2 g Unsaturated Fat; 5 g Monounsaturated Fat; 1 g Polyunsaturated Fat; 40 g Carb; 7 g Fiber; 13 g Sugar; 422 mg Phosphorus; 131 mg Calcium; 259 mg Sodium; 1408 mg Potassium; 6928 IU Vitamin A; 0 mg ATE Vitamin E; 87 mg Vitamin C; 52 mg Cholesterol

Mexican Stacks

Tasty tortillas layered with an extra lean beef mixture give you the flavor of Mexico without the calories. And that should make lots of people happy.

1 pound (455 g) extra lean ground beef

1 package taco seasoning

5 whole wheat tortillas, 6-inch (15 cm)

5 ounces (140 g) low fat cheddar cheese, grated

5 ounces (140 g) low fat Monterey Jack cheese, grated

4 ounces (115 g) olives, sliced

4 ounces (115 g) green chilies, chopped

½ cup (80 g) onion, chopped

1 teaspoon olive oil

Preheat oven to 350°F (180°C, or gas mark 4). Brown meat. Add taco seasoning according to directions on package. Layer tortillas in 9-inch (23 cm) pie pan sprayed with nonstick vegetable oil spray. Begin with tortillas. Spread with ¼ of meat, cheeses, olives, chilies, and onion. Repeat 4 times. Brush top tortilla with olive oil. Bake for 30 minutes or until top is golden brown.

6 SERVINGS

Each with: 420 Calories (47% from Fat, 28% from Protein, 25% from Carb); 29 g Protein; 22 g Total Fat; 8 g Unsaturated Fat; 10 g Monounsaturated Fat; 1 g Polyunsaturated Fat; 25 g Carb; 2 g Fiber; 1 g Sugar; 389 mg Phosphorus; 275 mg Calcium; 761 mg Sodium; 338 mg Potassium; 198 IU Vitamin A; 28 mg ATE Vitamin E; 7 mg Vitamin C; 62 mg Cholesterol

Fajita Tacos

The filling says fajita, but the corn tortilla says taco. In reality, it doesn't matter because there is way too much filling to stick in two tortillas anyway, so you'll probably end up eating it with a fork.

2 tablespoons (28 ml) olive oil

2 teaspoons ground cumin

1 teaspoon garlic, minced

1 pound (455 g) beef round steak, cut in strips

1½ cups (225 g) green bell pepper

1½ cups (225 g) red bell pepper

1 cup (160 g) onion, sliced

8 corn tortillas

½ cup (130 g) salsa

¼ cup (60 g) fat-free sour cream

In a skillet, sauté olive oil, cumin, and garlic for 1 minute. Add steak strips and cook about 5 minutes. Add green and red bell pepper and onion slices and cook for another 8 minutes. Place mixture in tortillas and fold. Top with salsa and sour cream.

4 SERVINGS

Each with: 365 Calories (34% from Fat, 33% from Protein, 33% from Carb); 31 g Protein; 14 g Total Fat; 4 g Unsaturated Fat; 8 g Monounsaturated Fat; 2 g Polyunsaturated Fat; 31 g Carb; 5 g Fiber; 7 g Sugar; 436 mg Phosphorus; 144 mg Calcium; 285 mg Sodium; 863 mg Potassium; 2244 IU Vitamin A; 15 mg ATE Vitamin E; 159 mg Vitamin C; 58 mg Cholesterol

Mexican Beef Stew

The inspiration for this recipe comes from an old *Better Homes and Gardens* Mexican cookbook. I always thought it was a very showy meal, with the large pieces of corn and zucchini. We made it lower in calories and healthier by using leaner meat and adding a lot more vegetables, while reducing the sodium.

2 pound (900 g) beef round steak, cubed

2 tablespoons (28 ml) oil

3 cups (700 ml) water

2 tablespoons (8 g) fresh parsley, chopped

2 cups (360 g) no-salt-added tomatoes

1 cup (160 g) onion, cut up

1 teaspoon red pepper flakes

1 ounce (28 g) sesame seeds

½ teaspoon garlic, minced

¼ teaspoon ground cumin

½ cup (120 ml) low sodium beef broth

2 cups (240 g) zucchini, cut in 1-inch (2.5 cm) pieces

2 cups (300 g) turnip, diced

3 ears corn, cut in 1-inch (2.5 cm) pieces

1 cup (122 g) carrot, sliced

2 medium potatoes, diced

 Tip: This can be cooked on the stove in a covered Dutch oven, but the long oven cooking makes the beef very tender.

Brown meat in oil, half at a time. Place meat, water, and parsley in covered roasting pan and cook at 350°F (180°C, or gas mark 4) until meat is tender, about 1½ hours. In a blender, combine tomatoes, onion, spices, and broth. Blend until nearly smooth. Add to beef mixture along with vegetables. Continue cooking until vegetables are done, about 40 minutes.

8 SERVINGS

Each with: 358 Calories (24% from Fat, 35% from Protein, 41% from Carb); 32 g Protein; 10 g Total Fat; 2 g Unsaturated Fat; 3 g Monounsaturated Fat; 3 g Polyunsaturated Fat; 37 g Carb; 6 g Fiber; 7 g Sugar; 417 mg Phosphorus; 122 mg Calcium; 135 mg Sodium; 1367 mg Potassium; 2361 IU Vitamin A; 0 mg ATE Vitamin E; 37 mg Vitamin C; 52 mg Cholesterol

Easy Slow Cooker Enchiladas Casserole

This is an easy to fix enchilada-style casserole that cooks in the slow cooker and leaves you with a house full of delicious aromas. Beans and vegetables kick up the nutrition and the taste of the Mexican-influenced treat.

1 pound (455 g) extra lean ground beef
1 cup (160 g) onion, chopped
1½ cups (225 g) red bell pepper, chopped
1½ cups (225 g) green bell pepper, chopped
10 ounces (280 g) frozen corn
2 cups (342 g) pinto beans
2 cups (344 g) black beans
2 cups (360 g) no-salt-added tomatoes
4 ounces (115 g) diced green chilies
1 teaspoon chili powder
1 teaspoon ground cumin
½ teaspoon black pepper
3 ounces (85 g) low fat cheddar cheese, shredded
3 ounces (85 g) low fat Monterey Jack cheese, shredded
6 whole wheat tortillas, 6-inch (15 cm)

In a nonstick skillet, brown beef, onion, and green and red bell peppers. Add remaining ingredients except cheese and tortillas, Bring to a boil. Reduce heat. Cover and simmer for 10 minutes. Combine cheeses in a bowl. In slow cooker, layer about ¾ cup beef mixture, one tortilla, and about ¼ cup (29 g) cheese. Repeat layers until all ingredients are used. Cover. Cook on low for 5 to 7 hours.

8 SERVINGS

Each with: 406 Calories (32% from Fat, 24% from Protein, 44% from Carb); 25 g Protein; 15 g Total Fat; 6 g Saturated Fat; 6 g Monounsaturated Fat; 1 g Polyunsaturated Fat; 45 g Carb; 8 g Fiber; 6 g Sugar; 351 mg Phosphorus; 183 mg Calcium; 405 mg Sodium; 769 mg Potassium; 1291 IU Vitamin A; 13 mg ATE Vitamin E; 93 mg Vitamin C; 44 mg Cholesterol

Mexican Steak Salad

If you have leftover London broil or other beef, this salad is a great tasting, healthy way to use it.
So you really should plan to have some leftover beef. The Mexican taste is a real pleaser,
and the nutrition will make everyone happy.

½ cup (115 g) sour cream
½ cup (130 g) salsa
2 tablespoons (2 g) cilantro,
divided
1 cup (256 g) kidney beans,
rinsed and drained
½ cup (56 g) low fat Monterey
Jack cheese
¼ cup (25 g) green onion, sliced
8 ounces (225 g) beef round
steak, cooked and sliced
1 small head iceberg lettuce,
shredded
5 radishes, thinly sliced
1 avocado, peeled and sliced
2 ounces (28 g) tortilla chips

In a small bowl, combine sour cream, salsa, and 1 tablespoon
(1 g) cilantro; set aside. In a medium bowl, combine beans,
cheese, green onion, and remaining 1 tablespoon (1 g)
cilantro. To serve, arrange bean mixture, beef, lettuce,
radishes, avocado, and tortilla chips on four individual plates.
Serve topped with the sour cream and salsa mixture.

4 SERVINGS

Each with: 368 Calories (38% from Fat, 27% from Protein, 35% from Carb);
26 g Protein; 16 g Total Fat; 5 g Saturated Fat; 7 g Monounsaturated Fat; 2 g
Polyunsaturated Fat; 33 g Carb; 9 g Fiber; 6 g Sugar; 418 mg Phosphorus; 201 mg
Calcium; 453 mg Sodium; 1111 mg Potassium; 1198 IU Vitamin A; 40 mg ATE
Vitamin E; 20 mg Vitamin C; 48 mg Cholesterol

Shout Olé for Mexican Beef Stew

This is a fairly traditional beef stew, with the flavor enhanced with Mexican spices.
It's a great meal for a cold day.

2 tablespoons (28 ml) olive oil

3 tablespoons (45 ml) red wine
vinegar

1½ pound (680 g) beef round
steak, cubed

1 cup (235 ml) red wine

1 cup (160 g) onion, minced

1 bay leaf

1 garlic clove, minced

½ teaspoon dried oregano

1 teaspoon ground cumin

¼ teaspoon black pepper, or to
taste

½ cup (123 g) no-salt-added
tomato sauce

4 medium potatoes, cubed

½ cup (61 g) carrot, sliced

 *Tip: For even easier
preparation, put everything in
a slow cooker and cook on low
for 8 to 10 hours.*

In a Dutch oven, sauté onion and garlic in oil. Add everything
else except potatoes and carrot. Cover tightly and simmer 1½
hours until meat is thoroughly tender. Half an hour before
meat is ready, add carrot and potatoes.

6 SERVINGS

Each with: 414 Calories (20% from Fat, 32% from Protein, 47% from Carb);
31 g Protein; 9 g Total Fat; 2 g Saturated Fat; 5 g Monounsaturated Fat; 1 g
Polyunsaturated Fat; 46 g Carb; 5 g Fiber; 6 g Sugar; 416 mg Phosphorus; 42 mg
Calcium; 193 mg Sodium; 1721 mg Potassium; 1386 IU Vitamin A; 0 mg ATE Vitamin
E; 29 mg Vitamin C; 65 mg Cholesterol

Spanish Steak and Vegetables

This is sort of like Swiss steak, only with a more southern European kind of flavor.

1 pound (455 g) beef round steak

1 cup (160 g) onion, sliced, divided

½ cup (50 g) celery, chopped, divided

1 cup (150 g) green bell pepper, sliced in rings, divided

2 teaspoons dried parsley

1 tablespoon (15 ml) Worcestershire sauce

1 tablespoon (9 g) dry mustard

1 tablespoon (8 g) chili powder

4 cups (720 g) no-salt-added tomatoes, divided

2½ teaspoons (8 g) minced garlic, divided

2 medium baking potatoes

1 pound (455 g) green beans, fresh

Cut steak into serving-size pieces. Place steak pieces in ovenproof casserole. Top with onion, celery, and green bell pepper. Combine the parsley, Worcestershire sauce, dry mustard, chili powder, 2 cups (360 g) tomatoes, and 2 teaspoons minced garlic. Pour over meat. Cover. Cook at 350°F (180°C, or gas mark 4) until steak is very tender, about 1½ hours. While steak is cooking, bake or microwave the potatoes. Combine beans, 2 cups (360 g) tomatoes, and ½ teaspoon minced garlic in a saucepan. Simmer until beans on done, about a half hour. Place ¼ of beans and steak and half of a potato on each plate. Serve sauce from steak over steak and potatoes.

4 SERVINGS

Each with: 374 Calories (11% from Fat, 35% from Protein, 54% from Carb); 33 g Protein; 5 g Total Fat; 1 g Saturated Fat; 2 g Monounsaturated Fat; 1 g Polyunsaturated Fat; 52 g Carb; 9 g Fiber; 11 g Sugar; 434 mg Phosphorus; 128 mg Calcium; 165 mg Sodium; 2004 mg Potassium; 1149 IU Vitamin A; 0 mg ATE Vitamin E; 113 mg Vitamin C; 65 mg Cholesterol

 Tip: Serve over noodles or rice.

Beef and Peppers German Style

Flavored and thickened with gingersnaps like sauerbraten, but with lots of added veggies and fruit, this beef is a nutritious meal all by itself.

2 pound (900 g) beef round roast, cut to 1-inch (2.5 cm) cubes

2 tablespoons (16 g) all purpose flour

¼ teaspoon black pepper

2 tablespoons (28 ml) olive oil

3 cups (700 ml) low sodium beef broth

⅓ cup (80 ml) cider vinegar

6 ounces (170 g) no-salt-added tomato paste

6 cups (900 g) green bell pepper, cut in 1-inch (2.5 cm) cubes

2 cups (244 g) carrot, cut into 2-inch (5 cm) chunks

1 tablespoon (7 g) caraway seed

1½ cups (300 g) apple, peeled and diced

¼ cup (15 g) fresh parsley, chopped

1½ cups (180 g) gingersnaps, crushed

2 tablespoons (2 g) brown sugar substitute, such as Splenda

Coat beef with flour mixed with black pepper. In a large heavy sauce pot or Dutch oven, heat oil. Add beef; brown well on all sides, a few pieces at a time. Remove the browned beef and set aside. Stir beef broth into the beef drippings in the sauce pot. Stir in vinegar and tomato paste. Cook and stir until mixture comes to a boil. Stir well to get drippings off the bottom of the pot. Return beef to pot. Bringing to a boil again. Reduce heat and simmer, covered, for 1½ hours. Add green bell pepper, carrot, and caraway seed. Bring mixture to a boiling point again. Reduce heat and simmer, covered, until meat and vegetables are fork tender, about 30 minutes. Stir in apple, parsley, gingersnaps, and brown sugar substitute. Cover and simmer for 5 minutes.

6 SERVINGS

Each with: 381 Calories (28% from Fat, 40% from Protein, 32% from Carb); 39 g Protein; 12 g Total Fat; 3 g Unsaturated Fat; 6 g Monounsaturated Fat; 1 g Polyunsaturated Fat; 31 g Carb; 6 g Fiber; 14 g Sugar; 435 mg Phosphorus; 100 mg Calcium; 289 mg Sodium; 1399 mg Potassium; 6345 IU Vitamin A; 0 mg ATE Vitamin E; 133 mg Vitamin C; 76 mg Cholesterol

Beef Stew Burgundy

Classy and classic, this beef and vegetables cooked in wine make the meal seem special even though the calories are low. Lean beef round steak becomes tender between the wine and the long slow cooking.

1 cup (235 ml) burgundy wine

3 pound (1⅓ kg) beef round steak, thinly sliced

28 ounces (785 g) no-salt-added tomatoes

¼ cup (38 g) tapioca, quick cooking

1 tablespoon (1.5 g) sugar substitute, such as Splenda

2 bay leaves

1 tablespoon (9 g) Mrs. Dash original blend

2 cups (244 g) carrot, sliced

2 large potatoes, cut up

10 ounces (280 g) frozen peas

1 cup (160 g) onion, chopped

Put wine and cut up beef in slow cooker on high for 1 hour. After 1 hour, add tomatoes, tapioca, sugar substitute, bay leaves, Mrs. Dash, and vegetables. Turn to low and cook for 6 to 8 hours. Remove bay leaves before serving.

8 SERVINGS

Each with: 398 Calories (15% from Fat, 48% from Protein, 38% from Carb); 45 g Protein; 6 g Total Fat; 2 g Unsaturated Fat; 2 g Monounsaturated Fat; 0 g Polyunsaturated Fat; 35 g Carb; 6 g Fiber; 5 g Sugar; 506 mg Phosphorus; 107 mg Calcium; 263 mg Sodium; 1495 mg Potassium; 4226 IU Vitamin A; 0 mg ATE Vitamin E; 30 mg Vitamin C; 78 mg Cholesterol

Easy to Fix, Easy on Your Diet Beef Burgundy

This is a great beef and noodles dish. It's easy to prepare in your slow cooker. And it's easy on your diet because the long slow cooking lets you use a cheaper, leaner cut of beef and still end up with a tender, delicious meal. This meal is a perfect example of how you can eat a lot of food that seems to be rich but is still low in calories.

4 slices low sodium bacon

2 pound (900 g) beef round steak, cut in 1-inch (2.5 cm) cubes

2 cups (244 g) carrot, cut into chunks

2 cups (320 g) onion, sliced

½ cup (63 g) all-purpose flour

½ teaspoon marjoram

¼ teaspoon garlic powder

¼ teaspoon black pepper

1½ cups (355 ml) low sodium beef broth

½ cup (120 ml) burgundy wine

1 tablespoon (15 ml) Worcestershire sauce

12 ounces (340 g) mushrooms, sliced

16 ounces (455 g) egg noodles, uncooked

2 tablespoons (8 g) fresh parsley

6 cups (600 g) green beans

Cook bacon until crisp; drain and crumble. Place beef, bacon, carrot, and onion in the bottom of the slow cooker. Whisk together flour, marjoram, garlic, and black pepper with broth, wine, and Worcestershire sauce. Pour mixture into cooker. Cook on high for 1 hour. Reduce to low and cook for 5 to 6 hours. Add mushrooms. Cook on high for 30 minutes or until mushrooms are tender. While mushrooms are cooking, prepare noodles and beans according to package directions. Serve beef over noodles with beans on the side.

8 SERVINGS

Each with: 352 Calories (17% from Fat, 41% from Protein, 41% from Carb); 36 g Protein; 7 g Total Fat; 2 g Unsaturated Fat; 2 g Monounsaturated Fat; 1 g Polyunsaturated Fat; 35 g Carb; 5 g Fiber; 5 g Sugar; 420 mg Phosphorus; 87 mg Calcium; 245 mg Sodium; 997 mg Potassium; 4518 IU Vitamin A; 4 mg ATE Vitamin E; 24 mg Vitamin C; 75 mg Cholesterol

Bulgogi

I first had bulgogi in Korea when I was stationed there in the Army many years ago. It was, and still is, my favorite Korean food. Bulgogi is thinly sliced beef, marinated in a spicy garlic sauce, and then broiled or barbecued. It is naturally low in calories and high in flavor. Here we team it with brown rice, which is also traditional, and cabbage, which is not unless it has been made into the pickled cabbage called Kimchee, which along with bulgogi are probably the best known Korean foods in the west.

2½ tablespoons (23 ml) low
  sodium soy sauce
¼ cup (25 g) green onion, sliced
½ teaspoon cloves garlic, minced
1 tablespoon (15 ml) sesame oil
2 tablespoons (26 g) sugar
¼ teaspoon black pepper
½ teaspoon ground ginger
1 tablespoon (8 g) sesame seeds
1 pound (455 g) beef round steak
2 cups (390 g) brown rice, cooked
4 cups (360 g) cabbage, steamed
  until crisp-tender

Combine soy sauce, onion, garlic, oil, sugar, black pepper, ginger, and sesame seeds in large bowl. Cut meat in thin 1-inch (2.5 cm) strips and place in bowl; coat well. Let stand at least 30 minutes. Broil or put on barbecue grill. Serve with cooked rice and steamed cabbage.

4 SERVINGS

Each with: 353 Calories (24% from Fat, 35% from Protein, 41% from Carb); 31 g Protein; 9 g Total Fat; 2 g Unsaturated Fat; 4 g Monounsaturated Fat; 2 g Polyunsaturated Fat; 36 g Carb; 4 g Fiber; 10 g Sugar; 378 mg Phosphorus; 106 mg Calcium; 423 mg Sodium; 770 mg Potassium; 221 IU Vitamin A; 0 mg ATE Vitamin E; 30 mg Vitamin C; 52 mg Cholesterol

Sweet and Sour Beef

Sweet and sour beef with lots of veggies provide great taste as well as top nutrition.

2 pound (900 g) beef round steak,
  cut into 1-inch (2.5 cm) cubes
2 tablespoons (28 ml) olive oil
16 ounces (455 g) no-salt-added
  tomato sauce
2 teaspoons chili powder
2 teaspoons paprika
¼ cup (6 g) sugar substitute, such
  as Splenda
½ cup (120 ml) cider vinegar
¼ cup (85 g) molasses
2 cups (244 g) carrot, sliced
  ¼-inch (6 mm) thick
2 cups (320 g) onion, chopped
3 cups (450 g) green bell pepper,
  cut into 1-inch (2.5 cm) squares

Brown meat in hot oil in skillet; transfer to slow cooker. Add all remaining ingredients; mix well. Cook for 6 to 7 hours on low setting.

6 SERVINGS

Each with: 366 Calories (25% from Fat, 41% from Protein, 34% from Carb); 38 g Protein; 10 g Total Fat; 2 g Unsaturated Fat; 6 g Monounsaturated Fat; 1 g Polyunsaturated Fat; 31 g Carb; 5 g Fiber; 18 g Sugar; 418 mg Phosphorus; 111 mg Calcium; 153 mg Sodium; 1448 mg Potassium; 6326 IU Vitamin A; 0 mg ATE Vitamin E; 77 mg Vitamin C; 70 mg Cholesterol

Stir-Fried Beef and Spinach

This stir-fry is full of super nutritious spinach, moving it ahead of many Asian entrees. And even with a generous serving of brown rice, it's still low in calories.

6 cups (1.2 kg) brown rice
1½ pound (680 g) beef round steak, fat trimmed off
2 tablespoons (28 ml) low sodium soy sauce
¼ teaspoon 5 spice powder
¼ cup (60 ml) low sodium beef broth
2 teaspoons cornstarch
1 tablespoon (15 ml) olive oil
1 teaspoon ginger root, grated
1 pound (455 g) fresh spinach
½ cup (62 g) water chestnuts, sliced

Cook rice according to package directions. Cut beef in thin bite-sized strips. Combine beef, soy sauce, and 5 spice powder; let stand at room temperature for 5 minutes. In small bowl, blend broth and cornstarch and set aside. Preheat wok or large skillet over high heat. Add oil. Stir-fry ginger root 30 seconds. Add half of beef and stir-fry 2 to 3 minutes until brown. Remove beef and stir-fry the rest. Return all the beef to wok, stir in cornstarch, and cook until thick and bubbly. Stir in spinach and chestnuts. Cook 1 to 2 minutes. Serve at once over rice.

6 SERVINGS

Each with: 419 Calories (17% from Fat, 32% from Protein, 50% from Carb); 33 g Protein; 8 g Total Fat; 2 g Unsaturated Fat; 4 g Monounsaturated Fat; 1 g Polyunsaturated Fat; 52 g Carb; 6 g Fiber; 1 g Sugar; 455 mg Phosphorus; 122 mg Calcium; 319 mg Sodium; 1076 mg Potassium; 7089 IU Vitamin A; 0 mg ATE Vitamin E; 22 mg Vitamin C; 52 mg Cholesterol

Steak and Vegetable Stir-Fry

This Asian dish is similar to pepper steak but with a greater
variety of vegetables for increased nutrition.

1½ pound (680 g) beef round
steak

3 tablespoons (45 ml) low sodium
soy sauce

2 tablespoons (28 ml) olive oil,
divided

¼ teaspoon black pepper

¼ teaspoon garlic, minced

½ teaspoon ground ginger

1 cup (150 g) green bell pepper,
cut in strips

2 cups (140 g) mushrooms, sliced

1 cup (160 g) onion, sliced

½ cup (120 ml) low sodium beef
broth

1 tablespoon (8 g) cornstarch

1 cup (180 g) tomatoes, cut in
wedges

2 cups (390 g) brown rice, cooked

Partially freeze beef. Slice diagonally into ¼-inch (6 mm) thick
slices. In a large bowl, combine soy sauce, 1 tablespoon oil
(15 ml), and black pepper. Add beef. Toss to coat well and
marinate for several hours in the refrigerator. In a wok or large
skillet, stir-fry the garlic and ginger in remaining oil for 1
minute. Add meat and stir-fry until browned, about 4 minutes.
Remove meat. Add all vegetables except tomatoes and stir-fry
until crisp-tender, about 2 minutes. Return beef to wok.
Combine remaining marinade, broth, and cornstarch. Pour
over beef. Cook and stir until thickened. Add tomatoes and
heat through. Serve over rice.

6 SERVINGS

Each with: 376 Calories (27% from Fat, 48% from Protein, 25% from Carb);
45 g Protein; 11 g Total Fat; 3 g Unsaturated Fat; 6 g Monounsaturated Fat; 1 g
Polyunsaturated Fat; 23 g Carb; 3 g Fiber; 2 g Sugar; 356 mg Phosphorus; 25 mg
Calcium; 334 mg Sodium; 669 mg Potassium; 248 IU Vitamin A; 0 mg ATE Vitamin E;
29 mg Vitamin C; 102 mg Cholesterol

Grilled Soy and Ginger Flank Steak with Vegetables

This is a sort of Asian flavored meal, with the soy sauce and ginger. But the ingredients, steak and corn on the cob, are classic American. But the important part is that it works, giving you a meal that is both healthy and flavorful.

1 pound (455 g) flank steak

1 tablespoon (6 g) fresh ginger, minced

2 teaspoons garlic, minced

¼ cup (60 ml) low sodium soy sauce

3 tablespoons (45 ml) dry red wine

1 tablespoon (20 g) honey

4 ears corn

4 red bell peppers, halved

8 ounces (225 g) mushrooms, whole

Rinse the meat and pat dry. Place steak in a 1 gallon (3.8 L) plastic freezer bag and add the remaining ingredients except the vegetables. Seal bag and turn to coat. Lightly oil a barbecue grill and preheat to very hot. Remove the steak from the bag, reserving marinade for vegetables. Cook steak, turning once, until done as you like it, about 15 minutes total for medium-rare. To serve, slice diagonally across the grain into thin slices. Add husked corn, halved and seeded red bell peppers, and mushrooms to the marinade after removing the steak and then cook on the grill, turning occasionally until slightly browned.

4 SERVINGS

Each with: 418 Calories (24% from Fat, 36% from Protein, 40% from Carb); 39 g Protein; 12 g Total Fat; 4 g Saturated Fat; 4 g Monounsaturated Fat; 1 g Polyunsaturated Fat; 43 g Carb; 7 g Fiber; 16 g Sugar; 427 mg Phosphorus; 37 mg Calcium; 620 mg Sodium; 1140 mg Potassium; 4667 IU Vitamin A; 0 mg ATE Vitamin E; 293 mg Vitamin C; 62 mg Cholesterol

Asian Pot Roast and Veggies

When you are looking for something a little different, how about as Asian-flavored meal from your slow cooker. This has a mild but distinctly Chinese flavor. The vegetables also take on Chinese flavor during the long slow cooking.

2 pound (900 g) beef chuck roast

1 tablespoon (15 ml) oil

2 teaspoons low sodium beef bouillon

½ cup (120 ml) low sodium soy sauce

2 tablespoons (28 ml) sherry

½ teaspoon garlic powder

¼ teaspoon ground ginger

1 cup (160 g) onion, sliced into strips

1 cup (150 g) red bell pepper, sliced into strips

1 cup (122 g) carrot, sliced

½ pound (225 g) green beans

3 tablespoons (24 g) cornstarch

3 tablespoons (45 ml) cold water

Trim excess fat from roast. In a skillet, brown beef on all sides in oil. Mix together broth, soy sauce, sherry, and spices. Place vegetables in bottom of slow cooker. Place meat on top. Pour sauce over. Cook on low for 8 to 10 hours or on high for 5 to 6 hours. Remove meat and vegetables. Turn heat to high. Stir cornstarch into water. Add to slow cooker. Cook until sauce is slightly thickened, about 15 to 20 minutes. Separate meat into serving size pieces. Spoon sauce over meat and vegetables.

6 SERVINGS

Each with: 415 Calories (32% from Fat, 53% from Protein, 16% from Carb); 53 g Protein; 14 g Total Fat; 5 g Saturated Fat; 5 g Monounsaturated Fat; 2 g Polyunsaturated Fat; 16 g Carb; 3 g Fiber; 5 g Sugar; 467 mg Phosphorus; 48 mg Calcium; 837 mg Sodium; 724 mg Potassium; 3611 IU Vitamin A; 0 mg ATE Vitamin E; 56 mg Vitamin C; 153 mg Cholesterol

Beef and Tomato Curry (Plus Other Good Stuff)

Beef, tomatoes, and other vegetables are simmered in a mild curry sauce to make this tasty dish. Like many soups and stews, it offers great nutrition and volume for the calories. Brown rice adds extra nutrition and filling power.

1 pound (455 g) beef round steak

½ cup (120 ml) low sodium beef broth

1½ cups (270 g) tomatoes, coarsely chopped

1 cup (150 g) green bell pepper, cut in 1-inch (2.5 cm) pieces

8 ounces (225 g) mushrooms, sliced

1½ cups (240 g) onion, coarsely chopped

1½ cups (180 g) zucchini, sliced

1 teaspoon curry powder

1 tablespoon (8 g) cornstarch

1 tablespoon (15 ml) water

1 cup (195 g) brown rice, cooked according to package directions

Cut meat into 1 × 2-inch (2.5 × 5 cm) strips. Spray skillet with nonstick vegetable oil spray. Cook meat in broth until tender. Add tomatoes, peeled and cut up, green bell pepper, onion, mushrooms, zucchini, and curry powder and heat to boiling. Cover and cook on medium for 3 to 5 minutes. Mix cornstarch and water. Stir into mixture and cook until thick and boiling. Serve over hot cooked rice.

4 SERVINGS

Each with: 391 Calories (13% from Fat, 34% from Protein, 53% from Carb); 34 g Protein; 6 g Total Fat; 2 g Saturated Fat; 2 g Monounsaturated Fat; 1 g Polyunsaturated Fat; 52 g Carb; 5 g Fiber; 6 g Sugar; 511 mg Phosphorus; 47 mg Calcium; 95 mg Sodium; 1137 mg Potassium; 585 IU Vitamin A; 0 mg ATE Vitamin E; 58 mg Vitamin C; 65 mg Cholesterol

Not Your Irish Corned Beef and Cabbage

Unlike the traditional version, this corned beef and cabbage cooks in a spicy tomato sauce.
But don't let that stop you. It tastes good, is full of nutrition, and is very low in calories.

1 large cabbage, sliced in ½-inch
  (1.3 cm) slices
½ cup (120 ml) water
1 cup (160 g) onion, cut in
  wedges
2 tablespoons (28 ml) olive oil
28 ounces (785 g) no-salt-added
  stewed tomatoes
¼ teaspoon cayenne pepper
¼ teaspoon black pepper
2 tablespoons (3 g) sugar
  substitute, such as Splenda
14 ounces (390 g) corned beef

In large pot, add sliced cabbage and ½ cup (120 ml) water.
Steam 10 minutes. In large skillet, sauté onion in oil until clear.
Add stewed tomatoes. Add cayenne pepper, black pepper, and
sugar substitute. Cook 20 minutes. Pour over cabbage. Cook
cabbage and tomato mixture 10 more minutes. Add corned
beef and cook about 6 minutes longer or until cabbage is
crisp-tender.

4 SERVINGS

Each with: 351 Calories (47% from Fat, 15% from Protein, 38% from Carb);
14 g Protein; 19 g Total Fat; 6 g Unsaturated Fat; 11 g Monounsaturated Fat; 1 g
Polyunsaturated Fat; 35 g Carb; 8 g Fiber; 16 g Sugar; 176 mg Phosphorus; 158 mg
Calcium; 1090 mg Sodium; 1011 mg Potassium; 621 IU Vitamin A; 0 mg ATE Vitamin
E; 62 mg Vitamin C; 35 mg Cholesterol

Dinners: Pork

Everything I said in the introduction to the beef chapter also applies here. Pork can be very high in fat content or if you are careful can fit easily into your diet. About the only pork we buy are whole pork loins, which I grab when they are on sale and cut into chops, roasts, cubes, and grind up the end pieces to make sausage. Pork loin is great because it is naturally low in fat and what fat it does have can be easily trimmed off. And it can be used in almost any kind of recipe, as this chapter proves. There also are a few recipes here that call for ham. We don't eat ham very often because of the high sodium content, but it is an occasional treat. There is also one lamb stew recipe thrown in so you lamb lovers don't feel left out.

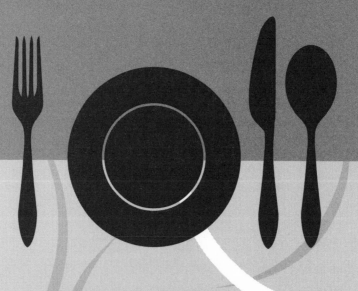

Down Home Southern Stuffed Pork Chops and Sweet Potatoes

For a taste of the southern United States, try these pork chops, filled with cornbread stuffing and flavored with orange and pecans. Sweet potatoes with an orange sauce make a perfect accompaniment while adding bulk and nutrition, particularly vitamin A.

4 pork loin chops, 1-inch (2.5 cm) thick

4 ounces (115 g) corn bread stuffing mix

2 tablespoons (28 ml) low sodium chicken broth

⅓ cup (80 ml) orange juice

1 tablespoon (7 g) pecans, finely chopped

½ teaspoon orange peel, grated

4 sweet potatoes

2 tablespoons (36 g) orange juice concentrate

¼ cup (4 g) brown sugar substitute, such as Splenda

With a sharp knife, cut a horizontal slit in side of each chop forming a pocket for stuffing. Combine stuffing with broth, orange juice, pecans and orange peel. Fill pockets with stuffing. Place in 9 × 13-inch (23 × 33 cm) glass baking dish. Peel sweet potatoes into 1-inch (2.5 cm) cubes. Place in 8-inch (10 cm) square baking dish. Combine orange juice concentrate and brown sugar substitute and pour over sweet potatoes. Place both pans in a 350°F (180°C, or gas mark 4) oven and bake until potatoes are tender and pork chops are cooked through, about 45 to 60 minutes.

4 SERVINGS

Each with: 391 Calories (16% from Fat, 28% from Protein, 56% from Carb); 27 g Protein; 7 g Total Fat; 2 g Saturated Fat; 3 g Monounsaturated Fat; 1 g Polyunsaturated Fat; 54 g Carb; 8 g Fiber; 12 g Sugar; 315 mg Phosphorus; 83 mg Calcium; 459 mg Sodium; 892 mg Potassium; 23 872 IU Vitamin A; 2 mg ATE Vitamin E; 41 mg Vitamin C; 64 mg Cholesterol

Barbecued Pork Chops Plate

A nice sweet/sour barbecue sauce gives these chops great flavor.
Baked potatoes and slaw complete the traditional barbecue plate.

Pork Chops
4 loin pork chops, 1-inch (2.5 cm)
   thick
1 cup (160 g) onion, finely
   chopped
2 tablespoons (28 ml) vinegar
1 tablespoon (15 ml) canola oil
½ teaspoon dry mustard
1 tablespoon (15 ml)
   Worcestershire sauce
1 teaspoon black pepper
1 tablespoon (13 g) sugar
½ teaspoon paprika

Baked Potatoes
2 medium potatoes

Coleslaw
2 cups (180 g) coleslaw mix
½ cup (115 g) peppercorn ranch
   dressing, see recipe in
   chapter 2

Score edges of chops to prevent curling. Place into a large baking pan, set aside. Combine remaining ingredients, mix well. Pour over chops to coat well. Cover and chill for 2 to 4 hours. Grill chops to desired doneness, basting often. Meanwhile, bake potatoes and split in half. Serve chop with half a baked potato and coleslaw, both topped with ranch dressing.

4 SERVINGS

Each with: 397 Calories (19% from Fat, 27% from Protein, 54% from Carb); 26 g Protein; 8 g Total Fat; 2 g Unsaturated Fat; 4 g Monounsaturated Fat; 2 g Polyunsaturated Fat; 53 g Carb; 5 g Fiber; 7 g Sugar; 379 mg Phosphorus; 78 mg Calcium; 462 mg Sodium; 1422 mg Potassium; 227 IU Vitamin A; 2 mg ATE Vitamin E; 48 mg Vitamin C; 64 mg Cholesterol

All In One Pork Chop Skillet

This meal in a pan gives you meat, vegetables, and fruit all cooked in the same pan. The ginger adds a spiciness that makes you forget it's supposed to be good for you.

1 cup (160 g) onion, chopped

1 tablespoon (15 ml) olive oil

3 pork loin chops

2 tablespoons (13 g) fresh ginger, thinly sliced

2 apples, peeled and thinly sliced

3 medium sweet potatoes, peeled and cubed

2 cups (280 g) butternut squash, peeled and cubed

½ cup (120 ml) water

Lightly brown the chopped onion in the olive oil using medium heat in a nonstick skillet, 2 to 4 minutes. Push the onion pieces to one side and brown the chops on each side. Spoon the onion pieces on top of each chop dividing evenly. Peel and slice the ginger and prepare the apple and vegetables while the chops are browning. Layer each chop with a topping of sliced ginger. Place apples and vegetables on top. Add the water to the skillet and cover tightly. Cook over low heat for 30 to 40 minutes, depending on the thickness of the pork chops.

3 SERVINGS

Each with: 402 Calories (21% from Fat, 25% from Protein, 55% from Carb); 25 g Protein; 9 g Total Fat; 2 g Unsaturated Fat; 5 g Monounsaturated Fat; 1 g Polyunsaturated Fat; 56 g Carb; 8 g Fiber; 22 g Sugar; 328 mg Phosphorus; 120 mg Calcium; 100 mg Sodium; 1252 mg Potassium; 33 780 IU Vitamin A; 2 mg ATE Vitamin E; 47 mg Vitamin C; 64 mg Cholesterol

Italian Pork Chops

Here are Italian-style pork chops, cooked to a tender goodness in tomato sauce. There's enough sauce here to serve over both the pork and the pasta.

2 tablespoons (28 ml) olive oil

4 pork loin chops

1 cup (160 g) onion, chopped

1 cup (150 g) green bell pepper, chopped

½ teaspoon garlic, minced

2 cups (360 g) no-salt-added tomatoes

1 teaspoon Italian seasoning

¼ teaspoon black pepper

8 ounces (225 g) whole wheat spaghetti

1 pound (455 g) frozen Italian vegetable mix

In a large skillet, heat the oil and brown the pork chops for 2 to 3 minutes per side. Remove the chops from the skillet and cover to keep warm. Add the onion, green bell pepper, and garlic to the skillet and sauté for 3 to 5 minutes until tender and lightly browned. Stir in the tomatoes, Italian seasoning, and black pepper. Return the pork chops to the skillet; reduce the heat to low, cover, and simmer for about 30 minutes or until the chops are cooked through. Prepare pasta and vegetable mix according to package directions. Serve pork chops and pasta with sauce over both and vegetables on the side.

4 SERVINGS

Each with: 373 Calories (28% from Fat, 31% from Protein, 41% from Carb); 30 g Protein; 12 g Total Fat; 3 g Unsaturated Fat; 7 g Monounsaturated Fat; 2 g Polyunsaturated Fat; 40 g Carb; 8 g Fiber; 6 g Sugar; 372 mg Phosphorus; 100 mg Calcium; 120 mg Sodium; 976 mg Potassium; 5943 IU Vitamin A; 2 mg ATE Vitamin E; 33 mg Vitamin C; 64 mg Cholesterol

Touch of the South Bourbon Pork Chops

This is a real southern United States treat with a bourbon flavored pecan onion relish topping, but it's still healthy and low in calories thanks to the use of lean loin chops.

2 tablespoons (28 g) unsalted butter

2 cups (320 g) onion, sliced

2 ounces (28 ml) bourbon

¼ cup (28 g) pecans, toasted and sliced

2 tablespoons (5 g) sage leaves, minced

2 tablespoons (28 ml) olive oil

4 pork loin chops

4 cups (496 g) frozen green beans

Melt butter in skillet over medium-high heat. Add onion. Sauté 1 minute and then cover and reduce heat to medium low. Simmer 10 minutes. Stir onion, scraping bits from bottom of pan. Continue cooking onion, uncovered, until they become caramelized. Add bourbon. Cook for 2 to 3 minutes or until almost all liquid is evaporated. Transfer onion to a bowl. Stir in pecans and sage. Keep warm. Wipe out pan with a paper towel. Add oil to pan. Add chops to pan. Turn burner to medium heat. Cook chops until browned, about 5 minutes. Flip chops, cover pan, reduce heat to low, and cook for another 7 to 10 minutes. When ready to serve, top each chop with a helping of the onion pecan mixture. Serve with prepared green beans.

4 SERVINGS

Each with: 393 Calories (54% from Fat, 27% from Protein, 19% from Carb); 25 g Protein; 22 g Total Fat; 7 g Unsaturated Fat; 11 g Monounsaturated Fat; 3 g Polyunsaturated Fat; 18 g Carb; 6 g Fiber; 5 g Sugar; 306 mg Phosphorus; 95 mg Calcium; 62 mg Sodium; 760 mg Potassium; 1008 IU Vitamin A; 50 mg ATE Vitamin E; 24 mg Vitamin C; 79 mg Cholesterol

Creole Pork Chops

Only mildly spicy, these chops cooked in a Creole style sauce should be popular even with people who don't usually like Cajun and Creole food. Served over brown rice, they make a complete meal that will please your taste buds but still be very low in calories.

6 pork loin chops
3 tablespoons (45 ml) olive oil
1 cup (160 g) onion, sliced
1 teaspoon garlic, minced
½ cup (75 g) green bell pepper,
   chopped
½ cup (120 ml) dry white wine
2 cups (360 g) no-salt-added
   tomatoes
3 tablespoons (45 ml) lemon juice
1½ tablespoons (23 ml)
   Worcestershire sauce
¼ teaspoon black pepper
1 bay leaf
3 cups (585 g) brown rice, cooked

Brown pork chops on both sides in 1½ tablespoons (23 ml) hot oil in skillet; drain chops and discard drippings. Add remaining 1½ tablespoons (23 ml) oil. Sauté onion and garlic in skillet for 3 minutes. Add green bell pepper. Sauté for 1 minute. Add wine. Bring to a boil; stirring to deglaze skillet. Return chops to skillet; spoon sauce over chops. Add tomatoes, lemon juice, seasonings, and enough water to cover chops if necessary. Simmer, lightly covered, for 1 hour or until chops are tender, turning occasionally. Remove chops to warming platter. Remove bay leaf. Cook sauce over high heat until thickened to desired consistency. Spoon over chops. Serve with rice.

6 SERVINGS

Each with: 346 Calories (32% from Fat, 30% from Protein, 38% from Carb); 25 g Protein; 12 g Total Fat; 3 g Unsaturated Fat; 7 g Monounsaturated Fat; 1 g Polyunsaturated Fat; 31 g Carb; 3 g Fiber; 4 g Sugar; 328 mg Phosphorus; 57 mg Calcium; 100 mg Sodium; 750 mg Potassium; 168 IU Vitamin A; 2 mg ATE Vitamin E; 35 mg Vitamin C; 64 mg Cholesterol

Pork and Squash Packets on the Grill

Pork, apples, and acorn squash wrapped in foil bake on the grill or in the oven for an easy meal and exceptional tenderness. The meal just says autumn in every way with its apples and winter squash, flavored with just a little brown sugar.

2 boneless pork loin chops, 1-inch (2.5 cm) thick

1 dash black pepper

3 cups (420 g) acorn squash, cut in ½-inch (1.3 cm) cubes

1 apple, cut in wedges

2 tablespoons (28 g) unsalted butter

2 tablespoons (2 g) brown sugar substitute, such as Splenda

Cut two 18 × 12-inch (46 × 30 cm) pieces of heavy foil; place pork chop in center of lower half of each piece of foil. Sprinkle with black pepper. Lay squash and apples on top of chop. Dot butter in center of each. Sprinkle with brown sugar substitute. Fold upper edge of foil over ingredients to meet bottom edge. Turn foil edges to form a ½-inch (1.3 cm) fold. Smooth fold. Double over again; press very tightly to seal, allowing room for expansion and heat circulation. Repeat folding and sealing at each end. Place packet on a baking sheet; bake at 425°F (220°C, or gas mark 7) or grill over medium heat for 25 to 30 minutes or until chops are done and vegetables are tender.

2 SERVINGS

Each with: 346 Calories (40% from Fat, 26% from Protein, 34% from Carb); 23 g Protein; 16 g Total Fat; 9 g Unsaturated Fat; 5 g Monounsaturated Fat; 1 g Polyunsaturated Fat; 30 g Carb; 4 g Fiber; 6 g Sugar; 306 mg Phosphorus; 89 mg Calcium; 59 mg Sodium; 1163 mg Potassium; 1157 IU Vitamin A; 97 mg ATE Vitamin E; 27 mg Vitamin C; 94 mg Cholesterol

Cowboy Skillet of Pork Chops and Beans

This is chuck wagon food from the American west. Or maybe it's just a great meal for a Saturday evening after working in the yard. This all in one pan meal will fill you up without filling you out thanks to lean pork loin, which cowboys probably never had.

6 boneless pork loin chops
1 tablespoon (15 ml) olive oil
1 cup (160 g) onion, chopped
1 cup (150 g) green bell pepper, chopped
½ teaspoon garlic, minced
½ cup (120 ml) low sodium chicken broth
½ cup (65 g) barbecue sauce
2 jalapeño peppers, chopped
4 cups (684 g) no-salt-added pinto beans, drained

In a large skillet, sear pork chops in oil until brown, about 5 minutes. Remove pork chops and place on plate. Add onion, green bell pepper, and garlic to skillet. Cook 10 minutes. Stir in broth, barbecue sauce, jalapeño pepper, and beans. Heat mixture to a boil. Return pork to skillet. Reduce heat. Cover and simmer 50 to 60 minutes, stirring sauce and turning chops occasionally until meat is fork-tender.

6 SERVINGS

Each with: 372 Calories (19% from Fat, 35% from Protein, 46% from Carb); 33 g Protein; 8 g Total Fat; 2 g Unsaturated Fat; 4 g Monounsaturated Fat; 1 g Polyunsaturated Fat; 43 g Carb; 10 g Fiber; 10 g Sugar; 393 mg Phosphorus; 71 mg Calcium; 273 mg Sodium; 813 mg Potassium; 137 IU Vitamin A; 2 mg ATE Vitamin E; 26 mg Vitamin C; 64 mg Cholesterol

Not Your Usual Pork Chop and Red Cabbage Skillet

We typically think of pork and red cabbage in the German sweet and sour style, but with its cumin, this one has more of a Southwestern flavor, even though it does still have vinegar and the sweetness of raisins. Whatever you call it, the flavor and nutrient content are high and the calories are low.

3 tablespoons (45 ml) olive oil

1 pound (455 g) boneless pork loin chops

1 teaspoon ground cumin

½ teaspoon black pepper, divided

1 cup (160 g) onion, sliced

6 cups (540 g) red cabbage, thinly sliced

½ cup (75 g) golden raisins

¼ cup (60 ml) red wine vinegar

¼ cup (60 ml) water

¼ cup (16 g) fresh dill, chopped

Heat 1 tablespoon (15 ml) of the oil in a large skillet over medium heat. Season the pork with the cumin and ¼ teaspoon black pepper and cook until browned and cooked through, 6 to 8 minutes per side. Meanwhile, heat the remaining oil in a second skillet over medium-high heat. Cook the onion, stirring occasionally, until softened, 3 to 4 minutes. To the second skillet, add the cabbage, raisins, vinegar, ¼ cup (60 ml) water, and ¼ teaspoon black pepper. Cook the cabbage mixture, covered, tossing occasionally, until just tender, 6 to 8 minutes. Stir in the dill. Serve the cabbage mixture with the pork.

4 SERVINGS

Each with: 368 Calories (36% from Fat, 29% from Protein, 35% from Carb); 28 g Protein; 16 g Total Fat; 3 g Unsaturated Fat; 10 g Monounsaturated Fat; 2 g Polyunsaturated Fat; 33 g Carb; 5 g Fiber; 20 g Sugar; 343 mg Phosphorus; 157 mg Calcium; 105 mg Sodium; 1085 mg Potassium; 1687 IU Vitamin A; 2 mg ATE Vitamin E; 82 mg Vitamin C; 71 mg Cholesterol

Apple Cranberry Stuffed Pork Roast with Sweet Potatoes

When I made this, my wife wondered about going to the trouble of butterflying the roast, but the results were worth what turned out to be not a lot of effort.

Filling
⅔ cup (160 ml) apple cider
¼ cup (60 ml) cider vinegar
½ cup (8 g) brown sugar substitute, such as Splenda
1 tablespoon (10 g) shallots, dried
1 cup (86 g) apples, dried
½ cup (60 g) dried cranberries
1 teaspoon ground ginger
½ teaspoon mustard seed
½ teaspoon allspice, ground
⅛ teaspoon cayenne pepper

Pork Roast
2 pound (900 g) boneless pork loin roast

Apple Sweet Potato Side Dish
6 sweet potatoes, peeled and cubed
6 apples, peeled, cored and cubed
½ cup (120 ml) apple juice
½ teaspoon cinnamon

Simmer filling ingredients in medium saucepan over medium-high heat. Cover, reduce heat, and cook until apples are very soft, about 20 minutes. Strain through a fine-mesh sieve, reserving the liquid. Return liquid to saucepan and simmer over medium-high heat until reduced to ½ cup (120 ml), about 5 minutes. Remove from heat, set aside, and reserve as a glaze. Preheat oven to 350°F (180°C, or gas mark 4). Lay the roast down, fat side up. Insert the knife into the roast ½ inch (1.3 cm) horizontally from the bottom of the roast, along the long side of the roast. Make a long cut along the bottom of the roast, stopping ½ inch (1.3 cm) before the edge. Open up the roast and continue to cut through the thicker half of the roast, keeping ½ inch (1.3 cm) from the bottom. Repeat until the roast is an even ½- inch (1.3 cm) thickness all over when laid out. Spread out the filling on the roast, leaving a ½-inch (1.3 cm) border from the edges. Starting with the short side of the roast, roll it up very tightly. Secure with kitchen twine at 1-inch (2.5 cm) intervals. Place roast on a rack in a roasting pan and place in oven on the middle rack. Cook for 45 to 60 minutes. Brush with half of the glaze and cook for 5 minutes longer. Remove the roast from the oven. Cover with foil to rest and keep warm for 15 minutes before slicing. Slice into ½-inch (1.3 cm) wide pieces, removing the cooking twine as you cut the roast. Serve with remaining glaze. After putting roast in the oven, peel and cube the apples and sweet potatoes. Transfer to an 8-inch (20 cm) square baking dish. Combine the apple juice and cinnamon and pour over. Place in oven and allow to cook until roast is done.

8 SERVINGS

Each with: 366 Calories (20% from Fat, 30% from Protein, 51% from Carb); 27 g Protein; 8 g Total Fat; 3 g Saturated Fat; 3 g Monounsaturated Fat; 1 g Polyunsaturated Fat; 46 g Carb; 5 g Fiber; 27 g Sugar; 290 mg Phosphorus; 50 mg Calcium; 84 mg Sodium; 902 mg Potassium; 17 937 IU Vitamin A; 2 mg ATE Vitamin E; 20 mg Vitamin C; 62 mg Cholesterol

Greek Gods Pork Loin

A Mediterranean-style sauce makes these thin pork slices a little different meal. Low in fat with the pork loin and high in flavor, this meal is sure to be popular.

---

12 ounce (340 g) pork loin, cut into ¼-inch (6 mm) thick slices

⅛ teaspoon black pepper

2 teaspoons olive oil

1½ cups (240 g) onion, cut into thin wedges

1 cup (150 g) green bell pepper, cut into thin bite-size strips

½ cup (35 g) mushrooms, sliced

2 cloves garlic, minced

½ teaspoon dried oregano

⅓ cup (47 g) pimento stuffed olives, sliced

4 cups (628 g) couscous, cooked

4 cups (400 g) green beans

Spray a large skillet with nonstick vegetable oil spray: heat over medium-high heat. Season pork with black pepper. Cook half of the pork slices at a time in skillet for 2 to 3 minutes or until meat is browned and no longer pink in center, turning once. Remove from heat: keep warm. Add olive oil to skillet. Heat over medium-high heat. Cook onion, green bell pepper, mushrooms, garlic, and oregano in skillet about 4 minutes or until crisp-tender. Stir in olives; heat through. Serve vegetable mixture and pork slices over couscous with beans on the side.

4 SERVINGS

Each with: 374 Calories (15% from Fat, 29% from Protein, 56% from Carb); 27 g Protein; 6 g Total Fat; 2 g Unsaturated Fat; 3 g Monounsaturated Fat; 1 g Polyunsaturated Fat; 53 g Carb; 8 g Fiber; 5 g Sugar; 293 mg Phosphorus; 84 mg Calcium; 61 mg Sodium; 818 mg Potassium; 913 IU Vitamin A; 2 mg ATE Vitamin E; 53 mg Vitamin C; 54 mg Cholesterol

Glazed Pork Roast with Vegetables

I grill this when it's warm enough. If you want to do that, it's best to grill using indirect heat. Place a pan of water under the roast and mound the charcoal around it or grill on the side with no flame on a gas grill. Close the grill to hold in the heat and smoke.

¼ cup (85 g) honey
1 tablespoon (9 g) dry mustard
¼ cup (60 ml) white wine vinegar
1 teaspoon chili powder
2 pound (900 g) pork tenderloin
4 medium potatoes
2 cups (244 g) carrot, sliced
4 medium turnips

Mix together honey, mustard, vinegar, and chili powder. Trim any excess fat from pork roast. Brush with glaze. Place in roasting pan surrounded by vegetables. Roast at 350°F (180°C, or gas mark 4) until done, 1 to 1½ hours, brushing with additional glaze occasionally.

8 SERVINGS

Each with: 356 Calories (11% from Fat, 33% from Protein, 56% from Carb); 29 g Protein; 4 g Total Fat; 1 g Unsaturated Fat; 2 g Monounsaturated Fat; 1 g Polyunsaturated Fat; 50 g Carb; 6 g Fiber; 14 g Sugar; 400 mg Phosphorus; 74 mg Calcium; 156 mg Sodium; 1537 mg Potassium; 3968 IU Vitamin A; 2 mg ATE Vitamin E; 42 mg Vitamin C; 74 mg Cholesterol

Pork Roast with Apples and Potatoes and Other Good Stuff

A pork loin roast, cooked with apples and vegetables, makes a great looking as well as great tasting meal. And the loin cut is low in fat. This recipe makes enough for a large get together, but if you have a smaller family, the leftovers are also good.

¾ teaspoon black pepper
2 pound (900 g) pork loin roast
8 small onions, peeled but left whole
8 medium potatoes
2 cups carrot, cut in 2-inch (5 cm) pieces
8 apples, cored
2 cups (475 g) apple cider

Sprinkle black pepper over pork roast and place in roasting pan. Roast at 325°F (170°C, or gas mark 3) for 1 hour. Pour off fat. Place vegetables and apples in alternate positions around roast. Add cider and roast an additional 1 to 1½ hours, basting often. Skim off fat when done.

8 SERVINGS

Each with: 429 Calories (20% from Fat, 44% from Protein, 36% from Carb); 47 g Protein; 9 g Total Fat; 3 g Saturated Fat; 4 g Monounsaturated Fat; 1 g Polyunsaturated Fat; 39 g Carb; 4 g Fiber; 26 g Sugar; 530 mg Phosphorus; 76 mg Calcium; 137 mg Sodium; 1261 mg Potassium; 3927 IU Vitamin A; 4 mg ATE Vitamin E; 18 mg Vitamin C; 135 mg Cholesterol

Lechon Asado Roast Pork

Lechon asado is a Cuban pork disk. The original uses sour orange juice, but in this case we substitute a combination of lime and orange juice for this ingredient that is often difficult to find. Vegetables, including some nontraditional ones like cauliflower, cook around it for a tasty and healthy one pan oven meal.

1 tablespoon (10 g) garlic, minced
1 bay leaf, ground
½ teaspoon dried oregano
½ teaspoon ground cumin
1 tablespoon (15 ml) olive oil
3 pound (1⅓ kg) pork loin roast
½ teaspoon black pepper, fresh ground
¼ cup (60 ml) orange juice
¼ cup (60 ml) lime juice
¼ cup (60 ml) dry white wine
1½ cups (240 g) onion, sliced
5 medium potatoes, peeled and quartered
2 pounds (900 g) cauliflower florets, steamed until crisp-tender

Mash the garlic into a paste and then add the ground bay leaf, oregano, cumin, and olive oil and mix together. Rub this all over the roast. Place roast in a large glass dish and then sprinkle with black pepper and pour orange and lime juice and wine over. Scatter the onion over the roast and then wrap entire roast in plastic and refrigerate. Marinate at least one hour or overnight, turning several times. Heat oven to 350°F (180°C, or gas mark 4). Put the meat in a roasting pan, saving the marinade, and place in the oven. Cook for an hour. Turn roast over, add marinated onion and other vegetables, and reduce heat to 325°F (170°C, or gas mark 3). Baste frequently with the pan juices and continue cooking until done (30 to 35 minutes to the pound, 180°F [82°C] internal temperature). Add water or wine if necessary to keep from burning.

10 SERVINGS

Each with: 360 Calories (20% from Fat, 38% from Protein, 42% from Carb); 34 g Protein; 8 g Total Fat; 2 g Unsaturated Fat; 4 g Monounsaturated Fat; 1 g Polyunsaturated Fat; 37 g Carb; 6 g Fiber; 4 g Sugar; 449 mg Phosphorus; 61 mg Calcium; 96 mg Sodium; 1537 mg Potassium; 47 IU Vitamin A; 3 mg ATE Vitamin E; 83 mg Vitamin C; 86 mg Cholesterol

Latin Style Pork and Potatoes

Cumin and citrus juice provide the flavor for this easy skillet meal. Low fat pork loin keeps it low enough in calories to make it a great meal in one pan.

1½ pound (680 g) pork loin roast, boneless, cut in 1-inch (2.5 cm) cubes
¼ cup (31 g) all purpose flour
3 tablespoons (45 ml) olive oil
½ cup (80 g) onion, chopped, 1 medium
2 slices low sodium bacon, cut up
½ cup (120 ml) water
2 tablespoons (28 ml) orange juice
2 tablespoons (28 ml) lime juice
2 tablespoons (14 g) ground cumin
1 teaspoon dried oregano
¼ teaspoon black pepper
4 cups (720 g) tomatoes, chopped
2 medium potatoes, diced
½ cup (115 g) fat-free sour cream

Coat pork with the flour. Heat oil in 10-inch (25 cm) skillet until hot. Cook and stir pork in oil over medium heat until brown. Remove pork with slotted spoon and drain. Cook and stir onion and bacon in the same skillet until bacon is crisp. Stir in the pork and the remaining ingredients except the sour cream. Heat to boiling and then reduce heat. Cover and simmer until pork is done, about 45 minutes. Stir in sour cream and heat until hot.

6 SERVINGS

Each with: 392 Calories (37% from Fat, 30% from Protein, 33% from Carb); 30 g Protein; 16 g Total Fat; 5 g Unsaturated Fat; 9 g Monounsaturated Fat; 2 g Polyunsaturated Fat; 32 g Carb; 4 g Fiber; 2 g Sugar; 400 mg Phosphorus; 80 mg Calcium; 115 mg Sodium; 1320 mg Potassium; 759 IU Vitamin A; 23 mg ATE Vitamin E; 56 mg Vitamin C; 82 mg Cholesterol

Very Low Calorie Roast Pork Tenderloin and Vegetables Meal

This is a great pork tenderloin meal in a pan, with roasted carrots and new potatoes surrounding it. The servings are generous, but the calorie count is still low because the tenderloin has so little fat.

2 pound (900 g) pork tenderloin

2 pounds (900 g) carrots, peeled and cut 2-inch (5 cm) slices

2 pounds (900 g) new potatoes, halved

2 cups (320 g) onion, cut wedges

1½ cups (150 g) celery, cut in chunks

1 tablespoon (15 ml) olive oil

2 teaspoons dried rosemary

1 teaspoon dried sage, crushed

¼ teaspoon black pepper

Preheat oven 450°F (230°C, or gas mark 8). Generously spray roasting pan with nonstick vegetable oil spray. Place tenderloins in pan. Place vegetables around. Drizzle oil evenly over all. Sprinkle spices over. Bake uncovered for 30 to 40 minutes or until thermometer inserted in thickest part reads 165°F (74°C) and vegetables are tender. Stir vegetables occasionally.

8 SERVINGS

Each with: 323 Calories (17% from Fat, 35% from Protein, 49% from Carb); 28 g Protein; 6 g Total Fat; 2 g Unsaturated Fat; 3 g Monounsaturated Fat; 1 g Polyunsaturated Fat; 40 g Carb; 7 g Fiber; 9 g Sugar; 392 mg Phosphorus; 80 mg Calcium; 166 mg Sodium; 1503 mg Potassium; 13 782 IU Vitamin A; 2 mg ATE Vitamin E; 22 mg Vitamin C; 74 mg Cholesterol

Pork Tenderloin with Cabbage and Apple Slaw

Tender lean pork tenderloin is simply prepared and teamed with a slaw containing Chinese cabbage and apple. The potatoes here show one of the tricks of low calorie cooking. By slicing them thinly, each serving contains more slices and looks bigger, but we hold down the calories.

3 tablespoons (45 ml) olive oil, divided
2½ pound (1.1 kg) pork tenderloin
¼ teaspoon black pepper
2 tablespoons (28 ml) rice vinegar
1 tablespoon (20 g) honey
1 pound (455 g) Napa cabbage, cored, and thinly sliced
1 apple, cut into thin wedges
¼ cup (4 g) fresh cilantro
2 red potatoes, sliced ¼-inch (6 mm) thick and boiled

Preheat oven to 400°F (200°C, or gas mark 6). Heat 1 tablespoon (15 ml) of the oil in a large ovenproof skillet over medium-high heat. Season the pork with black pepper and cook, turning occasionally, until browned, 6 to 8 minutes. Transfer the skillet to the oven and roast until the pork is cooked through, 12 to 14 minutes. Let rest at least 5 minutes before slicing. Meanwhile, in a large bowl, combine the vinegar, honey, and remaining 2 tablespoons (28 ml) of oil. Add the cabbage and apples and toss. Let sit for at least 5 minutes, tossing occasionally. Fold in the cilantro and serve with the pork and potatoes.

6 SERVINGS

Each with: 406 Calories (30% from Fat, 43% from Protein, 27% from Carb); 43 g Protein; 14 g Total Fat; 3 g Unsaturated Fat; 8 g Monounsaturated Fat; 1 g Polyunsaturated Fat; 27 g Carb; 2 g Fiber; 7 g Sugar; 521 mg Phosphorus; 47 mg Calcium; 112 mg Sodium; 1354 mg Potassium; 347 IU Vitamin A; 4 mg ATE Vitamin E; 30 mg Vitamin C; 123 mg Cholesterol

Sweet and Sour Pork Tenderloin

Hot, slightly sweet ginger gives the sauce a little bite. Fruit and vegetables add nutrition. This is a very tasty way to do pork tenderloin, and one that will not remind you that you are trying to lose weight.

2 tablespoons (28 ml) olive oil

1 tablespoon (6 g) fresh ginger, minced

½ teaspoon garlic, smashed

1 green bell pepper, cored, seeded, and cut in strips

1 pound (455 g) pork tenderloin, in 1-inch (2.5 cm) cubes

1 tablespoon (8 g) all purpose flour

1 cup (235 ml) low sodium beef broth

1 tablespoon (16 g) no-salt-added tomato paste

1 tablespoon (15 ml) low sodium soy sauce

1 tablespoon (15 ml) lemon juice

3 tablespoons (48 g) mango chutney

1 cup (165 g) pineapple chunks, in juice

2 cups (390 g) brown rice, cooked

Heat 1 tablespoon (15 ml) oil in medium nonstick skillet. Add ginger root, garlic, and green bell pepper and sauté over medium heat 5 minutes. Add remaining 1 tablespoon (15 ml) oil to skillet. Dust pork cubes with flour and add to skillet. Brown pork over high heat, turning to brown evenly. Pour in beef broth and stir up any browned bits in the skillet. Add tomato paste, soy sauce, lemon juice, and chutney. Stir mixture well. Cover skillet and simmer 10 minutes. Mixture will thicken. Stir in pineapple. Cover and simmer another 5 minutes. Serve over hot cooked rice.

4 SERVINGS

Each with: 384 Calories (28% from Fat, 29% from Protein, 43% from Carb); 28 g Protein; 12 g Total Fat; 3 g Unsaturated Fat; 7 g Monounsaturated Fat; 1 g Polyunsaturated Fat; 41 g Carb; 4 g Fiber; 6 g Sugar; 362 mg Phosphorus; 37 mg Calcium; 235 mg Sodium; 755 mg Potassium; 338 IU Vitamin A; 2 mg ATE Vitamin E; 39 mg Vitamin C; 74 mg Cholesterol

Pork Stroganoff with All the Trimmings

Even though beef is more traditional for stroganoff, this works well too. At least around here, you can buy a boneless pork loin for less than ground beef or any other beef cut for that matter. And it's a great deal nutritionally since it's so low in fat. So you can still have the noodles and broccoli.

1½ pound (680 g) pork loin, cubed

1 tablespoon (15 ml) olive oil

½ cup (80 g) onion, chopped

1 cup (235 ml) low sodium beef broth

8 ounces (225 g) mushrooms, sliced

¼ teaspoon garlic powder

1 teaspoon dill weed

⅛ teaspoon black pepper

½ cup (115 g) fat-free sour cream

¼ cup (60 ml) white wine

3 tablespoons (24 g) all purpose flour

2 cups (320 g) egg noodles, cooked

4 cups (284 g) broccoli florets, steamed until crisp-tender

In a skillet, brown the meat in the oil. Add the onion and cook until softened. Transfer to slow cooker. Combine broth, mushrooms, and spices. Pour over meat mixture. Cook on low for 8 to 10 hours or on high for 5 to 6 hours. Turn heat to high. Stir together sour cream, wine, and flour. Add to cooker. Cook until sauce is thickened, about 15 to 20 minutes. Serve over noodles with broccoli on the side.

6 SERVINGS

Each with: 416 Calories (48% from Fat, 29% from Protein, 23% from Carb); 30 g Protein; 22 g Total Fat; 8 g Unsaturated Fat; 10 g Monounsaturated Fat; 2 g Polyunsaturated Fat; 24 g Carb; 3 g Fiber; 3 g Sugar; 361 mg Phosphorus; 72 mg Calcium; 105 mg Sodium; 841 mg Potassium; 491 IU Vitamin A; 26 mg ATE Vitamin E; 55 mg Vitamin C; 94 mg Cholesterol

Pork and Chickpea Stir-Fry

This is a stir-fry in the cooking method but not in the usual ingredients.
It's a simple meal that's quickly cooked, full of nutrition, and great tasting.

1 pound (455 g) boneless pork loin chops, cut into 1½-inch (3.8 cm) thick strips

¼ cup (25 g) green onion, with tops, sliced

½ teaspoon garlic, crushed

2 teaspoons olive oil

2 cups (142 g) broccoli florets

3 cups (720 g) chickpeas, drained and rinsed

¼ cup (60 ml) low sodium beef broth

Stir-fry pork, green onion, and garlic in oil in wok or large skillet over high heat until pork is browned, 3 to 5 minutes. Add broccoli and stir-fry 2 to 3 minutes. Add chickpeas and broth and cook, covered, over medium heat until broccoli is crisp-tender, 3 to 4 minutes.

4 SERVINGS

Each with: 380 Calories (24% from Fat, 38% from Protein, 38% from Carb); 36 g Protein; 10 g Total Fat; 2 g Unsaturated Fat; 5 g Monounsaturated Fat; 2 g Polyunsaturated Fat; 36 g Carb; 10 g Fiber; 6 g Sugar; 482 mg Phosphorus; 98 mg Calcium; 86 mg Sodium; 920 mg Potassium; 1168 IU Vitamin A; 2 mg ATE Vitamin E; 37 mg Vitamin C; 71 mg Cholesterol

Stuffed Acorn Squash

This acorn squash stuffed with a ground pork mixture is a favorite around our house.

1 acorn squash, about 1 pound (455 g)

6 ounces (170 g) ground pork

¼ cup (25 g) celery, chopped

½ cup (80 g) onion, chopped

¼ teaspoon curry powder

¼ teaspoon cinnamon

½ cup (123 g) applesauce, unsweetened

1 slice whole wheat bread, cubed

 Tip: You could reduce the number of calories and amount of fat by using ground turkey.

Spray a 10 × 6 × 2-inch (25 × 15 × 5 cm) baking dish with nonstick vegetable oil spray. Halve squash; discard seeds. Place squash, cut side down, in baking dish. Bake, uncovered, in 350°F (180°C, or gas mark 4) oven for 50 minutes. Meanwhile, for stuffing, in a skillet, cook pork, celery, and onion until meat is no longer pink and vegetables are tender. Drain fat. Stir in curry powder and cinnamon; cook 1 minute more. Stir in applesauce and bread cubes. Turn squash cut side up in dish. Place stuffing in squash halves. Bake uncovered, 20 minutes more.

2 SERVINGS

Each with: 389 Calories (42% from Fat, 18% from Protein, 40% from Carb); 18 g Protein; 19 g Total Fat; 7 g Saturated Fat; 8 g Monounsaturated Fat; 2 g Polyunsaturated Fat; 40 g Carb; 6 g Fiber; 9 g Sugar; 265 mg Phosphorus; 118 mg Calcium; 135 mg Sodium; 1165 mg Potassium; 886 IU Vitamin A; 2 mg ATE Vitamin E; 28 mg Vitamin C; 61 mg Cholesterol

Cabbage Casserole

Ground turkey and sausage mix with brown rice and vegetables for an easy casserole that is full of flavor and nutrition without being full of calories.

½ pound (225 g) ground turkey

½ pound (225 g) sausage, cut into small pieces

2 cups (360 g) no-salt-added tomatoes

1 cup (160 g) onion, chopped

1 cup (190 g) brown rice, uncooked

1 tablespoon (8 g) chili powder

1 teaspoon garlic powder

1 cup (150 g) green bell pepper, chopped

4 cups (360 g) cabbage, shredded

¼ cup (60 ml) egg substitute

Mix all ingredients together in covered roasting pan. Bake at 350°F (180°C, or gas mark 4) for approximately 1½ hours. Stir a couple of times.

4 SERVINGS

Each with: 424 Calories (25% from Fat, 25% from Protein, 50% from Carb); 27 g Protein; 12 g Total Fat; 4 g Unsaturated Fat; 5 g Monounsaturated Fat; 2 g Polyunsaturated Fat; 54 g Carb; 7 g Fiber; 10 g Sugar; 375 mg Phosphorus; 131 mg Calcium; 352 mg Sodium; 1077 mg Potassium; 1060 IU Vitamin A; 0 mg ATE Vitamin E; 80 mg Vitamin C; 56 mg Cholesterol

Easy Does It Pork Stew

Easy to make in the slow cooker and chock full of vegetables, this is the kind of stew I'd want even if I weren't being careful about my diet.

1 pound (455 g) ground pork

1 cup (160 g) onion, chopped

1 cup (122 g) carrot, sliced

1 cup (150 g) turnip, diced

½ cup (50 g) celery, sliced

1 medium sweet potato, cubed and peeled

½ teaspoon dried rosemary

1 cup (235 ml) low sodium beef broth

Place meat and onion in nonstick skillet. Brown on stove top. Place drained meat and onion into slow cooker. Add remaining ingredients. Cover and cook on low for 6 to 8 hours.

4 SERVINGS

Each with: 372 Calories (59% from Fat, 23% from Protein, 18% from Carb); 21 g Protein; 24 g Total Fat; 9 g Unsaturated Fat; 11 g Monounsaturated Fat; 2 g Polyunsaturated Fat; 16 g Carb; 3 g Fiber; 7 g Sugar; 253 mg Phosphorus; 65 mg Calcium; 166 mg Sodium; 706 mg Potassium; 9883 IU Vitamin A; 2 mg ATE Vitamin E; 17 mg Vitamin C; 82 mg Cholesterol

Take Me to Jamaica Pork Stew

This is a flavorful pork stew with the taste of curry powder and lots of healthy vegetables.

1½ pound (680 g) pork loin roast, cubed

½ tablespoons minced garlic

1 tablespoon (15 ml) oil

1 cup (160 g) onion, coarsely chopped

2 cups (244 g) carrot, sliced

2 cups (360 g) no-salt-added tomatoes

1 medium sweet potato, peeled and cubed

½ cup (120 ml) water

2 tablespoons (12 g) curry powder

 Tip: If you have a market that sells Caribbean or Hispanic foods, look for mild Jamaican curry powder.

Brown pork and garlic in oil in a heavy skillet. Add vegetables, water, and curry powder. Cover and simmer until pork is tender, about 45 minutes.

4 SERVINGS

Each with: 354 Calories (29% from Fat, 44% from Protein, 27% from Carb); 39 g Protein; 11 g Total Fat; 3 g Unsaturated Fat; 4 g Monounsaturated Fat; 3 g Polyunsaturated Fat; 24 g Carb; 6 g Fiber; 10 g Sugar; 452 mg Phosphorus; 116 mg Calcium; 157 mg Sodium; 1304 mg Potassium; 13 857 IU Vitamin A; 3 mg ATE Vitamin E; 30 mg Vitamin C; 107 mg Cholesterol

Spicy Green Chili Pork

This is a chili variation that does not contain tomatoes and has pork instead of the more traditional beef.
Use of leftover pork loin roast keeps it low in fat and lots of vegetables add to the nutrition.
And the cayenne pepper and chilies gives it just enough heat.

3 cups (600 g) cannellini beans,
cooked according to package
directions
1 cup (160 g) onion, chopped
1 cup (150 g) green bell pepper,
chopped
1 teaspoon garlic, minced
4 ounces (115 g) chopped green
chiles
2 teaspoons dried oregano
1½ teaspoons ground cumin
¼ teaspoon ground cloves
¼ teaspoon cayenne pepper
4 cups (892 g) pork loin roast,
cooked and diced

Combine all ingredients in a large pot and simmer gently about
1 hour.

6 SERVINGS

Each with: 431 Calories (9% from Fat, 35% from Protein, 56% from Carb);
39 g Protein; 4 g Total Fat; 1 g Unsaturated Fat; 2 g Monounsaturated Fat; 1 g
Polyunsaturated Fat; 62 g Carb; 24 g Fiber; 5 g Sugar; 564 mg Phosphorus; 165 mg
Calcium; 65 mg Sodium; 1738 mg Potassium; 381 IU Vitamin A; 2 mg ATE Vitamin E;
73 mg Vitamin C; 48 mg Cholesterol

Southwestern Black Bean and Pork Stew

Cumin and cilantro give this stew a Southwestern flavor, while beans and squash provide a contrast in tastes and textures, as well as great nutrient density.

4 cups (950 ml) water
½ cup (125 g) dried black beans
2 ancho chilies
1 pound (455 g) pork loin roast
1½ (240 g) cups tomatoes, chopped
½ cup (80 g) onion, chopped
½ cup (120 ml) dry red wine
1 teaspoon dried sage
1 teaspoon dried marjoram
½ teaspoon ground cumin
¼ teaspoon ground cinnamon
½ teaspoon garlic, minced
2 cups (160 g) butternut squash, pared and cut in 1-inch (2.5 cm) cubes
1 cup (150 g) red bell pepper, diced
2 tablespoons (2 g) fresh cilantro, chopped

Heat water, beans, and ancho chilies to boiling in Dutch oven. Boil uncovered 2 minutes; remove from heat. Cover and let stand 1 hour. Remove chilies; reserve. Heat beans to boiling; reduce heat. Simmer covered for 1 hour. Seed and coarsely chop ancho chilies. Trim fat from pork. Cut pork into 1-inch (2.5 cm) cubes. Stir pork, ancho chilies, and remaining ingredients except squash, green bell pepper, and cilantro into beans. Heat to boiling; reduce heat. Cover and simmer 30 minutes, stirring occasionally. Stir in squash. Cover and simmer 30 minutes, stirring occasionally, until squash is tender. Stir in green bell pepper and cilantro. Cover and simmer about 5 minutes or until green bell pepper is crisp-tender.

4 SERVINGS

Each with: 337 Calories (17% from Fat, 39% from Protein, 44% from Carb); 32 g Protein; 6 g Total Fat; 2 g Unsaturated Fat; 2 g Monounsaturated Fat; 1 g Polyunsaturated Fat; 36 g Carb; 9 g Fiber; 5 g Sugar; 409 mg Phosphorus; 111 mg Calcium; 80 mg Sodium; 1513 mg Potassium; 10 814 IU Vitamin A; 2 mg ATE Vitamin E; 103 mg Vitamin C; 71 mg Cholesterol

Chinese Shredded Pork and Cabbage

If you replace the large amount of white rice with reasonable amounts of brown and feature lean meat and lots of vegetables, you can get a meal like this that tastes great, fills you up, and provides excellent nutrition.

1 pound (455 g) pork loin roast
4 tablespoons (60 ml) olive oil
2 cups (180 g) cabbage, shredded
1 cup (110 g) carrot, shredded
1 cup (160 g) onion, cut in strips
½ teaspoon oriental seasoning
¼ cup (60 ml) low sodium soy sauce
2 cups (390 g) cooked brown rice

Slice pork thinly and then shred the strips. Heat 2 tablespoons (28 ml) of the oil in a wok or heavy skillet. Stir-fry the pork until cooked through. Remove from wok. Add the other two tablespoons (28 ml) of oil and stir-fry the vegetables until crisp-tender. Return the pork to the wok. Add the seasoning and soy sauce. Heat through. Serve over rice.

4 SERVINGS

Each with: 421 Calories (41% from Fat, 27% from Protein, 32% from Carb); 28 g Protein; 19 g Total Fat; 4 g Saturated Fat; 12 g Monounsaturated Fat; 2 g Polyunsaturated Fat; 33 g Carb; 4 g Fiber; 3 g Sugar; 370 mg Phosphorus; 63 mg Calcium; 621 mg Sodium; 772 mg Potassium; 3937 IU Vitamin A; 2 mg ATE Vitamin E; 23 mg Vitamin C; 71 mg Cholesterol

Chinese Pork Stir-Fry

This is a fairly traditional Chinese style stir-fry, but it has a few more vegetables and a bit less rice to up the nutrition and lower the calories.

1 pound (455 g) pork loin
3 tablespoons (45 ml) olive oil
2 cups (180 g) cabbage, shredded
½ cup (55 g) carrot, shredded
1½ cups (107 g) broccoli florets
1 cup (160 g) onion, cut in strips
¼ cup (60 ml) low sodium soy sauce
½ teaspoon oriental seasoning
2 cups (390 g) brown rice, cooked

Slice pork thinly and then shred the strips. Heat 2 tablespoons (28 ml) of the oil in a wok or heavy skillet. Stir-fry the pork until cooked through. Remove from wok. Add the other tablespoon (15 ml) of oil and stir-fry the vegetables until crisp-tender. Return the pork to the wok. Add the seasoning and soy sauce. Heat through. Serve over rice.

4 SERVINGS

Each with: 394 Calories (36% from Fat, 29% from Protein, 34% from Carb); 29 g Protein; 16 g Total Fat; 3 g Unsaturated Fat; 10 g Monounsaturated Fat; 2 g Polyunsaturated Fat; 34 g Carb; 4 g Fiber; 4 g Sugar; 384 mg Phosphorus; 75 mg Calcium; 619 mg Sodium; 831 mg Potassium; 2842 IU Vitamin A; 2 mg ATE Vitamin E; 44 mg Vitamin C; 71 mg Cholesterol

Pork Loin Roast with Asian Vegetables

This is an Asian-style pork roast. It's almost more of a stew than a roast but good even if you call it that. And it's full of lots of good-for-you veggies.

1 teaspoon ground ginger

2 tablespoons (28 ml) olive oil

2½ pound (1.1 kg) pork loin roast

1 cup (235 ml) water

1 cup (160 g) onion, coarsely chopped

¼ cup (60 ml) low sodium soy sauce

¼ cup (60 ml) red wine vinegar

2 tablespoons (2 g) brown sugar substitute, such as Splenda

½ teaspoon garlic powder

¼ teaspoon black pepper

4 cups (580 g) snow pea pods

2 cups (360 g) no-salt-added tomatoes

8 ounces (225 g) water chestnuts

8 ounces (225 g) mushrooms, sliced

¼ cup (60 ml) water

2 tablespoons (16 g) cornstarch

4 cups (780 g) brown rice, cooked

In a large Dutch oven, sauté ginger in oil for 30 seconds. Add pork roast and brown meat on all sides. Add the water, onion, soy sauce, vinegar, brown sugar substitute, garlic, and black pepper. Cover and simmer about 1½ hours until tender. Add pea pods, undrained tomatoes, water chestnuts, and mushrooms. Cover and simmer until crisp-tender, 3 to 5 minutes. Remove vegetables and meat. Skim any fat from pan juices. Blend the ¼ cup (60 ml) water with the cornstarch and stir into pot. Cook and stir until bubbly. Serve sauce with vegetables and meat over rice.

8 SERVINGS

Each with: 408 Calories (23% from Fat, 35% from Protein, 41% from Carb); 36 g Protein; 11 g Total Fat; 3 g Unsaturated Fat; 6 g Monounsaturated Fat; 1 g Polyunsaturated Fat; 42 g Carb; 5 g Fiber; 7 g Sugar; 479 mg Phosphorus; 78 mg Calcium; 354 mg Sodium; 1139 mg Potassium; 622 IU Vitamin A; 3 mg ATE Vitamin E; 42 mg Vitamin C; 89 mg Cholesterol

Pork and Apple Curry

Curry flavor creates a new kind of pork dish.

2 tablespoons (28 ml) olive oil

1 pound (455 g) pork loin chops

1 cup (160 g) onion, thinly sliced

¼ teaspoon garlic, minced

1 apple, peeled and sliced

2 cups (280 g) butternut squash, peeled and cubed

1 cup (150 g) red bell pepper, cut in strips

½ cup (120 ml) low sodium chicken broth

1 teaspoon cornstarch

1 teaspoon curry powder

½ teaspoon ground cumin

¼ teaspoon black pepper, fresh ground

½ teaspoon cinnamon

2 cups (314 g) cooked whole wheat couscous

In a heavy fry pan, heat oil over medium-high heat. Cook pork chops until browned on both sides and almost cooked through; remove from pan and set aside. Over medium heat, cook the onion, garlic, apple, squash, and red bell pepper strips for 2 minutes or until softened. Blend chicken broth with cornstarch. Add to pan along with curry powder, cumin, black pepper, and cinnamon. Cook for 1 or 2 minutes until slightly reduced and thickened. Return pork chops to fry pan. Cook for 1 or 2 minutes or until heated through. Serve pork chops with sauce over couscous.

4 SERVINGS

Each with: 377 Calories (29% from Fat, 31% from Protein, 40% from Carb); 29 g Protein; 12 g Total Fat; 3 g Saturated Fat; 7 g Monounsaturated Fat; 1 g Polyunsaturated Fat; 39 g Carb; 5 g Fiber; 8 g Sugar; 324 mg Phosphorus; 78 mg Calcium; 77 mg Sodium; 919 mg Potassium; 8638 IU Vitamin A; 2 mg ATE Vitamin E; 91 mg Vitamin C; 71 mg Cholesterol

Old World Smoked Sausage Stew

This is the kind of meal I imagine my ancestors in Germany eating. It's a nice hearty stew of smoked sausage and beans that will both fill and warm you. In this version, we use turkey kielbasa, which helps to hold down the fat and calories, and there are plenty of vegetables to make it a meal in a bowl.

1 cup (160 g) onion, chopped

1 pound (455 g) turkey kielbasa, thinly sliced

2 tablespoons (28 ml) olive oil

30 ounces (840 g) great northern beans, no-salt-added, undrained

16 ounces (455 g) no-salt-added tomato sauce

4 ounces (115 g) diced green chilies

1 cup (122 g) carrot, thinly sliced

½ cup (75 g) green bell pepper, chopped

2 medium potatoes, diced

¼ teaspoon Italian seasoning

½ teaspoon dried thyme

¼ teaspoon black pepper

Sauté onion and kielbasa in oil in skillet until onions are soft. Transfer onions and kielbasa to slow cooker. Add all remaining ingredients to cooker and stir together well. Cover. Cook on low for 8 to 10 hours or until vegetables are tender.

8 SERVINGS

Each with: 393 Calories (32% from Fat, 19% from Protein, 50% from Carb); 18 g Protein; 14 g Total Fat; 4 g Unsaturated Fat; 7 g Monounsaturated Fat; 2 g Polyunsaturated Fat; 50 g Carb; 9 g Fiber; 4 g Sugar; 231 mg Phosphorus; 95 mg Calcium; 765 mg Sodium; 1109 mg Potassium; 2188 IU Vitamin A; 0 mg ATE Vitamin E; 41 mg Vitamin C; 40 mg Cholesterol

Full of Goodness Split Pea Soup with Ham

This is a little more than your usual split pea soup, with extra generous helpings of vegetables. Yet with all that taste and nutrition and the ability to fill you up and hold you over to the next meal, it still has less than 350 calories.

1 pound (455 g) ham, chopped
6 cups (1.4 L) water
1 pound (455 g) split peas
2 medium potatoes, peeled and diced
2½ cups (305 g) carrot, sliced
1½ cups (240 g) onion, chopped
1 cup (100 g) celery, chopped
½ teaspoon marjoram
¼ teaspoon black pepper

Place ham in slow cooker. Stir in water, peas, potatoes, carrot, onion, celery, marjoram, and black pepper. Cover and cook on low for 10 to 12 hours. Before serving, stir mixture.

6 SERVINGS

Each with: 346 Calories (18% from Fat, 29% from Protein, 53% from Carb); 25 g Protein; 7 g Total Fat; 2 g Unsaturated Fat; 3 g Monounsaturated Fat; 1 g Polyunsaturated Fat; 46 g Carb; 11 g Fiber; 8 g Sugar; 351 mg Phosphorus; 68 mg Calcium; 875 mg Sodium; 1380 mg Potassium; 6532 IU Vitamin A; 0 mg ATE Vitamin E; 31 mg Vitamin C; 31 mg Cholesterol

Pasta with Ham and Vegetables

This is a great pasta dish that can be eaten however you like it, hot, warm, or cold. Lots of zucchini and a little wine add interest, and spinach ups the nutrition index.

8 ounces (225 g) whole wheat pasta
4 tablespoons (60 ml) olive oil
½ pound (225 g) ham
6 cups (720 g) zucchini, sliced
1 cup (160 g) onion, sliced
½ cup (120 ml) white wine
6 ounces (170 g) spinach

Cook pasta according to directions. Add olive oil to a large nonstick pan. Add chopped ham and cook for about 5 minutes or until desired crispness. Add zucchini and onion to the pan with ham and oil and cook for about 10 more minutes, stirring occasionally until squash is golden brown. Add wine and cook about 5 more minutes. When done, add pasta and spinach and cook long enough for spinach to wilt.

4 SERVINGS

Each with: 361 Calories (48% from Fat, 21% from Protein, 31% from Carb); 19 g Protein; 19 g Total Fat; 4 g Unsaturated Fat; 12 g Monounsaturated Fat; 2 g Polyunsaturated Fat; 27 g Carb; 5 g Fiber; 6 g Sugar; 282 mg Phosphorus; 94 mg Calcium; 663 mg Sodium; 1030 mg Potassium; 4362 IU Vitamin A; 0 mg ATE Vitamin E; 46 mg Vitamin C; 23 mg Cholesterol

Ham Stuffed Eggplant

Ham may seem like an unusual meat to stuff eggplant with, but their flavors complement each other nicely. Tomatoes and other vegetables make this not just a filling meal, but one full of nutrition.

2 eggplants, each about 1 pound (455 g)

¼ cup (60 ml) olive oil

½ cup (80 g) onion, finely chopped

½ cup (50 g) scallions, finely chopped, including 3 inches (7.5 cm) of the green

1½ teaspoons garlic, minced

1 cup (180 g) no-salt-added tomatoes

1 teaspoon dried thyme

¼ teaspoon cayenne pepper

¼ teaspoon black pepper

½ pound (225 g) ham, finely ground

1½ cups (175 g) bread crumbs

¼ cup (15 g) fresh parsley, finely chopped

Cut the eggplants in half lengthwise and with a spoon, hollow out the center of each half to make a boat-like shell about ¼-inch (6 mm) thick. Finely chop the eggplant pulp and set aside. In a heavy skillet, heat the olive oil over moderate heat. Add the eggplant shells and turn them about with tongs until they are moistened on all sides. Then cover the skillet tightly and cook over moderate heat for 5 or 6 minutes. Turn the shells over and continue to cook, still tightly covered, for 5 minutes longer or until they are somewhat soft to the touch. Invert the shells on paper towels to drain and arrange them cut side up in a baking dish large enough to hold them snugly in one layer. Preheat the oven to 400°F (200°C, or gas mark 6). Add the onion, scallions, and garlic to the skillet and stirring frequently, cook for 5 minutes or until they are soft but not brown. Add the reserved chopped eggplant pulp, the tomatoes, thyme, cayenne pepper, and black pepper and stirring frequently, cook until most of the liquid in the pan evaporates and the mixture is thick enough to hold. Remove the skillet from the heat and stir in the ham, half of the bread crumbs, and the parsley. Spoon the filling into the eggplant shells, dividing it equally among them and mounding it slightly in the centers. Sprinkle shells with the remaining bread crumbs. Bake for 15 minutes or until the shells are tender and the filling lightly browned.

4 SERVINGS

Each with: 403 Calories (46% from Fat, 18% from Protein, 36% from Carb); 19 g Protein; 21 g Total Fat; 4 g Unsaturated Fat; 13 g Monounsaturated Fat; 3 g Polyunsaturated Fat; 36 g Carb; 3 g Fiber; 6 g Sugar; 219 mg Phosphorus; 123 mg Calcium; 914 mg Sodium; 518 mg Potassium; 576 IU Vitamin A; 0 mg ATE Vitamin E; 18 mg Vitamin C; 23 mg Cholesterol

Russian Vegetable Soup

This soup has a little bit of everything in it, and that really gives it a spark of flavor and a lot of nutrients.

3 quarts (2.8 L) water

1 pound (455 g) mixed dried beans

1 pound (455 g) ham hocks

2 tablespoons (28 ml) olive oil

1 cup (160 g) onion, diced

1 cup (100 g) celery, diced

½ cup (75 g) green bell pepper, diced

1 teaspoon garlic, crushed

2 cups (260 g) carrot, diced

2 cups (300 g) rutabaga, diced

2 cups (142 g) broccoli, diced

1 cup (200 g) pearl barley

2 tablespoons (2 g) dried parsley

1 tablespoon black pepper

1 teaspoon dried basil

1 teaspoon coriander

1 teaspoon nutmeg

Soak beans overnight. Put ham hocks and beans in large pot. Bring to a boil and then let it simmer for an hour. (It can be refrigerated overnight at this point to skim off grease.) Remove meat from ham bones and return to pot. Heat oil in a skillet and sauté onion, celery, green bell pepper, and garlic until softened, about 5 minutes. Add to pot. Simmer for another hour. Add carrot, rutabaga, broccoli, barley, and herbs. Simmer for another hour.

8 SERVINGS

Each with: 399 Calories (15% from Fat, 24% from Protein, 61% from Carb); 25 g Protein; 7 g Total Fat; 1 g Saturated Fat; 4 g Monounsaturated Fat; 1 g Polyunsaturated Fat; 62 g Carb; 16 g Fiber; 7 g Sugar; 361 mg Phosphorus; 211 mg Calcium; 418 mg Sodium; 1603 mg Potassium; 4199 IU Vitamin A; 0 mg ATE Vitamin E; 42 mg Vitamin C; 14 mg Cholesterol

Full Meal, Full You, Barley Salad

This makes a cool and crunchy salad with a vinaigrette dressing. Ham and barley add substance, as well as flavor.

1 cup (184 g) cooked pearl barley

½ cup (62 g) water chestnuts, drained, sliced

1 cup (100 g) celery, chopped

1 cup (150 g) green bell pepper, chopped

⅓ cup (64 g) pimento

¼ cup (40 g) onion, chopped

1 cup (150 g) ham, cubed

1 tablespoon (6 g) Italian seasoning

¼ cup (6 g) sugar substitute, such as Splenda

¼ cup (60 ml) olive oil

¼ cup (60 ml) red wine vinegar

4 cups (228 g) mixed greens

 Tip: Leave out the ham and serve with a piece of grilled meat.

Mix together cooked barley, water chestnuts, celery, green bell pepper, pimentos, onion, and ham. Cover and chill. In a screw-top jar, combine remaining ingredients except lettuce. Cover and shake well. Pour over salad and stir to mix just before serving. Place lettuce on plate and spoon salad on top.

4 SERVINGS

Each with: 385 Calories (40% from Fat, 15% from Protein, 45% from Carb); 15 g Protein; 18 g Total Fat; 3 g Saturated Fat; 12 g Monounsaturated Fat; 2 g Polyunsaturated Fat; 45 g Carb; 11 g Fiber; 5 g Sugar; 244 mg Phosphorus; 62 mg Calcium; 415 mg Sodium; 715 mg Potassium; 937 IU Vitamin A; 0 mg ATE Vitamin E; 48 mg Vitamin C; 14 mg Cholesterol

You Can Have a Little Lamb and Vegetable Stew

Lamb is often high in fat and calories. But if you are careful to pick a lean cut like an arm steak and trim the fat, you can still have it occasionally. This stew is rich in vegetables, which don't add that many calories but fill you up and keep you from getting hungry soon after eating.

2 tablespoons (28 ml) olive oil

1 pound (455 g) lamb steaks, bones removed and meat cut into 2-inch (5 cm) pieces

½ teaspoon black pepper

1 cup (122 g) carrot, cut into 3-inch (7.5 cm) sticks

1 cup (160 g) onion, sliced

1 tablespoon (8 g) all purpose flour

½ cup (60 ml) dry white wine

2 cups (475 ml) low sodium chicken broth

2 cups (360 g) no-salt-added tomatoes, drained

4 ounces (115 g) green beans, cut into small pieces

1 cup (60 g) fresh parsley, chopped

Heat 1 tablespoon (15 ml) of the oil in a large pot over medium-high heat. Season the lamb with black pepper. Cook, turning occasionally, until medium-rare, 6 to 8 minutes; transfer to a plate. Add the carrot, onion, and the remaining oil to the pot. Cook until beginning to soften, 3 to 4 minutes. Add the flour and cook for 1 minute. Add the wine and scrape up any brown bits. Add the broth, tomatoes, and green beans. Simmer until the vegetables are tender, 8 to 10 minutes. Stir in the lamb and parsley.

4 SERVINGS

Each with: 381 Calories (58% from Fat, 22% from Protein, 20% from Carb); 20 g Protein; 24 g Total Fat; 8 g Unsaturated Fat; 12 g Monounsaturated Fat; 2 g Polyunsaturated Fat; 19 g Carb; 4 g Fiber; 7 g Sugar; 245 mg Phosphorus; 107 mg Calcium; 135 mg Sodium; 915 mg Potassium; 5470 IU Vitamin A; 0 mg ATE Vitamin E; 46 mg Vitamin C; 60 mg Cholesterol

Dinners: Fish and Seafood

Fish and seafood are great choices for those people looking to lose a little weight and still eat healthy food. They are generally low in calories, and they contain many valuable nutrients like omega-3 fatty acids. Fortunately, it's not difficult to create great recipes using fish and seafood. This chapter contains some of our favorites.

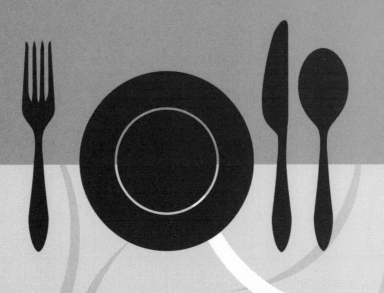

Oven Fried Fish

Nicely spiced fish is fried up in the oven with minimum fat.

2 tablespoons (28 g) unsalted
  butter, melted
1 tablespoon (15 ml) lemon juice
¼ teaspoon black pepper
¼ teaspoon paprika
¼ teaspoon dried basil
⅛ teaspoon garlic powder
1 pound (455 g) flounder
¼ cup (30 g) bread crumbs
2 tablespoons (28 ml) oil
2 medium potatoes

 Tip: Sprinkle the potatoes with garlic, black pepper, paprika, or other spices to suit your taste.

Combine butter, lemon juice, black pepper, paprika, basil, and garlic. Dredge fish in mixture and roll in bread crumbs. Spread oil in shallow baking dish and arrange fish in one layer. Spoon remaining mixture over fish. Cut potatoes into thin wedges and place on baking sheet. Spray with nonstick vegetable oil spray. Bake both uncovered at 475°F (240°C, or gas mark 9) for 15 minutes or until fish flakes easily with fork.

4 SERVINGS

Each with: 388 Calories (34% from Fat, 27% from Protein, 39% from Carb); 26 g Protein; 14 g Total Fat; 5 g Unsaturated Fat; 3 g Monounsaturated Fat; 5 g Polyunsaturated Fat; 37 g Carb; 4 g Fiber; 1 g Sugar; 329 mg Phosphorus; 63 mg Calcium; 154 mg Sodium; 1257 mg Potassium; 316 IU Vitamin A; 59 mg ATE Vitamin E; 23 mg Vitamin C; 70 mg Cholesterol

Not Your Mama's Tuna Casserole

This is a variation on the traditional tuna casserole. Brown rice contains more nutrients than the typical egg noodles, and yogurt provides flavor and creaminess. Plus extra vegetables add even more nutrition.

1¼ cup (238 g) brown rice, uncooked

3 cups (700 g) water

1 cup (100 g) chopped celery

½ cup (80 g) onion, finely diced

½ cup (115 g) plain fat-free yogurt

1 cup (235 ml) skim milk

1 cup (150 g) red bell pepper, chopped

½ teaspoon dried tarragon

14 ounces (390 g) tuna, water packed, drained

1½ cups (107 g) broccoli florets

20 ounces (570 g) frozen peas, thawed

¾ cup (86 g) low fat cheddar cheese, shredded

Combine rice and water in large saucepan. Bring to a boil. Reduce heat, cover, and cook 35 minutes. Remove from heat. Add celery, onion, yogurt, and skim milk. Add red bell pepper and tarragon; mix well. Add flaked tuna, broccoli, and thawed peas; mix well. Turn into 2-quart (1.9 L) casserole. Bake at 350°F (180°C, or gas mark 4) for 30 minutes. Top with shredded cheese.

6 SERVINGS

Each with: 372 Calories (8% from Fat, 35% from Protein, 56% from Carb); 33 g Protein; 3 g Total Fat; 1 g Saturated Fat; 1 g Monounsaturated Fat; 1 g Polyunsaturated Fat; 52 g Carb; 8 g Fiber; 4 g Sugar; 509 mg Phosphorus; 233 mg Calcium; 699 mg Sodium; 734 mg Potassium; 1803 IU Vitamin A; 47 mg ATE Vitamin E; 78 mg Vitamin C; 25 mg Cholesterol

More Like Your Mama's Tuna Casserole
(Only Better and Easier)

Here's a fairly traditional tuna noodle casserole, with added vegetables, that cooks in the slow cooker.

16 ounces (455 g) tuna, water packed

20 ounces (570 g) low sodium cream of mushroom soup

1 cup (235 ml) skim milk

2 tablespoons (8 g) fresh parsley, chopped

8 ounces (225 g) mushrooms, sliced

16 ounces (455 g) frozen mixed vegetables, thawed

16 ounces (455 g) frozen broccoli, carrot and cauliflower, thawed

10 ounces (280 g) egg noodles, cooked and drained

¼ cup (23 g) sliced almonds, toasted

Combine tuna, soup, skim milk, parsley, and vegetables. Fold in noodles. Pour into greased slow cooker. Top with almonds. Cover. Cook on low for 7 to 9 hours or on high for 3 to 4 hours.

6 SERVINGS

Each with: 364 Calories (19% from Fat, 31% from Protein, 50% from Carb); 29 g Protein; 8 g Total Fat; 2 g Saturated Fat; 3 g Monounsaturated Fat; 2 g Polyunsaturated Fat; 45 g Carb; 11 g Fiber; 7 g Sugar; 433 mg Phosphorus; 136 mg Calcium; 481 mg Sodium; 1045 mg Potassium; 6705 IU Vitamin A; 31 mg ATE Vitamin E; 8 mg Vitamin C; 35 mg Cholesterol

Fish and Wine Sauced Pasta

This makes a simple but flavorful sauce that is particularly good with whole wheat pasta. And the meal gets a great nutritional bonus both from the fish and the generous serving of broccoli on the side.

¼ cup (60 ml) olive oil

12 ounces (340 g) salmon fillets, cubed

12 ounces (340 g) fish fillets, cubed

1 teaspoon minced garlic

½ cup (120 ml) white wine

½ teaspoon dried oregano

½ teaspoon dried rosemary

1 teaspoon dried parsley

1 tablespoon (10 g) minced onion

12 ounces (340 g) whole wheat spaghetti

6 cups (426 g) broccoli florets, steamed until crisp-tender

Heat oil in a heavy skillet. Add fish and garlic and sauté for a minute or two until nearly cooked through. Add wine, minced onion, and spices and continue cooking until sauce has been reduced to about half. Serve over pasta with broccoli.

6 SERVINGS

Each with: 370 Calories (42% from Fat, 34% from Protein, 24% from Carb); 30 g Protein; 17 g Total Fat; 3 g Unsaturated Fat; 9 g Monounsaturated Fat; 4 g Polyunsaturated Fat; 22 g Carb; 4 g Fiber; 2 g Sugar; 404 mg Phosphorus; 141 mg Calcium; 120 mg Sodium; 741 mg Potassium; 662 IU Vitamin A; 16 mg ATE Vitamin E; 82 mg Vitamin C; 64 mg Cholesterol

Creamed Fish Fillets with Shrimp Sauce

Fish is poached in milk and then covered with a cheesy sauce containing shrimp in this recipe. It is the sort of thing to pull out and serve to company and then surprise them with the fact that it is *diet* food.

---

1 pound (455 g) cod, or other white fish

¼ cup (40 g) onion, minced

1½ cups (355 ml) skim milk

2 tablespoons (28 g) butter or margarine

2 tablespoons (16 g) all purpose flour

⅛ teaspoon black pepper

¼ cup (25 g) Parmesan cheese, grated

6 ounces (170 g) shrimp, cleaned, cooked, and chopped

2 tablespoons (28 ml) sherry

1 tablespoon (4 g) fresh parsley, minced

2 cups (390 g) brown rice, cooked

Slice fish in thin pieces. Place in greased baking dish and sprinkle with minced onion. Pour skim milk over fish. Bake in 400°F (200°C, or gas mark 6) oven until done. Fish may take anywhere from 15 to 30 minutes to bake, depending on thickness. When it is easily flaked with fork, it is ready. Meanwhile, melt butter in sauce pan; stir in flour and black pepper. When fish is done, remove from oven and turn up heat to 450°F (230°C, or gas mark 8). Pour milk out of fish pan and stir into butter mixture. Cook sauce, while stirring, until smooth and thickened. Add cheese and stir until melted. Add shrimp; heat. Stir in sherry. Pour sauce over fish; sprinkle with parsley and put back in oven to bake for 5 minutes or until very lightly browned. Serve over rice.

4 SERVINGS

Each with: 393 Calories (24% from Fat, 40% from Protein, 36% from Carb); 38 g Protein; 10 g Total Fat; 5 g Unsaturated Fat; 3 g Monounsaturated Fat; 1 g Polyunsaturated Fat; 34 g Carb; 2 g Fiber; 1 g Sugar; 551 mg Phosphorus; 258 mg Calcium; 318 mg Sodium; 832 mg Potassium; 596 IU Vitamin A; 148 mg ATE Vitamin E; 5 mg Vitamin C; 136 mg Cholesterol

Catfish Parmesan

Oven baked fish and potatoes are crunchy and full of flavor but not full of fat and calories.

2½ pounds (1.1 kg) catfish fillets, fresh or frozen

1 cup (115 g) bread crumbs

¾ cup (75 g) Parmesan cheese, grated

1 teaspoon paprika

½ teaspoon dried oregano

¼ teaspoon dried basil

½ teaspoon black pepper

2 tablespoons (28 g) unsalted butter, melted

2 medium potatoes, cut in wedges

1 lemon, cut in wedges

¼ cup (15 g) fresh parsley, chopped

20 ounces (570 g) green beans

Pat fish dry. Combine bread crumbs, cheese, and seasonings; stir well. Dip catfish in butter and roll each in crumb mixture. Arrange fish on baking sheet sprayed with nonstick vegetable oil spray. Place potato wedges around fish. Bake at 375°F (190°C, or gas mark 5) about 25 minutes or until fish flakes easily when tested with a fork. Garnish with lemon wedges and parsley. Serve with potatoes and green beans.

8 SERVINGS

Each with: 410 Calories (38% from Fat, 30% from Protein, 32% from Carb); 31 g Protein; 17 g Total Fat; 6 g Unsaturated Fat; 7 g Monounsaturated Fat; 3 g Polyunsaturated Fat; 32 g Carb; 5 g Fiber; 2 g Sugar; 462 mg Phosphorus; 191 mg Calcium; 330 mg Sodium; 1062 mg Potassium; 1179 IU Vitamin A; 56 mg ATE Vitamin E; 31 mg Vitamin C; 82 mg Cholesterol

Broccoli Fish Bake

A crispy bread crumb topping and a nice assortment of spices help make this fish and vegetable bake special. But it also provides lots of nutrition for not many calories.

1 cup (230 g) fat-free sour cream
1 cup (225 g) low fat mayonnaise
1 tablespoon (5 g) dried onion
2 teaspoons lemon pepper
¼ teaspoon white pepper
1 tablespoon (6 g) celery flakes
1 tablespoon (1 g) dried parsley
2 teaspoons lemon juice
⅛ teaspoon black pepper
20 ounces (570 g) broccoli
2 tablespoons (28 ml) lemon juice, divided
6 catfish fillets
¼ cup (30 g) bread crumbs

Mix first 9 ingredients and set aside. Spread broccoli in shallow casserole dish and drizzle with 1 tablespoon (15 ml) lemon juice. Layer fillets on broccoli and then spread the sour cream mixture. Top with sprinkled bread crumbs and remaining lemon juice. Bake covered at 350°F (180°C, or gas mark 4) for 45 minutes and then uncovered an additional 15 minutes until brown.

6 SERVINGS

Each with: 372 Calories (47% from Fat, 33% from Protein, 20% from Carb); 29 g Protein; 19 g Total Fat; 6 g Unsaturated Fat; 7 g Monounsaturated Fat; 3 g Polyunsaturated Fat; 18 g Carb; 4 g Fiber; 5 g Sugar; 444 mg Phosphorus; 119 mg Calcium; 486 mg Sodium; 885 mg Potassium; 921 IU Vitamin A; 64 mg ATE Vitamin E; 89 mg Vitamin C; 95 mg Cholesterol

Tuna Noodle (And Broccoli) Bake

Here's an updated version of the old familiar tuna noodle casserole. This one contains lots more vegetables and as a result lots more nutrition and fewer calories.

½ cup (80 g) onion, chopped
2 tablespoons (28 ml) olive oil
3 tablespoons (24 g) all purpose flour
2 cups (475 ml) skim milk
½ teaspoon savory
⅛ teaspoon black pepper
13 ounces (365 g) tuna, drained
10 ounces (280 g) broccoli, thawed
1 cup (110 g) Swiss cheese, shredded
8 ounces (225 g) egg noodles, cooked and drained

Cook onion in oil until tender; blend in flour. Add skim milk, savory, and black pepper. Cook until mixture boils and thickens. Combine all ingredients into 2-quart (1.9 L) casserole and bake uncovered at 350°F (180°C, or gas mark 4) for 30 minutes or until bubbly.

6 SERVINGS

Each with: 415 Calories (31% from Fat, 30% from Protein, 38% from Carb); 31 g Protein; 14 g Total Fat; 5 g Unsaturated Fat; 6 g Monounsaturated Fat; 2 g Polyunsaturated Fat; 40 g Carb; 3 g Fiber; 2 g Sugar; 478 mg Phosphorus; 375 mg Calcium; 106 mg Sodium; 581 mg Potassium; 696 IU Vitamin A; 107 mg ATE Vitamin E; 44 mg Vitamin C; 84 mg Cholesterol

Tuna Broccoli Rollups

These are sort of tuna enchiladas, full of a creamy tuna and broccoli mixture that tastes as good as it is good for you.

¼ cup (60 ml) skim milk

1 tablespoon (15 ml) lemon juice

1 can (10¾ ounces, or 305 g) low sodium cream of mushroom soup

7 ounces (200 g) tuna, drained

10 ounces (280 g) broccoli, thawed and drained

4 ounces (115 g) low fat cheddar cheese, shredded, divided

3 whole wheat tortillas, 8-inch (20 cm)

1 cup (180 g) tomato, chopped

Combine skim milk, lemon juice, and mushroom soup. Mix tuna, broccoli, and ½ of cheese in separate bowl. Stir ¾ cup (170 g) of soup mixture into tuna. Divide mixture evenly among tortillas and roll up. Stir tomatoes into remaining soup mixture and spoon over top of each rollup. Place rollup seam side down in greased baking dish. Bake covered at 350°F (180°C, or gas mark 4) for 35 to 40 minutes. Top center of each tortilla with remaining cheese. Return to oven and bake 5 minutes, uncovered.

3 SERVINGS

Each with: 398 Calories (22% from Fat, 34% from Protein, 44% from Carb); 34 g Protein; 10 g Total Fat; 4 g Unsaturated Fat; 3 g Monounsaturated Fat; 2 g Polyunsaturated Fat; 44 g Carb; 5 g Fiber; 5 g Sugar; 529 mg Phosphorus; 314 mg Calcium; 890 mg Sodium; 1055 mg Potassium; 1178 IU Vitamin A; 41 mg ATE Vitamin E; 93 mg Vitamin C; 39 mg Cholesterol

Pasta with Fish and Vegetables

Even though this recipe may seem higher in fat than most of the others, it's the good kind of fat that comes from olive oil and fish. So it won't hurt you to have it once in a while.

2 tablespoons (28 ml) olive oil

12 ounces (340 g) salmon fillets, cubed

12 ounces (340 g) cod fillets, cubed

1 teaspoon garlic, minced

½ cup (120 ml) white wine

½ cup (80 g) onion, minced

1 cup (150 g) red bell pepper, coarsely chopped

1 cup (150 g) green bell pepper, coarsely chopped

1 cup (71 g) broccoli florets

½ teaspoon dried oregano

½ teaspoon dried rosemary

1 teaspoon dried parsley

8 ounces (225 g) whole wheat fettuccine, cooked according to package directions

6 tablespoons (30 g) Parmesan cheese, shredded

Heat oil in a heavy skillet. Add fish and garlic and sauté for a minute or two until nearly cooked through. Add wine, vegetables, and spices and continue cooking until sauce has been reduced by about half. Serve over pasta, garnished with Parmesan cheese.

6 SERVINGS

Each with: 383 Calories (32% from Fat, 32% from Protein, 36% from Carb); 30 g Protein; 14 g Total Fat; 3 g Saturated Fat; 6 g Monounsaturated Fat; 3 g Polyunsaturated Fat; 34 g Carb; 1 g Fiber; 2 g Sugar; 417 mg Phosphorus; 118 mg Calcium; 169 mg Sodium; 703 mg Potassium; 1328 IU Vitamin A; 23 mg ATE Vitamin E; 82 mg Vitamin C; 63 mg Cholesterol

Salmon with Mediterranean Relish

A tomato and olive relish gives this cold water fish a warm water feel, reminiscent of Greece or the Mediterranean islands. Salmon is very high in omega-3 fatty acids, and the vegetables take care of other nutrition. Microwaving the rice and asparagus makes preparation even easier.

½ teaspoon black pepper, or to
taste
1 pound (455 g) salmon fillets
2 teaspoons ground cumin
2 cups (190 g) instant brown rice,
uncooked
2¼ cups (535 ml) water
½ pound (225 g) asparagus
2 cups (360 g) tomatoes, diced
¼ cup (25 g) green olives,
chopped
2 tablespoons (6 g) fresh basil,
chopped

Preheat oven to 425°F (220°C, or gas mark 7). Coat a large baking sheet with nonstick vegetable oil spray. Sprinkle black pepper on both sides of salmon fillets. Rub cumin (½ teaspoon per fillet) into flesh-side of salmon. Place salmon skin-side down on prepared baking sheet. Roast 10 minutes until fillets are fork-tender. Meanwhile, combine brown rice and 2¼ cups (535 ml) water in a microwave-safe bowl with a lid. Cover and microwave on high for 5 minutes. Let stand 5 minutes. Fluff with a fork. Place the asparagus in a microwave-safe dish with a lid. Cover and microwave on high for 3 minutes until crisp-tender. To make the relish, combine tomatoes, olives, and basil in a medium bowl. Toss to combine. Serve the salmon with the relish spooned over top and the rice and asparagus on the side.

4 SERVINGS

Each with: 360 Calories (36% from Fat, 30% from Protein, 34% from Carb); 27 g Protein; 15 g Total Fat; 3 g Unsaturated Fat; 6 g Monounsaturated Fat; 5 g Polyunsaturated Fat; 30 g Carb; 5 g Fiber; 1 g Sugar; 398 mg Phosphorus; 81 mg Calcium; 151 mg Sodium; 825 mg Potassium; 1095 IU Vitamin A; 17 mg ATE Vitamin E; 28 mg Vitamin C; 67 mg Cholesterol

Salmon, Vegetables, and Everything in One Packet

On hot days, it's sometimes a good idea to not use the stove at all. This recipe gives you meat, veggies, and starch in one easy grilled packet. And it gives you enough that you are going to need a big piece of foil.

2 cups (190 g) instant brown rice, uncooked

2 cups (475 ml) low sodium chicken broth

1½ cups (180 g) zucchini, thinly sliced

1½ cups (165 g) carrot, shredded

1½ cups (225 g) red bell pepper, sliced

8 ounces (225 g) mushrooms, sliced

1 pound (455 g) salmon fillets

½ teaspoon black pepper

1 lemon, sliced

Heat grill to medium. Spray four large pieces of heavy duty aluminum foil with nonstick vegetable oil spray. In a bowl, mix together rice and broth. Let stand until most of broth is absorbed, about 5 minutes. Stir in vegetables. Place salmon fillet in center of each piece of foil. Sprinkle with black pepper and place lemon slices on top. Place rice mixture around fish. Fold up foil and bring edges together. Fold over several times to seal. Fold in ends, allowing some room for rice expansion. Place on grill and grill until salmon is done, 10 to 15 minutes.

4 SERVINGS

Each with: 395 Calories (32% from Fat, 31% from Protein, 37% from Carb); 31 g Protein; 14 g Total Fat; 3 g Saturated Fat; 5 g Monounsaturated Fat; 5 g Polyunsaturated Fat; 37 g Carb; 6 g Fiber; 7 g Sugar; 475 mg Phosphorus; 62 mg Calcium; 145 mg Sodium; 1185 mg Potassium; 7680 IU Vitamin A; 17 mg ATE Vitamin E; 130 mg Vitamin C; 67 mg Cholesterol

Spice It Up, Fill You Up Catfish Creole

This is actually a very simple, Creole-style recipe. Any white fish can be substituted for the catfish.

2 tablespoons (28 g) unsalted butter

1½ cups (240 g) onion, chopped

1 cup (100 g) celery, chopped

1 cup (150 g) green bell pepper, chopped

½ teaspoon garlic, minced

2 cups (360 g) no-salt-added tomatoes

1 lemon, sliced

1 tablespoon (15 ml) Worcestershire sauce

1 tablespoon (7 g) paprika

1 bay leaf

¼ teaspoon dried thyme

¼ teaspoon Tabasco sauce

2 pounds (900 g) catfish fillets

1½ cups (293 g) brown rice, cooked

2 pounds (900 g) cauliflower florets, steamed until crisp-tender

Melt the butter in a large skillet over medium heat. Add the onion, celery, green bell pepper, and garlic. Cook until soft. Add tomatoes and their liquid. Break the tomatoes with a spoon. Add lemon slices, Worcestershire sauce, paprika, bay leaf, thyme, and Tabasco sauce. Cook, stirring occasionally, for about 15 minutes or until the sauce is slightly thickened. Press fish pieces down into sauce and spoon some of the sauce over the top of the fish. Cover the pan and simmer gently until the fish flakes when prodded with a fork. Remove bay leaf. Serve over hot cooked rice with steamed cauliflower.

6 SERVINGS

Each with: 360 Calories (25% from Fat, 18% from Protein, 57% from Carb); 17 g Protein; 10 g Total Fat; 4 g Saturated Fat; 3 g Monounsaturated Fat; 2 g Polyunsaturated Fat; 53 g Carb; 9 g Fiber; 8 g Sugar; 355 mg Phosphorus; 90 mg Calcium; 107 mg Sodium; 874 mg Potassium; 1066 IU Vitamin A; 40 mg ATE Vitamin E; 112 mg Vitamin C; 35 mg Cholesterol

Quick Tuna Gumbo

Low in fat and high in taste and nutrition, this gumbo goes together quickly.

2 cups (390 g) brown rice, cooked
13 ounces (370 g) tuna, in water
10 ounces (280 g) okra, cut
2 cups (510 g) no-salt-added
   stewed tomatoes
8 ounces (225 g) no-salt-added
   tomato paste
4 ounces (115 g) green chilies,
   diced
1 cup (160 g) onion, cut fine
1 cup (235 ml) water

Cook rice according to package directions. Mix all other ingredients. Cook in a large sauce pan until okra is done. Serve over rice.

4 SERVINGS

Each with: 351 Calories (11% from Fat, 33% from Protein, 56% from Carb); 30 g Protein; 4 g Total Fat; 1 g Unsaturated Fat; 1 g Monounsaturated Fat; 2 g Polyunsaturated Fat; 51 g Carb; 9 g Fiber; 14 g Sugar; 412 mg Phosphorus; 164 mg Calcium; 509 mg Sodium; 1404 mg Potassium; 1406 IU Vitamin A; 6 mg ATE Vitamin E; 50 mg Vitamin C; 40 mg Cholesterol

Salmon and Vegetables Teriyaki

This recipe gives you so much great tasting salmon and vegetables that you won't even think about the fact that dishes like this are usually made much less healthy by putting them over white rice.

¼ cup (60 ml) low sodium soy sauce

¼ cup (60 ml) rice wine vinegar

¼ cup (6 g) sugar substitute, such as Splenda

¼ teaspoon garlic powder

½ teaspoon ground ginger

¼ teaspoon black pepper

1 pound (455 g) salmon fillets, cubed

2 cups (240 g) zucchini, sliced

1½ cups (240 g) onion, quartered

1½ cups (225 g) red bell pepper, cubed

2 cups (200 g) cauliflower florets

1 pound (455 g) mushrooms, sliced in half

2 tablespoons (28 ml) oil

2 tablespoons (16 g) cornstarch

Combine soy sauce, vinegar, sugar substitute, and spices. Stir until sugar is dissolved. Place fish in one plastic zipper bag and vegetables in another. Divide sauce between the 2 bags. Seal and marinate in refrigerator at least one hour, turning occasionally. Drain, reserving sauce. Heat oil in wok. Add vegetables and stir-fry 5 minutes. Add fish and stir-fry one more minute. Stir cornstarch into reserved marinade, add to wok, and cook and stir until thickened.

4 SERVINGS

Each with: 375 Calories (47% from Fat, 30% from Protein, 23% from Carb); 29 g Protein; 20 g Total Fat; 4 g Saturated Fat; 6 g Monounsaturated Fat; 9 g Polyunsaturated Fat; 23 g Carb; 6 g Fiber; 10 g Sugar; 438 mg Phosphorus; 55 mg Calcium; 91 mg Sodium; 1241 mg Potassium; 1939 IU Vitamin A; 17 mg ATE Vitamin E; 155 mg Vitamin C; 67 mg Cholesterol

Sweet Spicy Fish

This salmon is a real taste treat as well as being at the top of the nutritional ladder. Teamed with brown rice and steamed veggies, it makes a great meal.

1½ pounds (680 g) salmon fillets, cut ¾-inch (1.9 cm) thick

¼ cup (85 g) honey

¼ cup (60 ml) low sodium soy sauce

2 tablespoons (28 ml) lemon juice

1 tablespoon (15 ml) sesame oil

¼ teaspoon red pepper flakes

½ teaspoon black pepper

3 cups (585 g) brown rice, cooked

3 cups (257 g) broccoli and cauliflower mix, steamed until crisp-tender

Place fish in glass or ceramic baking dish. Combine honey, soy, lemon juice, sesame oil, red pepper flakes, and black pepper and pour over fish to coat. Cover with plastic wrap and marinate 30 minutes before cooking. Light barbecue grill. When coals are ready, oil grill with cooking spray and put in place. Place fish on grill, skin side down. Cover and cook 5 minutes. Drizzle fish with marinade and cook 3 minutes more or until fish turns opaque. Serve with cooked rice and steamed vegetables.

6 SERVINGS

Each with: 401 Calories (35% from Fat, 27% from Protein, 38% from Carb); 27 g Protein; 16 g Total Fat; 3 g Unsaturated Fat; 6 g Monounsaturated Fat; 6 g Polyunsaturated Fat; 38 g Carb; 3 g Fiber; 13 g Sugar; 387 mg Phosphorus; 48 mg Calcium; 441 mg Sodium; 628 mg Potassium; 379 IU Vitamin A; 17 mg ATE Vitamin E; 46 mg Vitamin C; 67 mg Cholesterol

Teriyaki Fish with Rice and Broccoli

This is an Teriyaki flavored catfish dish. For those of you (like me) who love Chinese food, it doesn't get any better than this.

¼ cup (31 g) all purpose flour

⅛ teaspoon black pepper

12 ounces (340 g) catfish fillets, cut in 1-inch (2.5 cm) cubes

2 tablespoons (28 ml) olive oil

¼ cup (60 ml) low sodium soy sauce

¼ cup (6 g) sugar substitute, such as Splenda

½ teaspoon sesame oil

¼ cup (12 g) chives, chopped

6 cups (426 g) broccoli florets, steamed until crisp-tender

3 cups (585 g) brown rice, cooked

Combine the flour and black pepper in a zipper bag. Add the fish and shake to coat. Heat the oil in a large skillet. Add the fish and cook until done. Remove from skillet. Add the soy sauce and sugar substitute to the pan. Cook and stir until the sugar substitute is melted. Stir in the sesame oil. Add the fish and chives and stir to coat. Serve with broccoli over rice.

4 SERVINGS

Each with: 426 Calories (33% from Fat, 20% from Protein, 47% from Carb); 22 g Protein; 16 g Total Fat; 3 g Saturated Fat; 9 g Monounsaturated Fat; 3 g Polyunsaturated Fat; 51 g Carb; 6 g Fiber; 3 g Sugar; 399 mg Phosphorus; 91 mg Calcium; 622 mg Sodium; 834 mg Potassium; 1045 IU Vitamin A; 13 mg ATE Vitamin E; 120 mg Vitamin C; 40 mg Cholesterol

Salmon and Pasta Caesar Salad

Perfect for a summer lunch or dinner, this tasty salad full of good things will be a real pleaser. And it will please you even more when you noticed that it only contains about 350 calories per serving.

8 ounces (225 g) whole wheat
  pasta
16 ounces (455 g) canned
  salmon, broken into pieces
¼ cup (30 g) zucchini, thinly
  sliced
¼ cup (25 g) celery, thinly sliced
¼ cup (48 g) pimento
¼ cup (60 ml) olive oil
1 tablespoon (15 ml) white wine
  vinegar
½ teaspoon Dijon mustard
½ teaspoon lemon juice
⅛ teaspoon garlic powder
lettuce leaves

Cook pasta according to package directions. Cool. In bowl, combine the next four ingredients. In blender container, combine the next four ingredients. Blend until smooth. Pour over salad ingredients. Cover and chill several hours. To serve, line salad plates with lettuce. Spoon salad onto leaves.

4 SERVINGS

Each with: 356 Calories (51% from Fat, 31% from Protein, 18% from Carb); 28 g Protein; 20 g Total Fat; 4 g Unsaturated Fat; 12 g Monounsaturated Fat; 3 g Polyunsaturated Fat; 16 g Carb; 2 g Fiber; 1 g Sugar; 460 mg Phosphorus; 297 mg Calcium; 103 mg Sodium; 427 mg Potassium; 440 IU Vitamin A; 20 mg ATE Vitamin E; 12 mg Vitamin C; 44 mg Cholesterol

Fish Mexicali

With the flavor of salsa and loaded with healthy red and yellow bell peppers,
this Mexican casserole is sure to please.

1½ cups (143 g) instant brown
  rice
16 ounces (455 g) salsa
1 teaspoon dried thyme
1 cup (150 g) red bell pepper,
  sliced
1 cup (150 g) yellow bell pepper,
  sliced
1½ pounds (680 g) catfish fillets
¼ teaspoon black pepper
½ teaspoon paprika
4 tablespoons (4 g) fresh cilantro

In a microwaveable casserole dish, stir rice, salsa, and thyme. Cover and microwave on high for 7 minutes, stirring once or twice. Stir in red bell pepper. Place fish fillets on top of rice. Sprinkle with black pepper and paprika. Cover and microwave on high 4 or 5 minutes. Let stand 5 minutes. Garnish with cilantro.

4 SERVINGS

Each with: 367 Calories (35% from Fat, 33% from Protein, 32% from Carb); 31 g Protein; 14 g Total Fat; 3 g Unsaturated Fat; 6 g Monounsaturated Fat; 3 g Polyunsaturated Fat; 30 g Carb; 5 g Fiber; 7 g Sugar; 458 mg Phosphorus; 72 mg Calcium; 589 mg Sodium; 983 mg Potassium; 2448 IU Vitamin A; 26 mg ATE Vitamin E; 175 mg Vitamin C; 80 mg Cholesterol

Tuscan Shrimp with White Beans

This is one of those recipes that sounds a bit strange, with the mixture of shrimp and beans. But the first time we had it, it became an instant hit. Veggies and beans and low calorie shrimp make it lean but full of fiber and nutrients.

3 cups (786 g) cannellini beans
4 tablespoons (60 ml) olive oil
¾ pound (340 g) shrimp, peeled
1 teaspoon garlic, minced
½ cup (75 g) green bell pepper, diced
2 cups (360 g) no-salt-added tomatoes, diced
10 basil leaves
2 tablespoons (28 ml) lemon juice
2 tablespoons (8 g) fresh parsley

Drain the beans over a bowl and reserve the liquid. Put the white beans in a large skillet with just enough of their liquid to cover them. Add 2 tablespoons (28 ml) of the olive oil and bring the beans to a low simmer. Keep warm while you prepare the shrimp. Heat remaining oil in a large skillet over high heat. Add the shrimp and cook for about 1 minute, tossing frequently. Remove the shrimp with tongs to a bowl. Add the garlic to the pan and sauté until the garlic browns. Add the green bell pepper and cook for 1 minute. Add the tomato and basil and stir briefly and then add the lemon juice. Cook for about 1 minute and then stir in the shrimp. Toss well and cook briefly to reheat the shrimp. Spoon the white beans on a platter or individual plates. Top with the shrimp. Sprinkle with parsley.

4 SERVINGS

Each with: 434 Calories (33% from Fat, 28% from Protein, 40% from Carb); 31 g Protein; 16 g Total Fat; 2 g Unsaturated Fat; 10 g Monounsaturated Fat; 2 g Polyunsaturated Fat; 44 g Carb; 10 g Fiber; 4 g Sugar; 419 mg Phosphorus; 184 mg Calcium; 141 mg Sodium; 993 mg Potassium; 607 IU Vitamin A; 46 mg ATE Vitamin E; 41 mg Vitamin C; 129 mg Cholesterol

Roasted Shrimp and Peppers

The great thing about seafood is that it is naturally low in calories so you can eat more than you would of some other meats. Well, that is just one of the great things. The other is that it tastes great, especially when you team shrimp and peppers in a flavorful sauce like in this dish.

2 cups (390 g) brown rice, cooked
1 cup (150 g) red bell pepper,
   thinly sliced
1 cup (150 g) green bell pepper,
   thinly sliced
1 lemon, thinly sliced
¼ cup (16 g) fresh thyme
¼ cup (25 g) scallions, halved
   lengthwise and sliced into
   1-inch (2.5 cm) pieces
¼ teaspoon red pepper flakes
2 tablespoons (28 ml) olive oil,
   divided
1½ pounds (680 g) large shrimp,
   peeled and deveined
½ teaspoon paprika
¼ teaspoon black pepper

Preheat oven to 450°F (230°C, or gas mark 8). Cook the rice according to the package directions. Meanwhile, in a large bowl, toss the red and green bell pepper, lemon, thyme, scallions, crushed red pepper, and 1 tablespoon (15 ml) of the oil. Spread on a baking sheet. Add the shrimp to the bowl and toss with the paprika, the remaining tablespoon (15 ml) of oil, and black pepper. Nestle the shrimp in the red and green bell pepper on the baking sheet. Roast until the shrimp are cooked through and the bell peppers are tender, 10 to 12 minutes. Serve over the rice.

4 SERVINGS

Each with: 382 Calories (26% from Fat, 40% from Protein, 34% from Carb); 38 g Protein; 11 g Total Fat; 2 g Unsaturated Fat; 6 g Monounsaturated Fat; 2 g Polyunsaturated Fat; 32 g Carb; 5 g Fiber; 3 g Sugar; 453 mg Phosphorus; 170 mg Calcium; 258 mg Sodium; 607 mg Potassium; 1993 IU Vitamin A; 92 mg ATE Vitamin E; 115 mg Vitamin C; 259 mg Cholesterol

Shrimp Tacos with Citrus Cabbage Slaw

Mexican meals are often high in calories and fat, but this one proves they don't need to be. Shrimp and a cabbage slaw, reminiscent of the ones found in Baja fish tacos, start the meal off on the right nutritional foot. And reduced fat refried beans finish it off.

¼ cup (60 ml) orange juice

2 tablespoons (28 ml) lime juice

2 tablespoons (30 g) low fat sour cream

¼ teaspoon black pepper

½ pound (225 g) cabbage, shredded

1 cup (164 g) corn

2 tablespoons (18 g) jalapeño pepper, chopped

1 tablespoon (15 ml) olive oil

1 pound (455 g) medium shrimp, peeled and deveined

8 whole wheat tortillas, 6-inch (15 cm), warmed

2 cups (476 g) refried beans, see recipe in chapter 14

In a large bowl, whisk the orange and lime juices, sour cream, and black pepper. Add the cabbage, corn, and jalapeño and toss to combine. Let sit for 10 minutes. Meanwhile, heat the oil in a large skillet over medium-high heat. Cook the shrimp until opaque throughout, 2 to 3 minutes. Serve the shrimp with the tortillas, the slaw, and the refried beans.

4 SERVINGS

Each with: 388 Calories (18% from Fat, 33% from Protein, 49% from Carb); 34 g Protein; 8 g Total Fat; 2 g Unsaturated Fat; 4 g Monounsaturated Fat; 2 g Polyunsaturated Fat; 51 g Carb; 11 g Fiber; 4 g Sugar; 507 mg Phosphorus; 198 mg Calcium; 274 mg Sodium; 886 mg Potassium; 319 IU Vitamin A; 61 mg ATE Vitamin E; 38 mg Vitamin C; 182 mg Cholesterol

Shrimp Pasta Salad

This is a great salad, full of shrimp and vegetables, which is still extremely low in calories.

2 pounds (900 g) shrimp

1 pound (455 g) whole wheat
pasta, shells, bows, or shape of
your choice

1 tablespoon (4 g) dill weed

1 tablespoon (3 g) fresh basil,
chopped

2¼ cups (510 g) low fat
mayonnaise

2 tablespoons (28 ml) tarragon
vinegar

¼ cup (36 g) capers

2 cups (260 g) peas, cooked

2 cups (238 g) cucumber, diced

1½ cups (225 g) red bell pepper,
diced

¾ cup (75 g) scallions, finely
chopped

 *Tip: This is better made the
day before to allow the flavors
to develop.*

Cook, peel, and devein shrimp. Cut in bite size pieces. Cook pasta according to package directions. Drain. Cool slightly. Grind dill and basil together. Mix mayonnaise, vinegar, and capers with dill and basil. In large bowl, mix shrimp, pasta, peas, cucumbers, red bell pepper, and scallions. Pour dressing over mixture. Toss gently. Refrigerate.

8 SERVINGS

Each with: 320 Calories (14% from Fat, 39% from Protein, 47% from Carb); 29 g Protein; 5 g Total Fat; 1 g Unsaturated Fat; 0 g Monounsaturated Fat; 1 g Polyunsaturated Fat; 35 g Carb; 6 g Fiber; 7 g Sugar; 360 mg Phosphorus; 109 mg Calcium; 970 mg Sodium; 488 mg Potassium; 1593 IU Vitamin A; 61 mg ATE Vitamin E; 62 mg Vitamin C; 180 mg Cholesterol

Shrimp Fried Rice

Yes, it's acceptable to have fried rice. This version works because the shrimp is low calorie and the brown rice and extra vegetables provide the bulk and nutrition to keep you going.

3 cups (585 g) brown rice, cooked

2 tablespoons (28 ml) sesame oil

2 tablespoons (28 ml) low sodium soy sauce

1 teaspoon garlic, minced

1 tablespoon (8 g) fresh ginger, grated

¾ pound (340 g) shrimp

4 cups (280 g) bok choy

1 cup (145 g) snow pea pods, chopped

½ cup (120 g) water chestnuts, diced

1 cup (110 g) carrot, shredded

Sauté first 5 ingredients for 3 minutes. Add remaining ingredients and cook for 5 minutes more until shrimp are pink and vegetables are crisp-tender.

4 SERVINGS

Each with: 395 Calories (23% from Fat, 23% from Protein, 54% from Carb); 23 g Protein; 10 g Total Fat; 2 g Unsaturated Fat; 3 g Monounsaturated Fat; 4 g Polyunsaturated Fat; 54 g Carb; 6 g Fiber; 3 g Sugar; 350 mg Phosphorus; 117 mg Calcium; 675 mg Sodium; 641 mg Potassium; 4321 IU Vitamin A; 46 mg ATE Vitamin E; 24 mg Vitamin C; 129 mg Cholesterol

Seafood Continental

OK, I don't know why I called it that. It just seemed to fit somehow. This is a rich, creamy shrimp dish that tastes like it has a lot more calories than it does.

20 ounces (570 g) low sodium cream of celery soup

½ cup (120 ml) skim milk

2 tablespoons (28 ml) dry white wine

1½ pounds (680 g) shrimp

1 cup (110 g) Swiss cheese, grated

2 tablespoons (8 g) fresh parsley, chopped

2 tablespoons (28 g) unsalted butter

¼ cup (30 g) bread crumbs

3 cups (585 g) brown rice, cooked

3 cups (213 g) broccoli florets, steamed until crisp-tender

Blend soup, skim milk, and wine. Mix with shrimp, cheese, and parsley. Spoon into shallow baking dish. Dot with butter. Sprinkle with bread crumbs. Bake at 400°F (200°C, or gas mark 6) for 20 minutes or until crumbs are golden. Serve over rice with steamed broccoli.

6 SERVINGS

Each with: 425 Calories (33% from Fat, 34% from Protein, 33% from Carb); 35 g Protein; 15 g Total Fat; 8 g Unsaturated Fat; 4 g Monounsaturated Fat; 3 g Polyunsaturated Fat; 35 g Carb; 3 g Fiber; 2 g Sugar; 523 mg Phosphorus; 357 mg Calcium; 604 mg Sodium; 521 mg Potassium; 1059 IU Vitamin A; 171 mg ATE Vitamin E; 43 mg Vitamin C; 209 mg Cholesterol

Greek Shrimp Bake

Feta cheese and ripe olives give this baked shrimp dish the flavor of Greece.
Lots of veggies make it nutritious.

1 cup (190 g) brown rice,
uncooked

2 cups (475 g) low sodium
chicken broth

1 cup (100 g) celery, sliced

½ cup (80 g) onion, chopped

2 tablespoons (28 ml) olive oil

16 ounces (455 g) no-salt-added
stewed tomatoes

1½ pounds (680 g) shrimp,
shelled

¾ cup (113 g) feta cheese,
crumbled

½ cup (70 g) ripe olives, sliced

1 teaspoon dill weed

Prepare rice according to package directions using chicken broth in place of the water. In a large pan, cook celery and onion in oil until tender. Add tomatoes, stir in rice, ½ of shrimp, cheese, ½ of olives, and dill weed. Turn into 2-quart (1.9 L) casserole. Top with rest of shrimp. Bake uncovered at 350°F (180°C, or gas mark 4) for 25 minutes. Garnish with the rest of the olives.

6 SERVINGS

Each with: 378 Calories (31% from Fat, 33% from Protein, 36% from Carb); 31 g Protein; 13 g Total Fat; 4 g Unsaturated Fat; 6 g Monounsaturated Fat; 2 g Polyunsaturated Fat; 34 g Carb; 3 g Fiber; 5 g Sugar; 446 mg Phosphorus; 211 mg Calcium; 685 mg Sodium; 593 mg Potassium; 560 IU Vitamin A; 85 mg ATE Vitamin E; 10 mg Vitamin C; 189 mg Cholesterol

Seafood Alfredo That You Can Eat

Generally when we think of Alfredo, we think of a dish loaded with fat because of oil, butter, cream, and cheese. But it doesn't have to be so. Our version is still creamy and gets its flavor from generous amounts of seafood, salmon, and vegetables. So you can eat it and still stay on your diet.

8 ounces (225 g) shrimp

8 ounces (225 g) scallops

½ pound (225 g) salmon fillets, cubed

1 teaspoon garlic, chopped

3 tablespoons (45 ml) olive oil

1 cup (160 g) onion, cut in wedges

1 cup (150 g) red bell pepper, sliced

1 cup (71 g) broccoli florets

3 tablespoons (24 g) all purpose flour

1½ cups (355 ml) skim milk

1 teaspoon Italian seasoning

¼ cup (25 g) Parmesan cheese

8 ounces (225 g) whole wheat spaghetti, cooked according to package directions

In a large saucepan, sauté shrimp, scallops, salmon, and garlic in 2 tablespoons (28 ml) olive oil until just cooked through. Remove and sauté vegetables in remaining oil. Shake together flour and skim milk. Add to pan along with Italian seasoning. Cook and stir until thickened and just beginning to boil. Stir in cheese. Serve over pasta.

6 SERVINGS

Each with: 402 Calories (29% from Fat, 31% from Protein, 40% from Carb); 32 g Protein; 13 g Total Fat; 3 g Saturated Fat; 7 g Monounsaturated Fat; 3 g Polyunsaturated Fat; 41 g Carb; 4 g Fiber; 2 g Sugar; 435 mg Phosphorus; 194 mg Calcium; 273 mg Sodium; 647 mg Potassium; 1408 IU Vitamin A; 79 mg ATE Vitamin E; 64 mg Vitamin C; 111 mg Cholesterol

Shrimp Pasta Primavera

The lemon juice gives this a distinctive flavor while complementing the shrimp nicely.
It contains a healthy amount of vegetables (in both senses of the phrase),
while still staying within our diet, so why not enjoy it?

8 ounces (225 g) whole wheat
fettuccine

1 tablespoon (15 ml) olive oil

2 cups (142 g) broccoli florets

4 ounces (115 g) fresh green
beans

½ cup (75 g) red bell pepper, cut
in strips

1 pound (455 g) shrimp, peeled
and deveined

¼ cup (60 ml) lemon juice

½ cup (120 ml) low sodium
chicken broth

1 tablespoon (1.5 g) sugar
substitute, such as Splenda

1 tablespoon (8 g) cornstarch

Cook fettuccini according to package directions and drain. Heat oil in a large skillet. Add vegetables and cook for 3 to 4 minutes, stirring frequently. Stir in shrimp and continue to cook for 4 more minutes. In a small bowl, combine remaining ingredients. Stir into shrimp mixture. Cook 1 to 2 minutes longer until thickened and bubbly. Stir in cooked fettuccini and cook until heated through.

4 SERVINGS

Each with: 384 Calories (14% from Fat, 34% from Protein, 52% from Carb); 33 g Protein; 6 g Total Fat; 1 g Saturated Fat; 3 g Monounsaturated Fat; 2 g Polyunsaturated Fat; 52 g Carb; 1 g Fiber; 1 g Sugar; 422 mg Phosphorus; 117 mg Calcium; 255 mg Sodium; 567 mg Potassium; 2013 IU Vitamin A; 61 mg ATE Vitamin E; 79 mg Vitamin C; 172 mg Cholesterol

Crab Salad in Zucchini Bowls

This salad is naturally low in calories, while providing nutrients from the vegetables and the seafood. Curry flavored dressing adds interest, and spicy olive oil provides even more kick to dip the bread in or drizzle over the salad.

¼ cup (60 g) low fat mayonnaise

1 tablespoon (1 g) fresh cilantro, chopped

1 teaspoon curry powder

¼ teaspoon black pepper

1 pound (455 g) crabmeat

1 cup (150 g) green bell pepper, diced

8 zucchini, halved lengthwise and seeds removed

8 teaspoons (40 g) olive oil

½ teaspoon crushed red pepper flakes

4 slices French bread, toasted

 Tip: You can change the oil flavoring by adding other herbs and spices such as Italian seasoning or curry powder, with or without the red pepper flakes.

In a medium bowl, combine mayonnaise, cilantro, curry powder, and black pepper. Add crabmeat and green bell pepper and mix gently to combine. Spoon mixture into carved-out zucchini halves. In a small bowl, combine olive oil and red pepper flakes. Serve crab-stuffed zucchini and bread with olive-oil mixture on the side.

4 SERVINGS

Each with: 348 Calories (32% from Fat, 34% from Protein, 34% from Carb); 30 g Protein; 12 g Total Fat; 2 g Unsaturated Fat; 7 g Monounsaturated Fat; 2 g Polyunsaturated Fat; 29 g Carb; 5 g Fiber; 6 g Sugar; 438 mg Phosphorus; 184 mg Calcium; 719 mg Sodium; 1201 mg Potassium; 799 IU Vitamin A; 2 mg ATE Vitamin E; 76 mg Vitamin C; 103 mg Cholesterol

Crawfish Pie

Or you can call it crayfish if you prefer (and aren't from Louisiana). This relatively uncommon seafood livens up this pie, which is also filled with lots of healthy veggies.

¾ cup (113 g) red bell pepper, chopped

1 cup (160 g) onion, chopped

½ cup (50 g) celery, chopped

2 tablespoons (28 g) unsalted butter

1½ pounds (680 g) crawfish tails

½ cup (50 g) green onion, chopped

½ cup (30 g) fresh parsley, minced

½ teaspoon black pepper

⅛ teaspoon cayenne pepper papper

½ teaspoon garlic powder

2 pie crusts

Sauté red bell pepper, onion, and celery in butter until tender. Add crawfish tails, green onion, parsley, and seasonings. Place half of the pie crust dough in a 9-inch (23 cm) pie pan. Fill with the cooled filling. Place top crust on pie, moisten edges, and seal edges. Cut two or three 1-inch long (2.5 cm) slits in the top crust. Bake for 10 minutes at 450°F (230°C, or gas mark 8); lower oven to 375°F (190°C, or gas mark 5) and cook for 35 minutes longer or until crust is golden brown.

6 SERVINGS

Each with: 442 Calories (51% from Fat, 19% from Protein, 30% from Carb); 21 g Protein; 25 g Total Fat; 8 g Unsaturated Fat; 10 g Monounsaturated Fat; 6 g Polyunsaturated Fat; 33 g Carb; 4 g Fiber; 3 g Sugar; 309 mg Phosphorus; 60 mg Calcium; 396 mg Sodium; 495 mg Potassium; 1324 IU Vitamin A; 49 mg ATE Vitamin E; 46 mg Vitamin C; 132 mg Cholesterol

Oven Fish Chowder

This delicious and nutritious fish chowder bakes in the oven while you do other things.

1 pound (455 g) haddock

2 potatoes, peeled and cubed

1 cup (160 g) onion, chopped

½ teaspoon garlic, sliced

¼ teaspoon dill weed

½ cup (120 ml) dry white wine

½ cup (120 ml) boiling water

1 bay leaf

½ cup (61 g) carrot, sliced

1 tablespoon (14 g) unsalted butter, in chunks

⅛ teaspoon black pepper

14 ounces (425 ml) fat-free evaporated milk

Put all ingredients, except evaporated milk, into large casserole. Cover and bake at 375°F (190°C, or gas mark 5) for 1 hour. Heat evaporated milk to scalding and add to chowder. Stir to break up fish or cut up with knife.

4 SERVINGS

Each with: 391 Calories (10% from Fat, 36% from Protein, 53% from Carb); 33 g Protein; 4 g Total Fat; 2 g Unsaturated Fat; 1 g Monounsaturated Fat; 0 g Polyunsaturated Fat; 49 g Carb; 4 g Fiber; 14 g Sugar; 535 mg Phosphorus; 372 mg Calcium; 218 mg Sodium; 1641 mg Potassium; 2493 IU Vitamin A; 160 mg ATE Vitamin E; 24 mg Vitamin C; 76 mg Cholesterol

Quick and Easy Salmon Stew

This is an easy way to make stew using canned salmon. It can easily be put together when you get home from work and still have dinner on the table at a reasonable hour.

1 cup (122 g) carrot, sliced
1½ cups (240 g) onion, chopped
16 ounces (455 g) canned salmon
10 ounces (280 g) frozen corn
¼ teaspoon black pepper
14 ounces (425 ml) fat-free
  evaporated milk
3 cups (700 ml) skim milk

Cook carrots and onion until tender. In large pot, combine carrot, onion, salmon with juice, corn, black pepper, and evaporated milk. Add skim milk and bring to a boil, stirring constantly. Turn burner off and continue to stir until mixture stops boiling.

4 SERVINGS

Each with: 413 Calories (17% from Fat, 41% from Protein, 42% from Carb); 42 g Protein; 8 g Total Fat; 2 g Unsaturated Fat; 3 g Monounsaturated Fat; 2 g Polyunsaturated Fat; 44 g Carb; 4 g Fiber; 18 g Sugar; 892 mg Phosphorus; 860 mg Calcium; 343 mg Sodium; 1387 mg Potassium; 4688 IU Vitamin A; 250 mg ATE Vitamin E; 14 mg Vitamin C; 52 mg Cholesterol

Salmon and Peanut Butter Stew

This is vaguely Thai, with its ginger and peanut flavors, but really hard to define. Whatever you call it, it tastes good and is full of nutrition.

⅓ cup (53 g) onion, chopped
⅓ cup (33 g) celery, chopped
½ cup (75 g) red bell pepper,
  sliced
2½ tablespoons (35 g) butter
¼ teaspoon ground ginger
¼ teaspoon turmeric
½ teaspoon black pepper
14 ounces (390 g) no-salt-added
  tomatoes, chopped
⅔ cup (160 ml) water
½ pound (225 g) salmon steaks
¾ cup (195 g) peanut butter,
  chunky
3 cups (585 g) brown rice, cooked
1 teaspoon lemon juice

Sauté onion, celery, and red bell pepper in the butter. Add ginger, turmeric, black pepper, tomatoes, and water; bring to boil. Cover. Simmer for 20 minutes at medium heat. Season and broil salmon until done. Heat peanut butter until it's melted and add to mixture. Place salmon on bed of rice. Squeeze lemon juice on salmon and cover with stew and serve.

6 SERVINGS

Each with: 426 Calories (52% from Fat, 17% from Protein, 31% from Carb); 18 g Protein; 25 g Total Fat; 7 g Unsaturated Fat; 10 g Monounsaturated Fat; 6 g Polyunsaturated Fat; 34 g Carb; 4 g Fiber; 6 g Sugar; 246 mg Phosphorus; 53 mg Calcium; 76 mg Sodium; 618 mg Potassium; 681 IU Vitamin A; 45 mg ATE Vitamin E; 36 mg Vitamin C; 35 mg Cholesterol

Fisherman's Pride Stew

This is a great fish stew, full of fish and vegetables and delicious as well as nutritious.

6 slices low sodium bacon, chopped

2 cups (320 g) onion, sliced

2 pounds (900 g) haddock, cut in 2½-inch (6.3 cm) pieces

3 medium potatoes, cut in ¾-inch (1.9 cm) cubes

1½ cups (183 g) carrot, cut in ¾-inch (1.9 cm) cubes

½ teaspoon celery seed

½ cup (75 g) green bell pepper, diced

½ teaspoon black pepper

3 cups (700 ml) water

28 ounces (785 g) no-salt-added crushed tomatoes

2 tablespoons (8 g) fresh parsley, chopped

 Tip: You can substitute any white fish for the haddock.

In a deep kettle or Dutch oven, sauté bacon until lightly browned; remove bacon, set aside. In same kettle, sauté onion until tender. Add fish, potatoes, carrot, celery seed, green bell pepper, black pepper, and water. Simmer, covered, until vegetables are tender, about 25 minutes. Add tomatoes; heat. Garnish with parsley and crumbled bacon bits.

6 SERVINGS

Each with: 375 Calories (13% from Fat, 40% from Protein, 48% from Carb); 37 g Protein; 5 g Total Fat; 1 g Unsaturated Fat; 2 g Monounsaturated Fat; 1 g Polyunsaturated Fat; 45 g Carb; 7 g Fiber; 6 g Sugar; 501 mg Phosphorus; 107 mg Calcium; 236 mg Sodium; 1860 mg Potassium; 4938 IU Vitamin A; 27 mg ATE Vitamin E; 88 mg Vitamin C; 95 mg Cholesterol

Thick and Rich Fish Chowder

This makes great chowder, flavorful and filling.

2 tablespoons (28 ml) olive oil
2 cups (320 g) chopped onion
1 cup (70 g) mushrooms, sliced
1 cup (100 g) celery, chopped
5 cups (1.1 L) low sodium
   chicken broth, divided
4 medium potatoes, diced
2 pounds (900 g) cod, diced into
   ½-inch (1.3 cm) cubes
⅛ teaspoon seafood seasoning
¼ teaspoon black pepper
¼ cup (31 g) all purpose flour
3 cups (700 ml) fat-free
   evaporated milk

 Tip: You can substitute other
fish or a combination of
different types of fish for
the cod.

In a large stockpot, heat oil over medium heat. Sauté onion, mushrooms, and celery until tender. Add 4 cups (950 ml) chicken broth and potatoes; simmer for 10 minutes. Add fish and simmer another 10 minutes. Season to taste with seafood seasoning and black pepper. Mix together remaining broth and flour until smooth; stir into soup. Cook until slightly thickened. Remove from heat and stir in evaporated milk. Serve.

8 SERVINGS

Each with: 390 Calories (13% from Fat, 36% from Protein, 51% from Carb); 35 g Protein; 6 g Total Fat; 1 g Saturated Fat; 3 g Monounsaturated Fat; 1 g Polyunsaturated Fat; 50 g Carb; 4 g Fiber; 15 g Sugar; 601 mg Phosphorus; 337 mg Calcium; 241 mg Sodium; 1885 mg Potassium; 505 IU Vitamin A; 127 mg ATE Vitamin E; 42 mg Vitamin C; 53 mg Cholesterol

Alaska Salmon Chowder

They know how to make hearty, warming, filling soups in Alaska.
And this chowder is a prime example. But it's loaded with so much salmon
and so many vegetables that you won't believe its low calorie count.

1 cup (160 g) onion, chopped
2 tablespoons (28 ml) olive oil
2 medium potatoes, diced
1 cup (122 g) carrot, sliced
20 ounces (570 g) frozen broccoli
2 cups (475 ml) low sodium
  chicken broth
32 ounces (900 g) salmon
14 ounces (425 g) fat-free
  evaporated milk
2 tablespoons (16 g) cornstarch
4 cups (950 ml) skim milk

Sauté chopped onion in olive oil in saucepan. Add vegetables and broth. Simmer until vegetables are tender. Add flaked salmon and evaporated milk mixed with cornstarch and heat. Add the 4 cups (950 ml) of skim milk just before serving and reheat.

8 SERVINGS

Each with: 408 Calories (24% from Fat, 38% from Protein, 39% from Carb); 38 g Protein; 11 g Total Fat; 3 g Unsaturated Fat; 5 g Monounsaturated Fat; 2 g Polyunsaturated Fat; 39 g Carb; 4 g Fiber; 8 g Sugar; 765 mg Phosphorus; 661 mg Calcium; 274 mg Sodium; 1495 mg Potassium; 2916 IU Vitamin A; 154 mg ATE Vitamin E; 77 mg Vitamin C; 49 mg Cholesterol

Full of Seafood Cioppino

Cioppino is a traditional fisherman's stew made from a combination of whatever the catch was that day. Our version contains fish, shrimp, crab, and clams, but feel free to use other seafood or to use multiple varieties of fish. This soup is flavorful and filling.

1 pound (455 g) catfish

1 cup (150 g) green bell pepper, cut into ½-inch (2.5 cm) squares

1 cup (160 g) onion, finely chopped

1 cup (122 g) carrot, sliced

1 cup (100 g) celery, sliced

½ teaspoon garlic, minced

1 tablespoon (15 ml) cooking oil

2 cups (360 g) no-salt-added tomatoes, cut up

8 ounces (225 g) no-salt-added tomato sauce

½ cup (120 ml) dry white wine

3 tablespoons (12 g) fresh parsley, chopped

¼ teaspoon dried oregano

¼ teaspoon dried basil

¼ teaspoon black pepper

12 ounces (340 g) shrimp, frozen or fresh

16 ounces (455 g) crab meat

7 ounces (200 g) minced clams

Cut fillets into 1-inch (2.5 cm) pieces; set aside. In a 3-quart (2.8 L) saucepan cook green bell pepper, onion, carrot, celery, and garlic in hot oil until onion is tender, not brown. Add undrained tomatoes, tomato sauce, wine, parsley, oregano, basil, and black pepper. Bring to a boil. Reduce heat. Cover; simmer 20 minutes. Add fish pieces, shrimp, undrained clams, and crab. Bring just to boiling. Reduce heat; cover and simmer 5 to 7 minutes or until fish and shrimp are done.

6 SERVINGS

Each with: 369 Calories (28% from Fat, 54% from Protein, 18% from Carb); 48 g Protein; 11 g Total Fat; 2 g Saturated Fat; 4 g Monounsaturated Fat; 4 g Polyunsaturated Fat; 15 g Carb; 3 g Fiber; 7 g Sugar; 610 mg Phosphorus; 193 mg Calcium; 429 mg Sodium; 1341 mg Potassium; 3482 IU Vitamin A; 100 mg ATE Vitamin E; 54 mg Vitamin C; 203 mg Cholesterol

Warm You Up Fish Stew

Hearty and warm and full of vegetables, this stew will fill you up, warm you up, and keep you that way.

8 slices low sodium bacon

1½ cups (240 g) onion, sliced

1½ pounds (680 g) haddock, cut
in 2½-inch (6.3 cm) pieces

3 medium potatoes, cut in ¾-inch
(1.9 cm) cubes

2 cups (142 g) broccoli florets

½ teaspoon celery seed

1½ cups (183 g) carrot, cut in
¾-inch (1.9 cm) cubes

¼ cup (38 g) green bell pepper,
diced

½ teaspoon black pepper

3 cups (700 ml) water, boiling

28 ounces (785 g) no-salt-added
crushed tomatoes

2 tablespoons (8 g) fresh parsley,
chopped

In a deep kettle or Dutch oven, sauté bacon until lightly browned; remove bacon and set aside. In the same kettle, sauté onion until tender. Add fish, potatoes, broccoli, celery seed, carrot, green bell pepper, black pepper, and boiling water. Simmer, covered, until vegetables are tender, about 25 minutes. Add tomatoes; heat. Garnish with parsley and crumbled bacon bits.

6 SERVINGS

Each with: 369 Calories (14% from Fat, 35% from Protein, 51% from Carb); 32 g Protein; 6 g Total Fat; 2 g Unsaturated Fat; 2 g Monounsaturated Fat; 1 g Polyunsaturated Fat; 47 g Carb; 7 g Fiber; 8 g Sugar; 446 mg Phosphorus; 146 mg Calcium; 249 mg Sodium; 1809 mg Potassium; 4439 IU Vitamin A; 20 mg ATE Vitamin E; 76 mg Vitamin C; 76 mg Cholesterol

Asian Fish Soup

The fish is actually almost an afterthought here. It is cooked until it falls apart and becomes part of the broth that it filled with tofu and vegetables.

½ pound (225 g) catfish
2 quarts (1.9 L) water
1 teaspoon olive oil
1 bay leaf
1 teaspoon garlic, minced
1 teaspoon low sodium soy sauce
1 cup (130 g) carrot, chopped
1 cup (100 g) celery, chopped
¼ cup (25 g) scallions, chopped
¼ cup (15 g) fresh parsley, chopped
1 teaspoon dried oregano
1 teaspoon mustard
¼ cup (25 g) Parmesan cheese, grated
8 ounces (225 g) firm tofu, diced
4 cups (780 g) brown rice, cooked

Cut fish into thumb sized pieces. Add pieces to 2 quarts (1.9 L) water. Add olive oil, bay leaf, garlic, and soy sauce. Bring to boil and then reduce to low boil. Add chopped carrot, celery, scallions, and parsley. Continue on low boil until carrots are soft and then lower heat to simmer. Add oregano, mustard, and cheese. Cover and stir occasionally. Let cook until fish pieces have broken apart. Add tofu. Let simmer for 5 minutes. Stir occasionally. Remove bay leaf. Divide rice among four bowls. Ladle soup over top.

4 SERVINGS

Each with: 391 Calories (25% from Fat, 21% from Protein, 54% from Carb); 21 g Protein; 11 g Total Fat; 3 g Unsaturated Fat; 4 g Monounsaturated Fat; 3 g Polyunsaturated Fat; 53 g Carb; 5 g Fiber; 3 g Sugar; 387 mg Phosphorus; 160 mg Calcium; 251 mg Sodium; 672 mg Potassium; 4439 IU Vitamin A; 16 mg ATE Vitamin E; 10 mg Vitamin C; 32 mg Cholesterol

Thai Fish Soup

The flavors of Thailand fill this fish soup, which doesn't taste at all like diet food.

1 cup (190 g) brown rice, uncooked

2 cups (475 ml) water

2 tablespoons (28 ml) lemon juice

4 cups (950 ml) low sodium chicken broth, or low sodium vegetable broth

1 pound (455 g) tilapia fillets, or other firm white fish

4 cups (80 g) arugula, tough stems removed

1 cup (130 g) carrot, finely shredded

¼ cup (24 g) fresh mint, thinly sliced

¼ cup (25 g) scallions, finely chopped

Combine rice and water in a medium saucepan. Bring to a simmer over medium heat; cover and cook until the water is absorbed, about 20 minutes. Stir in lemon juice. Meanwhile, bring broth to a simmer in another medium saucepan over medium-high heat. Reduce the heat so the broth remains steaming but not simmering. Add fish and cook until just tender, about 5 minutes. Remove and break into bite-size chunks. Divide the lemon rice among 4 bowls. Top with equal portions of the fish, arugula (or watercress), carrot, mint, and scallions. Ladle 1 cup (235 ml) of the warm broth into each bowl and serve.

4 SERVINGS

Each with: 360 Calories (14% from Fat, 37% from Protein, 49% from Carb); 33 g Protein; 6 g Total Fat; 1 g Unsaturated Fat; 2 g Monounsaturated Fat; 2 g Polyunsaturated Fat; 44 g Carb; 3 g Fiber; 2 g Sugar; 477 mg Phosphorus; 140 mg Calcium; 168 mg Sodium; 1073 mg Potassium; 4799 IU Vitamin A; 53 mg ATE Vitamin E; 10 mg Vitamin C; 36 mg Cholesterol

Dinners: Vegetarian

Vegetarian meals are another great choice for healthy, reduced calorie eating. They are naturally low in fats in general and saturated fats in particular. This makes it easy to achieve that high nutrient, low calorie balance that we are looking for. They also offer a tremendous variety of flavors, adding variety to your mega meal plan. We try to have at least one vegetarian dinner a week, and I often eat meatless lunches.

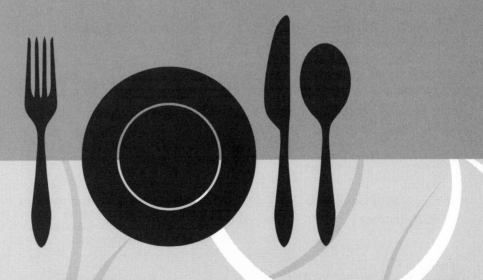

Meal in a Potato

You'll really get your veggies in this recipe. And you'll also get so much taste and volume that you won't even think about the fact that it is meatless.

1 pound (455 g) cauliflower florets, steamed until crisp-tender

1 pound (455 g) broccoli florets, steamed until crisp-tender

1 cup (160 g) onion, steamed until crisp-tender

1 cup (150 g) red bell pepper, steamed until crisp-tender

4 large potatoes, baked

1 cup (110 g) low fat Swiss cheese

Steam vegetables. Cook potatoes in oven or microwave until done. Split and top with hot vegetables. Sprinkle with cheese.

4 SERVINGS

Each with: 408 Calories (6% from Fat, 19% from Protein, 74% from Carb); 21 g Protein; 3 g Total Fat; 1 g Saturated Fat; 1 g Monounsaturated Fat; 1 g Polyunsaturated Fat; 80 g Carb; 13 g Fiber; 10 g Sugar; 451 mg Phosphorus; 424 mg Calcium; 157 mg Sodium; 1675 mg Potassium; 1988 IU Vitamin A; 13 mg ATE Vitamin E; 247 mg Vitamin C; 12 mg Cholesterol

A Little Different Stuffed Pepper

Peas and carrots, as well as finely chopped walnuts, give these stuffed peppers not only a nutritional boost, but a flavor boost as well.

4 green bell peppers

1 tablespoon (15 ml) olive oil

1 cup (160 g) onion, chopped

½ teaspoon garlic, minced

1 teaspoon dried oregano

1 teaspoon dried basil

½ cup (61 g) carrot, julienned

1 cup (150 g) peas, fresh or frozen

1 cup (180 g) tomato, diced

⅓ cup (40 g) walnuts, finely chopped

1½ cups (293 g) brown rice, cooked

2 cups (490 g) low sodium spaghetti sauce

Preheat oven to 350°F (180°C, or gas mark 4). Wash and clean green bell peppers. Cut off tops and remove seeds and membrane. Steam peppers 3 to 4 minutes. Meanwhile, heat oil in wok or large skillet and add onion and garlic. Sauté 1 minute. Add herbs, carrot, and peas. Continue to cook 3 to 5 minutes or until carrots are tender, stirring constantly. Reduce heat and add the tomato, walnuts, brown rice, and ½ cup (123 g) tomato sauce. Heat through. Stuff mixture into peppers. Spread ½ cup (123 g) sauce in bottom of baking dish. Stand peppers upright. Pour remaining sauce over the tops of peppers. Bake in oven for 30 minutes.

4 SERVINGS

Each with: 405 Calories (35% from Fat, 10% from Protein, 55% from Carb); 11 g Protein; 17 g Total Fat; 2 g Unsaturated Fat; 8 g Monounsaturated Fat; 5 g Polyunsaturated Fat; 58 g Carb; 12 g Fiber; 22 g Sugar; 248 mg Phosphorus; 99 mg Calcium; 186 mg Sodium; 1129 mg Potassium; 3861 IU Vitamin A; 0 mg ATE Vitamin E; 147 mg Vitamin C; 0 mg Cholesterol

Stuffed Tomatoes

Cheese, rice, and fresh herbs make the filling of these stuffed tomatoes tasty as well as nutritious. It's perfect for a summer meal when fresh tomatoes are plentiful.

10 large tomatoes
2 cups (390 g) brown rice, cooked
1 cup (160 g) onion, chopped
1 teaspoon garlic, minced
¼ cup (16 g) fresh dill
¼ cup (15 g) fresh parsley, chopped
¼ cup (65 g) no-salt-added tomato paste
¼ cup (60 ml) water
1 cup (115 g) low fat cheddar cheese
¼ cup (60 ml) olive oil
¼ teaspoon black pepper

Slice tops from tomatoes and scoop out centers. Discard the hard center. Place in baking pan. Mix all ingredients together and spoon into tomato cups. Replace tops. Pour in enough boiling water to cover bottom of pan. Cover and bake at 350°F (180°C, or gas mark 4) degrees for about 45 minutes and then uncover and bake until brown and done.

5 SERVINGS

Each with: 367 Calories (55% from Fat, 6% from Protein, 40% from Carb); 5 g Protein; 23 g Total Fat; 3 g Unsaturated Fat; 16 g Monounsaturated Fat; 3 g Polyunsaturated Fat; 38 g Carb; 6 g Fiber; 3 g Sugar; 154 mg Phosphorus; 41 mg Calcium; 44 mg Sodium; 926 mg Potassium; 2344 IU Vitamin A; 0 mg ATE Vitamin E; 87 mg Vitamin C; 0 mg Cholesterol

Vegetable Noodle Bake

This is sort of like the old familiar noodle casserole, with lots of vegetables and no meat.
But the taste is so good, you won't even miss it.

½ cup (50 g) celery, chopped

1 cup (160 g) onion, chopped

1 cup (150 g) red bell pepper, chopped

2 tablespoons (28 ml) olive oil

8 ounces (225 g) whole wheat noodles, cooked and drained

½ cup (58 g) low fat Monterey Jack cheese

1 cup (71 g) broccoli florets, cooked and drained

½ cup (120 ml) skim milk

⅛ teaspoon black pepper

¼ cup (30 g) bread crumbs

2 tablespoons (14 g) low fat cheddar cheese, grated

1 tablespoon (7 g) wheat germ

1 tablespoon (14 g) unsalted butter, melted

Sauté first three ingredients in oil until tender but not brown. Stir in noodles, Monterey Jack cheese, broccoli, skim milk, and black pepper. Turn into an ungreased 1½-quart (1.4 L) casserole. Bake, covered, at 350°F (180°C, or gas mark 4) for 15 minutes. Combine bread crumbs, cheddar, wheat germ, and butter; sprinkle around the edge of casserole. Bake, uncovered, for 10 minutes.

4 SERVINGS

Each with: 400 Calories (27% from Fat, 17% from Protein, 56% from Carb); 17 g Protein; 13 g Total Fat; 4 g Unsaturated Fat; 6 g Monounsaturated Fat; 2 g Polyunsaturated Fat; 59 g Carb; 3 g Fiber; 5 g Sugar; 351 mg Phosphorus; 194 mg Calcium; 220 mg Sodium; 467 mg Potassium; 1578 IU Vitamin A; 55 mg ATE Vitamin E; 94 mg Vitamin C; 13 mg Cholesterol

Stuffed Cabbage Fingers

Unlike more traditional stuffed cabbage, this vegetarian version is formed into small rolls with individual leaves and then cooked in a cheesy tomato sauce. Tofu adds protein and an assortment of vegetables add other nutrients to this tasty meal.

1 head cabbage
2 tablespoons (28 ml) olive oil
1 teaspoon garlic, minced
1 cup (122 g) carrot, sliced thin
½ pound (225 g) mushrooms, sliced
1 cup (160 g) onion, chopped
2 cups (390 g) brown rice, cooked
8 ounces (225 g) firm tofu, cubed
1 tablespoon (7 g) caraway seeds
⅛ teaspoon dried thyme
¼ teaspoon dried basil
¼ teaspoon dried oregano
¼ teaspoon black pepper
3 cups (735 g) no-salt-added tomato sauce
½ cup (50 g) Parmesan cheese, grated

Rinse cabbage. Fill a pot with enough water to cover cabbage. Bring water to a boil. Place whole cabbage in water and blanch for 3 minutes, turning occasionally. Remove from pot and separate leaves from cabbage carefully. Place cabbage back in water for 2 to 3 minutes, if necessary, to remove inner leaves easily. Set aside. Heat oil in a large skillet. Add garlic and sauté for 1 minute. Add carrot, mushrooms, and onion and stir-fry for 3 minutes. Add rice; stir to combine. Add tofu, caraway seeds, thyme, basil, oregano, and black pepper; stir gently. Turn off heat. Spread cabbage leaves out and place 2 tablespoons (28 g) rice mixture in center of each. Roll up and secure with toothpicks. Cover bottom of two heatproof 9 × 9-inch (23 × 23 cm) baking dishes with tomato sauce. Carefully place rolls in. Top with remaining sauce and cheese. Place baking dishes in a preheated 350°F (180°C, or gas mark 4) oven and bake for 30 minutes.

4 SERVINGS

Each with: 397 Calories (30% from Fat, 17% from Protein, 53% from Carb); 17 g Protein; 14 g Total Fat; 4 g Unsaturated Fat; 7 g Monounsaturated Fat; 2 g Polyunsaturated Fat; 54 g Carb; 10 g Fiber; 16 g Sugar; 378 mg Phosphorus; 271 mg Calcium; 275 mg Sodium; 1469 mg Potassium; 4711 IU Vitamin A; 15 mg ATE Vitamin E; 59 mg Vitamin C; 11 mg Cholesterol

Savory Lentil Pie

This crustless pie has a crunchy topping from cracker crumbs, which are lower in calories and fat than pie crust. Lentils add fiber and protein and vegetables up the nutrition but not the calorie count. Nicely spicy, it's a great choice for a cool night.

⅔ cup (128 g) lentils, rinsed
2 cups (475 ml) water
1 cup (160 g) onion, chopped
1 cup (122 g) carrot, sliced
½ cup (50 g) celery, sliced
6 cups (1.4 L) low sodium vegetable broth
3 medium potatoes, cubed
½ teaspoon dried sage
½ teaspoon dried parsley
3 tablespoons (42 g) unsalted butter
3 tablespoons (24 g) all purpose flour
1 cup (100 g) cracker crumbs

Cook lentils in 2 cups (475 ml) of water on low heat. Cook onion, carrot, and celery in broth for 10 minutes. Add potatoes and cook vegetables 20 more minutes. Meanwhile, add sage and parsley to lentils. Prepare a thickening agent by melting butter in a skillet, adding flour, and then 1 cup (235 ml) of liquid from the cooking vegetables. Drain vegetables (keeping extra liquid for possible use if the filling is too thick). Mix everything in a baking dish, put cracker crumbs on top, and bake at 350°F (180°C, or gas mark 4) until brown.

6 SERVINGS

Each with: 435 Calories (26% from Fat, 10% from Protein, 64% from Carb); 11 g Protein; 13 g Total Fat; 5 g Unsaturated Fat; 4 g Monounsaturated Fat; 2 g Polyunsaturated Fat; 70 g Carb; 8 g Fiber; 4 g Sugar; 253 mg Phosphorus; 115 mg Calcium; 309 mg Sodium; 1174 mg Potassium; 2822 IU Vitamin A; 48 mg ATE Vitamin E; 27 mg Vitamin C; 15 mg Cholesterol

Marinated Vegetable Salad

This hearty salad is a full meal. It's full of beans and cheese for protein, as well as a generous helping of lots of vegetables, and is the perfect meal for a warm evening.

4 cups (360 g) red cabbage, shredded

4 cups (440 g) carrot, shredded

2 cups (512 g) kidney beans, drained

2 cups (200 g) green beans, cooked and cooled

2 cups (480 g) chickpeas, drained

32 cherry tomatoes, halved

⅓ cup (8 g) sugar substitute, such as Splenda

⅓ cup (60 ml) olive oil

½ cup (120 ml) cider vinegar

¼ cup (40 g) onion, minced

1½ cups (173 g) low fat cheddar cheese, shredded

In a 2½-quart (2.4 L) bowl, place a layer of cabbage, carrot, kidney beans, green beans, chickpeas, and tomatoes. In a jar with tight lid, place sugar substitute, oil, vinegar, and onion. Cover and shake until well mixed. Pour over vegetables. Cover bowl with plastic wrap. Refrigerate at least 4 hours to marinate vegetables. Top with cheese before serving.

6 SERVINGS

Each with: 415 Calories (34% from Fat, 20% from Protein, 46% from Carb); 21 g Protein; 16 g Total Fat; 3 g Unsaturated Fat; 10 g Monounsaturated Fat; 2 g Polyunsaturated Fat; 50 g Carb; 16 g Fiber; 11 g Sugar; 398 mg Phosphorus; 278 mg Calcium; 286 mg Sodium; 1153 mg Potassium; 11 836 IU Vitamin A; 20 mg ATE Vitamin E; 64 mg Vitamin C; 7 mg Cholesterol

Great Grilled Vegetable Meal

Grilled vegetables are teamed with tomatoes and fresh mozzarella for a warm salad that is perfect for warm weather.

4 red bell peppers

8 Japanese eggplants

2 heads radicchio

2 bulbs fennel

2 tablespoons (28 ml) olive oil

4 medium tomatoes, sliced

8 ounces (225 g) fresh mozzarella

2 tablespoons (28 ml) balsamic vinegar

 Tip: You can substitute other vegetables like onions and zucchini.

Heat a grill and place the red bell peppers on to cook. Grill until the skin of the peppers is blackened and appears blistered. Remove peppers from the grill and place in a brown paper bag. Roll bag up and allow to set for about 10 minutes in order to enhance flavor. Split the eggplant, radicchio, and fennel in halves; brush radicchio, fennel, and fleshy parts of eggplant with a bit of the olive oil. Place eggplant, radicchio, and fennel on the grill and grill until done, about 8 to 10 minutes. While vegetables are grilling, peel the peppers by placing under cold water and scraping the blistered skin off. It should come off easily. Divide the grilled vegetables among 4 plates. Add slices of the fresh tomatoes and cheese. Drizzle with vinegar.

4 SERVINGS

Each with: 394 Calories (37% from Fat, 20% from Protein, 43% from Carb); 22 g Protein; 18 g Total Fat; 7 g Unsaturated Fat; 8 g Monounsaturated Fat; 2 g Polyunsaturated Fat; 46 g Carb; 18 g Fiber; 11 g Sugar; 508 mg Phosphorus; 595 mg Calcium; 498 mg Sodium; 2137 mg Potassium; 6225 IU Vitamin A; 70 mg ATE Vitamin E; 356 mg Vitamin C; 36 mg Cholesterol

Good for You Good Tasting Veggie Rice Dinner

About as simple as a meal can get, an assortment of vegetables are sautéed and served over brown rice, with cheese sprinkled over. But don't be too fast to write it off. This meal has great taste appeal as well as great nutrition, all while holding down the calories.

¾ cup (143 g) brown rice

1 cup (160 g) onion, chopped

1 teaspoon garlic, minced

2 tablespoons (28 ml) olive oil

1 cup (120 g) zucchini, chopped

1 cup (150 g) green bell pepper, chopped

½ teaspoon dried oregano

⅛ teaspoon black pepper

1 cup (180 g) tomatoes, chopped

16 ounces (455 g) kidney beans, drained

½ cup (58 g) low fat cheddar cheese, shredded

Cook rice as per package directions. Sauté chopped onion and minced garlic in oil. Add zucchini and green bell pepper and seasonings. Sauté until crispy tender. Add tomatoes and beans and heat through. Serve over rice with shredded cheese on top.

4 SERVINGS

Each with: 396 Calories (21% from Fat, 18% from Protein, 61% from Carb); 18 g Protein; 9 g Total Fat; 2 g Unsaturated Fat; 6 g Monounsaturated Fat; 1 g Polyunsaturated Fat; 62 g Carb; 14 g Fiber; 3 g Sugar; 370 mg Phosphorus; 177 mg Calcium; 116 mg Sodium; 873 mg Potassium; 482 IU Vitamin A; 10 mg ATE Vitamin E; 49 mg Vitamin C; 3 mg Cholesterol

Eggplant Zucchini Casserole

Called it baked spaghetti, vegetable lasagna, or whatever you want, this vegetarian dish is healthy, tasty, and filling. Spaghetti teams with vegetables, primarily eggplant and zucchini, in an Italian-style baked casserole.

1 medium eggplant, peeled and sliced

2 cups (240 g) zucchini, sliced

28 ounces (758 g) low sodium spaghetti sauce

½ cup (50 g) celery, chopped

1 cup (150 g) green bell pepper, chopped

8 ounces (225 g) part skim mozzarella, grated

8 ounces (225 g) whole wheat spaghetti, broken into 1-inch (2.5 cm) pieces

Layer ½ eggplant slices in greased 9 × 13-inch (23 × 33 cm) baking dish, then ½ zucchini, then ½ spaghetti, ½ celery, and green bell pepper. Sprinkle with ½ cheese and ½ spaghetti sauce. Repeat layers. Bake, covered, at 350°F (180°C, or gas mark 4) for 1½ hours.

6 SERVINGS

Each with: 403 Calories (28% from Fat, 18% from Protein, 54% from Carb); 19 g Protein; 13 g Total Fat; 5 g Unsaturated Fat; 6 g Monounsaturated Fat; 1 g Polyunsaturated Fat; 58 g Carb; 11 g Fiber; 19 g Sugar; 362 mg Phosphorus; 367 mg Calcium; 291 mg Sodium; 974 mg Potassium; 1234 IU Vitamin A; 47 mg ATE Vitamin E; 44 mg Vitamin C; 24 mg Cholesterol

Zucchini Corn Casserole

A simple zucchini and corn bake becomes a full meal when layered with two kinds of cheese.

3 cups (360 g) zucchini, thinly sliced

1½ cups (338 g) fat-free cottage cheese

¾ cup (86 g) bread crumbs

¼ cup (28 g) wheat germ

2 tablespoons (8 g) fresh parsley, minced

1 tablespoon (5 g) fresh basil, minced

3 cups (492 g) frozen corn

2 cups (360 g) tomatoes, sliced

4 ounces (115 g) low fat cheddar cheese, shredded

Pat zucchini dry with a paper towel. Set aside. Preheat oven to 350°F (180°C, or gas mark 4). In medium sized bowl, combine cottage cheese, bread crumbs, wheat germ, parsley, and basil. Set aside. Line bottom of a greased 2-quart (1.9 L) baking dish with zucchini. Using half of the cottage cheese mixture, spoon on top of zucchini and press on the mixture with a fork or spatula to spread it around. Cover with corn. Sprinkle the remaining cottage cheese mixture on top of the corn. Cover the casserole with the tomato slices and sprinkle the cheese on top of the tomatoes. Cover the casserole with foil, put in hot oven, and bake it for 15 minutes. Remove foil and bake casserole for another 15 minutes. Remove the casserole from the oven and let the casserole stand for about 10 minutes before serving.

4 SERVINGS

Each with: 349 Calories (16% from Fat, 30% from Protein, 54% from Carb); 28 g Protein; 6 g Total Fat; 2 g Unsaturated Fat; 2 g Monounsaturated Fat; 2 g Polyunsaturated Fat; 50 g Carb; 7 g Fiber; 10 g Sugar; 525 mg Phosphorus; 243 mg Calcium; 701 mg Sodium; 947 mg Potassium; 1198 IU Vitamin A; 26 mg ATE Vitamin E; 46 mg Vitamin C; 9 mg Cholesterol

Zippy Stuffed Eggplant

You won't believe how much food this is for how few calories. Eggplant halves are stuffed with a spicy cheese and vegetable mixture that not only tastes great but is full of nutrition and fiber.

3 large eggplants

1 pound (455 g) mushrooms, chopped

½ teaspoon garlic, minced

3 cups (540 g) tomatoes, diced

1 cup (160 g) onion, chopped

¼ teaspoon black pepper

3 tablespoons (45 ml) olive oil

1½ cups (338 g) fat-free cottage cheese

¼ cup (4 g) brown sugar substitute, such as Splenda

2 cups (230 g) low fat cheddar cheese, grated

1 cup (240 g) garbanzo beans

½ teaspoon dried thyme

¼ teaspoon Tabasco sauce

¼ cup (15 g) sunflower seeds, toasted

1 teaspoon paprika

¼ cup (15 g) fresh parsley, chopped

Preheat oven to 350°F (180°C, or gas mark 4). Slice eggplant lengthwise. Scoop out centers, leaving ¼-inch (6 mm) shells. Reserve and chop centers. Sauté reserved eggplant with mushrooms, garlic, tomatoes, onion, and black pepper in oil until onion is tender. Stir in next 6 ingredients. Stuff eggplant shells with mixture; sprinkle with toasted sunflower seeds, paprika, and parsley. Arrange on baking dish. Bake for 40 minutes.

6 SERVINGS

Each with: 356 Calories (35% from Fat, 28% from Protein, 37% from Carb); 26 g Protein; 15 g Total Fat; 4 g Unsaturated Fat; 7 g Monounsaturated Fat; 3 g Polyunsaturated Fat; 35 g Carb; 13 g Fiber; 10 g Sugar; 536 mg Phosphorus; 273 mg Calcium; 637 mg Sodium; 1186 mg Potassium; 1071 IU Vitamin A; 33 mg ATE Vitamin E; 33 mg Vitamin C; 12 mg Cholesterol

Warm Bean and Pasta Toss

A sort of warm pasta salad, this dish features beans and vegetables tossed
with pasta and heated but not cooked.

8 ounces (225 g) whole wheat
    pasta, such as penne
2 cups (524 g) white beans,
    rinsed and drained
40 cherry tomatoes, halved
1 cup (150 g) green bell pepper,
    chopped
2 tablespoons (28 ml) olive oil
½ cup (20 g) fresh basil, chopped
½ teaspoon garlic cloves, minced
¼ cup (25 g) Parmesan cheese,
    grated

*Tip: You could serve over
lettuce if desired.*

Cook noodles, drain, and return to pot. Toss with next 6
ingredients and warm for 5 minutes. Top with Parmesan
cheese.

4 SERVINGS

Each with: 341 Calories (25% from Fat, 17% from Protein, 57% from Carb);
16 g Protein; 10 g Total Fat; 2 g Unsaturated Fat; 6 g Monounsaturated Fat; 1 g
Polyunsaturated Fat; 52 g Carb; 12 g Fiber; 1 g Sugar; 267 mg Phosphorus; 244 mg
Calcium; 102 mg Sodium; 958 mg Potassium; 1623 IU Vitamin A; 7 mg ATE Vitamin
E; 66 mg Vitamin C; 6 mg Cholesterol

Veggie Burgers You Can Love

Ever long for a big juicy burger but worry about the number of calories and the amount of fat? Worry no more. These burgers are big and juicy and lean. Mushrooms add extra moisture to the protein rich tofu and oat base. So enjoy.

2 cups (320 g) onion, chopped
¾ pound (340 g) mushrooms, chopped
1 teaspoon garlic, crushed
2 pounds (900 g) tofu
3 cups (240 g) rolled oats
10 ounces (280 g) frozen spinach, thawed and drained
2 tablespoons (28 ml) low sodium soy sauce
4 tablespoons (60 ml) Worcestershire sauce
½ teaspoon black pepper
1 teaspoon paprika
1 teaspoon lemon juice
8 whole wheat rolls
2 cups (320 g) tomatoes, sliced
8 leaves romaine lettuce
8 dill pickle halves

Sauté onion, mushrooms, and garlic in a small amount of water until they are softened and water is absorbed. Mash tofu in a large bowl. Add oats, spinach (make sure all excess water is removed), seasonings, and lemon juice. Mix well. Stir in onion–mushroom mixture. Shape into patties and place on nonstick cookie sheet. Bake at 350°F (180°C, or gas mark 4) for 20 minutes; turn over and then cook an additional 10 minutes. Serve on rolls with lettuce and tomato and pickle on the side.

8 SERVINGS

Each with: 352 Calories (20% from Fat, 20% from Protein, 60% from Carb); 18 g Protein; 8 g Total Fat; 1 g Unsaturated Fat; 2 g Monounsaturated Fat; 3 g Polyunsaturated Fat; 55 g Carb; 8 g Fiber; 9 g Sugar; 365 mg Phosphorus; 148 mg Calcium; 904 mg Sodium; 995 mg Potassium; 4362 IU Vitamin A; 0 mg ATE Vitamin E; 40 mg Vitamin C; 0 mg Cholesterol

Vegetarian Stuffed Zucchini

A cheesy vegetable mixture makes these stuffed zucchini a pleasure to eat
as well as a nutritious, healthy alternative.

3 large zucchini

2 tablespoons (28 ml) olive oil

½ pound (225 g) mushrooms,
chopped

1 cup (160 g) onion, chopped

1 teaspoon garlic clove, crushed

2 tablespoons (18 g) sunflower
seeds

¼ teaspoon dried rosemary

¼ teaspoon dried basil

¼ teaspoon dried thyme

¾ cup (175 ml) egg substitute,
beaten

3 cups (675 g) fat-free cottage
cheese

½ cup (58 g) wheat germ

3 tablespoons (45 ml) low sodium
soy sauce

1 cup (115 g) low fat cheddar
cheese, grated

2 cups (390 g) brown rice, cooked

Cut zucchini in halves lengthwise. Scoop out insides and sauté
in oil with the next 4 ingredients until translucent. Remove
from heat and add seasonings. Mix beaten egg substitute with
next 5 ingredients. Combine with cooked vegetables. Stuff
the empty zucchini shells with the mixture. Bake at 350°F
(180°C, or gas mark 4) for 40 minutes.

6 SERVINGS

Each with: 354 Calories (29% from Fat, 35% from Protein, 37% from Carb);
31 g Protein; 11 g Total Fat; 3 g Unsaturated Fat; 5 g Monounsaturated Fat; 3 g
Polyunsaturated Fat; 33 g Carb; 5 g Fiber; 8 g Sugar; 581 mg Phosphorus; 219 mg
Calcium; 931 mg Sodium; 878 mg Potassium; 469 IU Vitamin A; 26 mg ATE Vitamin
E; 24 mg Vitamin C; 9 mg Cholesterol

Vegetarian Stroganoff

I know it may sound weird, but trust me here. This dish is definitely a stroganoff in flavor, but an assortment of vegetables take the place of the meat, keeping the calories low and the nutrition high.

1 pound (455 g) whole wheat noodles

2 tablespoons (28 ml) olive oil

2 cups (300 g) green bell pepper, diced

2½ cups (400 g) tomatoes, cut into wedges

2 cups (240 g) zucchini, diced

1 cup (82 g) eggplant, diced

1 cup (100 g) celery, diced

1 cup (100 g) green beans

¼ teaspoon black pepper

½ teaspoon ground cumin

1 tablespoon (10 g) chopped onion

1 teaspoon chili powder

2 tablespoons (3 g) fresh parsley, chopped

3 cups (690 g) fat-free sour cream

Boil the noodles. In the meantime, sauté the next 7 ingredients. When vegetables are translucent, add the next 4 ingredients and sauté a few minutes longer. As soon as the eggplant is cooked, add the last 2 ingredients as well as noodles that have been boiled and drained.

8 SERVINGS

Each with: 383 Calories (34% from Fat, 12% from Protein, 53% from Carb); 13 g Protein; 15 g Total Fat; 7 g Unsaturated Fat; 6 g Monounsaturated Fat; 1 g Polyunsaturated Fat; 54 g Carb; 3 g Fiber; 2 g Sugar; 277 mg Phosphorus; 144 mg Calcium; 67 mg Sodium; 596 mg Potassium; 1166 IU Vitamin A; 91 mg ATE Vitamin E; 53 mg Vitamin C; 35 mg Cholesterol

Vegetarian Skillet Meal

This is like a frittata, but it's cooked in a covered skillet on top of the stove. Cast iron works really well for this. This great combination of vegetables held together by egg makes a really nutritious meal.

2 tablespoons (28 ml) olive oil

1 teaspoon garlic, minced

1½ cups (240 g) onion, thinly sliced

½ cup (120 ml) low sodium vegetable broth

1 cup (150 g) green bell pepper, diced

2 medium potatoes, cubed

2 cups (360 g) tomatoes, diced

2 cups (240 g) zucchini, diced

½ teaspoon black pepper

1 cup (82 g) eggplant, unpeeled, diced

2 cups (475 ml) egg substitute

Heat olive oil in large skillet. Add garlic. Cook until golden. Discard garlic. Add onion to hot oil. Sauté until tender. Add broth or water, green bell pepper, potatoes, tomatoes, zucchini, black pepper, and eggplant. Mix well. Pour egg substitute over. Cover and cook over low heat until vegetables are tender and eggs are set, about 30 minutes.

4 SERVINGS

Each with: 388 Calories (28% from Fat, 22% from Protein, 50% from Carb); 22 g Protein; 12 g Total Fat; 2 g Unsaturated Fat; 7 g Monounsaturated Fat; 3 g Polyunsaturated Fat; 49 g Carb; 7 g Fiber; 6 g Sugar; 337 mg Phosphorus; 132 mg Calcium; 397 mg Sodium; 1781 mg Potassium; 1201 IU Vitamin A; 0 mg ATE Vitamin E; 84 mg Vitamin C; 1 mg Cholesterol

Vegetarian Rice Skillet

Seeds and nuts provide additional flavor and protein to this skillet meal of rice and vegetables.

2 cups (390 g) brown rice, cooked
1 cup (100 g) celery, sliced
1 cup (100 g) scallion, sliced
1 cup (150 g) green bell pepper, sliced
¼ cup (35 g) raisins
½ ounce (15 g) cashews, chopped
2 tablespoons (28 ml) olive oil
¼ cup (60 ml) low sodium vegetable broth
1 tablespoon (8 g) sesame seeds
1 tablespoon (9 g) sunflower seeds
2 teaspoons Italian seasoning
1 cup (180 g) plum tomatoes, cut into wedges
8 ounces (225 g) low fat Monterey Jack cheese, coarsely grated, divided

In large skillet, mix all ingredients, except tomatoes and ¼ of the cheese. Toss well to combine. Top with tomatoes and sprinkle with remaining cheese. Cover and cook over low heat just until heated through, about 12 to 15 minutes.

4 SERVINGS

Each with: 378 Calories (37% from Fat, 20% from Protein, 43% from Carb); 19 g Protein; 16 g Total Fat; 4 g Unsaturated Fat; 8 g Monounsaturated Fat; 3 g Polyunsaturated Fat; 42 g Carb; 5 g Fiber; 9 g Sugar; 452 mg Phosphorus; 321 mg Calcium; 456 mg Sodium; 549 mg Potassium; 907 IU Vitamin A; 34 mg ATE Vitamin E; 46 mg Vitamin C; 12 mg Cholesterol

Did I Say Tofu Quiche?

Yes, I did, for want of a better term. And it works well, the tofu blending into the eggs and mayonnaise until it's not even noticeable as a separate ingredient. But it supercharges the dish, giving it great nutrient value for very few calories.

12 ounces (340 g) firm tofu,
drained
1 cup (122 g) carrot, sliced
2 cups (240 g) zucchini, sliced
6 ounces (170 g) water chestnuts,
sliced
¼ cup (25 g) green onion, sliced
1 cup (225 g) low fat mayonnaise
1½ cups (355 ml) egg substitute

Drain tofu by wrapping in cheesecloth and setting a weight on top of it. (A couple of dinner plates work well.) Let sit approximately 20 minutes. Chop vegetables. Mash tofu in large bowl with pastry blender or potato masher. Stir in mayonnaise until blended. Stir in egg substitute until just mixed. Stir in vegetables. Grease 9-inch (23 cm) baking dish. Pour mixture into dish and bake 1 hour at 350°F (180°C, or gas mark 4).

3 SERVINGS

Each with: 360 Calories (27% from Fat, 31% from Protein, 43% from Carb); 25 g Protein; 10 g Total Fat; 2 g Unsaturated Fat; 2 g Monounsaturated Fat; 4 g Polyunsaturated Fat; 35 g Carb; 6 g Fiber; 14 g Sugar; 362 mg Phosphorus; 147 mg Calcium; 950 mg Sodium; 1384 mg Potassium; 5920 IU Vitamin A; 0 mg ATE Vitamin E; 20 mg Vitamin C; 10 mg Cholesterol

Dinner in a Dish Artichoke Pie

Meatless meals don't have to be tasteless, not do they have to be something that leaves you feeling like you haven't had a full dinner. This Italian-style pie is loaded with vegetables to give you a full feeling that will last.

¾ cups (175 ml) egg substitute

3 ounces (85 g) fat-free cream cheese, softened

¾ teaspoon garlic powder

1 tablespoon dried chives

¼ teaspoon black pepper

1½ cups (173 g) part skim mozzarella, shredded

1 cup (150 g) ricotta cheese

½ cup (115 g) low fat mayonnaise

1 can (6 ounces, or 170 g) artichoke hearts

8 ounces (225 g) mushrooms, sliced

1 cup (240 g) garbanzo beans, cooked

½ cup (70 g) black olives, sliced

2 ounces (55 g) pimento, drained and diced

2 tablespoons (8 g) fresh parsley, chopped

One 9-inch (23 cm) pie shell, unbaked

⅓ cup (33 g) Parmesan cheese, grated

In a mixing bowl, beat egg substitute. Stir in cream cheese, garlic powder, chives, and black pepper. Stir in 1 cup (115 g) mozzarella, ricotta, and mayonnaise. Quarter 2 artichoke hearts and set aside 6 pieces. Chop remaining artichoke hearts; fold into cheese mixture. Fold in mushrooms, garbanzo beans, olives, pimento, and parsley. Turn mixture into pie shell. Bake in a 350°F (180°C, or gas mark 4) oven for 30 minutes. Top with remaining ½ cup (60 g) mozzarella and the Parmesan cheese. Bake about 15 minutes more until set. Let stand for 10 minutes. Top with quartered artichokes.

6 SERVINGS

Each with: 405 Calories (52% from Fat, 17% from Protein, 30% from Carb); 18 g Protein; 24 g Total Fat; 8 g Saturated Fat; 7 g Monounsaturated Fat; 2 g Polyunsaturated Fat; 31 g Carb; 5 g Fiber; 5 g Sugar; 295 mg Phosphorus; 246 mg Calcium; 771 mg Sodium; 540 mg Potassium; 932 IU Vitamin A; 75 mg ATE Vitamin E; 15 mg Vitamin C; 33 mg Cholesterol

Black Bean and Zucchini Quesadilla

This may sound like an unusual combination, but the zucchini takes on the Mexican flavor and it all works very well together. It also provides great nutrition.

2 cups (240 g) zucchini, chopped

1 cup (172 g) black beans, rinsed and drained

1 tablespoon (15 ml) olive oil

1 tablespoon (7 g) ground cumin

4 whole wheat tortillas, 8-inch (20 cm)

½ cup (58 g) cheddar cheese, shredded

¼ cup (65 g) salsa

Sauté first 4 ingredients for 5 minutes. Place mixture on tortillas; sprinkle with cheese. Fold in half and heat in skillet until cheese melts and tortilla is toasted. Top with salsa.

4 SERVINGS

Each with: 386 Calories (28% from Fat, 19% from Protein, 53% from Carb); 19 g Protein; 12 g Total Fat; 5 g Unsaturated Fat; 6 g Monounsaturated Fat; 1 g Polyunsaturated Fat; 52 g Carb; 10 g Fiber; 3 g Sugar; 330 mg Phosphorus; 219 mg Calcium; 337 mg Sodium; 1001 mg Potassium; 417 IU Vitamin A; 43 mg ATE Vitamin E; 13 mg Vitamin C; 17 mg Cholesterol

Tamale Pie

A tasty chili flavored cornmeal crust wraps around a bean based filling with lots of vegetables in this pie. The result is the kind of thing you can serve to anyone and not worry about it being diet food.

Filling

¼ cup (38 g) green bell pepper, chopped

¼ cup (25 g) celery, chopped

½ cup (80 g) onion, chopped

1 tablespoon (15 ml) olive oil

2 teaspoons chili powder

1 teaspoon ground cumin

1 teaspoon garlic, minced

2 cups (512 g) kidney beans, drained

2 tablespoons (32 g) no-salt-added tomato paste

½ cup (70 g) ripe olives

½ cup (82 g) corn

Crust

1½ cups (210 g) cornmeal

1 cup (235 ml) cold water

2 cups (475 ml) boiling water

½ teaspoon chili powder

⅓ cup (38 g) low fat cheddar cheese, grated

Sauté vegetables for filling. When onions become translucent, add spices and crushed garlic. Mash beans. Mix beans and tomato paste into vegetables. Add olives and corn. Set aside. Stir cornmeal into 1 cup (235 ml) cold water. Then stir cornmeal mixture into 2 cups (475 ml) boiling water. Add chili powder. Cook and stir until thick. Press ⅔ of the cornmeal mixture into the bottom and sides of an 8 × 8-inch (20 × 20 cm) pan. Pour the bean mixture into the crust. Top with remaining cornmeal mixture. Sprinkle with cheese and bake at 350°F (180°C, or gas mark 4) for 30 minutes.

4 SERVINGS

Each with: 410 Calories (16% from Fat, 16% from Protein, 68% from Carb); 17 g Protein; 8 g Total Fat; 1 g Unsaturated Fat; 4 g Monounsaturated Fat; 1 g Polyunsaturated Fat; 70 g Carb; 15 g Fiber; 3 g Sugar; 260 mg Phosphorus; 147 mg Calcium; 257 mg Sodium; 705 mg Potassium; 867 IU Vitamin A; 7 mg ATE Vitamin E; 15 mg Vitamin C; 2 mg Cholesterol

Taco Buffet

A nice choice for family or entertaining, this recipe lets people choose their own fillings for their tacos. The fact that there is no meat isn't even an issue with the beans and other tasty filling choices.

2 cups (344 g) black beans, drained

10 ounces (280 g) frozen corn, cooked and cooled

4 ounces (115 g) green chilies, chopped

1½ cups (270 g) tomatoes, chopped

2 tablespoons (2 g) fresh cilantro, chopped

3 tablespoons (45 ml) lime juice, divided

½ teaspoon black pepper, divided

3 cups (270 g) red cabbage, shredded

6 cups (432 g) iceberg lettuce, shredded

2 avocados, peeled and chopped

1 tablespoon (15 ml) olive oil

8 ounces (225 g) low fat cheddar cheese, shredded

12 taco shells

Rinse and drain beans. Drain corn and chopped green chilies. Chop tomatoes. In medium bowl, mix beans, corn, chilies, tomato, cilantro, 2 tablespoons (28 ml) lime juice, ¼ teaspoon black pepper, finely sliced cabbage, and lettuce; toss in a bowl. Cut avocados in half. Remove seeds and peel. Cut into small chunks. In a bowl, gently mix avocados, olive oil, 1 tablespoon (15 ml) lime juice, and ¼ teaspoon black pepper. To serve, arrange bowls of bean mixture, lettuce mixture, avocados, and cheese on a large tray. Let everyone fill their own shells.

6 SERVINGS

Each with: 434 Calories (40% from Fat, 17% from Protein, 43% from Carb); 19 g Protein; 20 g Total Fat; 4 g Unsaturated Fat; 10 g Monounsaturated Fat; 4 g Polyunsaturated Fat; 49 g Carb; 13 g Fiber; 8 g Sugar; 475 mg Phosphorus; 265 mg Calcium; 1027 mg Sodium; 1163 mg Potassium; 1162 IU Vitamin A; 23 mg ATE Vitamin E; 54 mg Vitamin C; 8 mg Cholesterol

Veggie Burritos

With the flavor of traditional burritos, but not the calorie count, these burritos are a great choice for lunch or dinner. Filled with an assortment of vegetables, they will leave you satisfied both by the taste and the volume.

1 cup (160 g) onion, finely chopped

1 teaspoon garlic, minced

2 tablespoons (28 ml) olive oil

1 teaspoon dried oregano

1 cup (150 g) green bell pepper, chopped

1 cup (120 g) zucchini, chopped

1 cup (110 g) carrot, grated

4 ounces (115 g) green chilies, chopped

1 teaspoon ground cumin

6 whole wheat tortillas, 8-inch (20 cm)

2 cups (476 g) refried beans, see recipe in chapter 14

1½ cups (173 g) low fat cheddar cheese, grated

½ cup (130 g) salsa

¼ cup (60 g) fat-free sour cream

Sauté onion and garlic in hot oil in a frying pan with oregano. Add the green bell pepper, zucchini, carrot, and chili peppers. Sauté 5 minutes until tender but not overcooked. Remove from heat and add cumin. Microwave the tortillas for 10 to 15 seconds to soften them. Spread about 2 tablespoons (28 g) refried beans in center of tortilla, add about ½ cup (115 g) of vegetable mixture, and sprinkle with cheese. Fold up sides and then roll the rest of the tortilla. Place seam side down on a cookie sheet. Bake at 350°F (180°C, or gas mark 4) for about 10 minutes until golden brown. Serve with salsa and sour cream.

6 SERVINGS

Each with: 366 Calories (30% from Fat, 19% from Protein, 51% from Carb); 18 g Protein; 13 g Total Fat; 4 g Unsaturated Fat; 7 g Monounsaturated Fat; 1 g Polyunsaturated Fat; 49 g Carb; 8 g Fiber; 4 g Sugar; 336 mg Phosphorus; 272 mg Calcium; 632 mg Sodium; 601 mg Potassium; 2991 IU Vitamin A; 30 mg ATE Vitamin E; 41 mg Vitamin C; 18 mg Cholesterol

Bean and Guacamole Burritos

This is a delicious vegetarian Mexican meal, high in fiber and nutrition and low in saturated fat.

1 cup (190 g) brown rice, uncooked

¼ cup (38 g) green bell pepper, diced

¼ cup (45 g) onion, diced

4 ounces (115 g) green chilies, diced

¾ cup (195 g) salsa, divided

½ cup (119 g) refried beans, see recipe in chapter 14

6 tablespoons (88 g) guacamole

1 cup (47 g) romaine lettuce, shredded

2 whole wheat tortillas, 8-inch (20 cm)

Cook rice according to package directions, adding green bell pepper, onion, green chilies, and ¼ cup (65 g) salsa. Stir together beans and ½ cup (65 g) salsa. Microwave for 1 to 2 minutes. Place warm bean mixture, guacamole, and lettuce on tortillas and roll up. Serve with rice on the side.

2 SERVINGS

Each with: 408 Calories (20% from Fat, 12% from Protein, 68% from Carb); 13 g Protein; 9 g Total Fat; 2 g Unsaturated Fat; 5 g Monounsaturated Fat; 2 g Polyunsaturated Fat; 73 g Carb; 12 g Fiber; 6 g Sugar; 249 mg Phosphorus; 157 mg Calcium; 886 mg Sodium; 843 mg Potassium; 2459 IU Vitamin A; 0 mg ATE Vitamin E; 62 mg Vitamin C; 5 mg Cholesterol

10 Layer Taco Dinner

Kind of a combination of 7 layer dip (only 3 layers better) and taco salad, this dinner sized, Mexican flavored stack of goodness will not only fill you up but make your taste buds sit up and take notice.

1 package taco seasoning, reduced sodium

8 ounces (225 g) fat-free sour cream

3 cups (216 g) iceberg lettuce, shredded

1½ cups (357 g) refried beans, see recipe in chapter 14

2 ripe avocados, mashed with lemon

½ cup (58 g) Monterey Jack cheese, shredded

½ cup (58 g) low fat cheddar cheese, shredded

2 cups (360 g) tomatoes, chopped fine

½ cup (50 g) green onion, sliced

15 ounces (425 g) black olives, sliced

4 ounces (115 g) chopped green chilies

 Tip: If you like your Mexican food spicy, feel free to add more chilies. Each 4 ounce (115 g) can only adds 4 calories per serving.

Mix the taco seasoning into the sour cream. Layer on a large serving plate in the following order: lettuce, refried beans, avocados, sour cream mixture, Monterey Jack cheese, cheddar cheese, tomatoes, green onion, black olives, and chilies.

6 SERVINGS

Each with: 402 Calories (59% from Fat, 13% from Protein, 28% from Carb); 13 g Protein; 26 g Total Fat; 8 g Saturated Fat; 14 g Monounsaturated Fat; 2 g Polyunsaturated Fat; 28 g Carb; 11 g Fiber; 2 g Sugar; 249 mg Phosphorus; 282 mg Calcium; 927 mg Sodium; 735 mg Potassium; 1902 IU Vitamin A; 66 mg ATE Vitamin E; 25 mg Vitamin C; 32 mg Cholesterol

Pizza Salad, Now There's a Combination

If you have a taste for pizza but are trying to get your recommended vegetables in for the day, this salad topped pizza may be the solution you are looking for.

---

3 large tomatoes

8 ounces (225 g) fresh mozzarella, shredded

2 tablespoons (10 g) Parmesan cheese

1 pizza crust, unbaked

2 cups (94 g) romaine lettuce, shredded

1 cup (150 g) green bell pepper, thinly sliced

1 cup (160 g) red onion, thinly sliced

1 cup (120 g) zucchini, thinly sliced

1 cup (71 g) broccoli florets

¼ cup (35 g) ripe olives, sliced

2 tablespoons (28 ml) *Reduced Fat Italian Dressing*, see recipe in chapter 2

Preheat oven to 450°F (230°C, or gas mark 8). Core tomatoes; slice into ¼-inch (6 mm) thick slices and set aside. Sprinkle mozzarella and Parmesan cheeses evenly over pizza crust. Top with tomato slices, slightly overlapping. Bake about 8 minutes or until cheese melts. Meanwhile, in medium bowl, combine romaine, green bell pepper, and olives. Sprinkle with Italian dressing. Toss to coat. Remove pizza from oven. Top with romaine mixture. Cut into wedges. Serve immediately.

6 SERVINGS

Each with: 385 Calories (29% from Fat, 19% from Protein, 52% from Carb); 18 g Protein; 12 g Total Fat; 5 g Saturated Fat; 5 g Monounsaturated Fat; 2 g Polyunsaturated Fat; 51 g Carb; 2 g Fiber; 3 g Sugar; 242 mg Phosphorus; 351 mg Calcium; 961 mg Sodium; 423 mg Potassium; 2252 IU Vitamin A; 49 mg ATE Vitamin E; 60 mg Vitamin C; 26 mg Cholesterol

Italian Oven Meal in a Pot

This Italian vegetarian dish, halfway between a soup and a casserole, cooks in the oven while you do other things. The cheeses add richness, and the beans and veggies take care of the nutrition.

1 cup (120 g) zucchini, sliced

1½ cups (240 g) onion, sliced

2 cups (480 g) garbanzo beans

2 cups (360 g) no-salt-added tomatoes, chopped

8 ounces (225 g) whole wheat pasta, cooked according to package directions

1½ cups (355 ml) dry white wine

2 teaspoons garlic, minced

1 teaspoon dried basil

1 bay leaf

2 ounces (55 g) Monterey Jack cheese, shredded

2 ounces (55 g) Romano cheese, grated

Combine zucchini, onion, beans, tomatoes and their liquid, pasta, wine, garlic, basil, and bay leaf in 3-quart (2.8 L) baking dish. Cover and bake at 400°F (200°C, or gas mark 6) for 1 hour, stirring once halfway through. Remove bay leaf. Stir in cheeses and bake 10 minutes longer.

6 SERVINGS

Each with: 376 Calories (18% from Fat, 19% from Protein, 64% from Carb); 16 g Protein; 7 g Total Fat; 4 g Saturated Fat; 2 g Monounsaturated Fat; 1 g Polyunsaturated Fat; 56 g Carb; 8 g Fiber; 5 g Sugar; 327 mg Phosphorus; 257 mg Calcium; 421 mg Sodium; 583 mg Potassium; 289 IU Vitamin A; 27 mg ATE Vitamin E; 21 mg Vitamin C; 18 mg Cholesterol

Pasta with Mushroom and Sun-Dried Tomato Sauce

A quick and very flavorful mushroom sauce with sun-dried tomatoes makes this pasta special. You'll love the way it tastes and fills, even without any meat.

1 pound (455 g) mushrooms, sliced

½ teaspoon garlic, minced

1 cup (55 g) sun-dried tomatoes, chopped

½ cup (120 ml) dry white wine

½ cup (120 ml) low sodium vegetable broth

¼ cup (15 g) Italian parsley, chopped

10 ounces (280 g) whole wheat pasta

¼ cup (25 g) Parmesan cheese

Combine all ingredients except pasta and cheese in a large saucepan. Cover and simmer for 1 hour. Cook pasta according to package directions. Serve with sauce, sprinkled with cheese.

4 SERVINGS

Each with: 392 Calories (17% from Fat, 18% from Protein, 65% from Carb); 18 g Protein; 8 g Total Fat; 2 g Saturated Fat; 3 g Monounsaturated Fat; 1 g Polyunsaturated Fat; 66 g Carb; 9 g Fiber; 2 g Sugar; 377 mg Phosphorus; 126 mg Calcium; 329 mg Sodium; 1004 mg Potassium; 698 IU Vitamin A; 7 mg ATE Vitamin E; 36 mg Vitamin C; 6 mg Cholesterol

Three Greens Lasagna

Many lasagna recipes contain spinach. But not many contain the nutritional boost of three greens, spinach, kale, and arugula, like this one does. It's so good that even confirmed meat eaters will agree that vegetarian meals can be delicious and satisfying.

1 pound (455 g) lasagna noodles, preferably whole wheat

16 ounces (455 g) fat-free cottage cheese

1 teaspoon dried thyme

1 teaspoon dried basil

1 teaspoon dried oregano

2 teaspoons garlic, minced

28 ounces (785 ml) low sodium spaghetti sauce

5 cups (335 g) kale

5 cups (100 g) arugula

5 cups (150 g) spinach

1 cup (180 g) roasted red peppers, diced

¼ cup (25 g) Parmesan cheese, grated

Cook lasagna noodles according to package directions. Preheat oven to 375°F (190°C, or gas mark 5). Mix cottage cheese, thyme, basil, oregano, and garlic in a medium bowl. Spread 1 cup (245 g) pasta sauce on the bottom of a 13 × 9-inch (33 × 23 cm) baking dish. Add one layer of cooked lasagna noodles. Top lasagna with greens and roasted red peppers. Spread spoonfuls of the cheese mixture over vegetables. Repeat layers, finishing with pasta and sauce. Sprinkle grated Parmesan on top of the lasagna and bake uncovered for about 40 minutes or until bubbly around the edges. Let the lasagna stand 10 minutes to make cutting easier. Slice into 8 pieces and serve.

8 SERVINGS

Each with: 408 Calories (17% from Fat, 19% from Protein, 64% from Carb); 20 g Protein; 8 g Total Fat; 2 g Unsaturated Fat; 4 g Monounsaturated Fat; 1 g Polyunsaturated Fat; 67 g Carb; 6 g Fiber; 14 g Sugar; 180 mg Phosphorus; 209 mg Calcium; 349 mg Sodium; 909 mg Potassium; 9736 IU Vitamin A; 10 mg ATE Vitamin E; 104 mg Vitamin C; 5 mg Cholesterol

Stuffed Shells Florentine

This is a vegetarian Italian meal that is low in fat, but high in nutrition, with the addition of extra vegetables to the mixture used to stuff the shells.

10 ounces (280 g) jumbo pasta shells

1 cup (70 g) mushrooms, chopped

1 cup (160 g) onion, chopped

1 cup (150 g) green bell pepper, chopped

½ teaspoon garlic, minced

½ teaspoon onion powder

½ teaspoon dried parsley

¼ teaspoon black pepper

16 ounces (455 g) low fat cottage cheese

20 ounces (570 g) frozen spinach, thawed and well drained

½ cup (120 ml) egg substitute

15 ounces (425 g) low sodium marinara sauce

Preheat oven to 350°F (180°C, or gas mark 4). Cook pasta according to package instructions. Sauté mushrooms, onion, green bell pepper, garlic, and seasonings in a skillet sprayed with nonstick vegetable oil spray. Remove from heat and stir in cottage cheese, spinach, and egg substitute. Spoon the mix into the shells. Spread ½ cup (123 g) of the sauce into the bottom of a 13 × 9-inch (33 × 23 cm) baking dish and place the shells in the dish. Top with the rest of the sauce and bake 35 to 40 minutes.

5 SERVINGS

Each with: 412 Calories (14% from Fat, 27% from Protein, 59% from Carb); 28 g Protein; 6 g Total Fat; 2 g Unsaturated Fat; 2 g Monounsaturated Fat; 2 g Polyunsaturated Fat; 61 g Carb; 6 g Fiber; 3 g Sugar; 358 mg Phosphorus; 227 mg Calcium; 828 mg Sodium; 1218 mg Potassium; 11 212 IU Vitamin A; 19 mg ATE Vitamin E; 65 mg Vitamin C; 8 mg Cholesterol

Fettuccine with Many Vegetables

Fresh vegetables and Romano cheese make the pasta dish special. If you think you don't like meatless meals, this might be the place to start.

½ pound (225 g) asparagus

2 tablespoons (28 ml) olive oil

½ teaspoon garlic, minced

1 cup (120 g) zucchini, seeds removed, diced small

1 cup (160 g) onion, sliced

1 cup (150 g) red bell peppers, sliced

¼ cup (25 g) green onion, thinly sliced

½ cup (65 g) peas, defrosted and drained

¼ teaspoon black pepper

8 ounces (225 g) whole wheat fettuccine, cooked according to package directions

¼ cup (15 g) fresh parsley, minced

3 tablespoons (9 g) fresh chives, minced

2 ounces (55 g) Romano cheese, grated

Cut the asparagus on the diagonal into ½-inch (1.3 cm) pieces. Bring a pan of water to a boil, add asparagus, and time for 2 minutes. Drain, rinse with cold water, and pat dry. In a large skillet, heat oil over medium heat. Add garlic and sauté for 1 minute. Stir in zucchini, onion, red bell pepper, and green onion, sautéing for 2 minutes. Add asparagus, peas, and black pepper, heating for 2 minutes. Drain fettuccine and put back into hot pan. Add vegetables, parsley, chives, and cheese, stirring to coat.

4 SERVINGS

Each with: 375 Calories (27% from Fat, 17% from Protein, 57% from Carb); 17 g Protein; 12 g Total Fat; 4 g Saturated Fat; 6 g Monounsaturated Fat; 1 g Polyunsaturated Fat; 56 g Carb; 4 g Fiber; 5 g Sugar; 340 mg Phosphorus; 221 mg Calcium; 249 mg Sodium; 547 mg Potassium; 2327 IU Vitamin A; 13 mg ATE Vitamin E; 91 mg Vitamin C; 15 mg Cholesterol

Vegetable Sauced Spaghetti

Both creamy and tomatoey, this sauce tastes like it should be rich and full of calories.
But it's not and its nutrition is boosted by generous helpings of a number of vegetables,
so you can enjoy the taste without the guilt.

8 ounces (225 g) whole wheat
spaghetti
1 cup (160 g) onion, chopped
2 cups (240 g) zucchini, chopped
2 cups (240 g) yellow squash,
chopped
8 ounces (225 g) mushrooms,
chopped
½ cup (65 g) carrot, chopped
2 tablespoons (28 ml) olive oil
16 ounces (455 g) no-salt-added
tomatoes
12 ounces (340 g) no-salt-added
tomato paste
1 can (10¾ ounces, or 305 g) low
sodium cream of mushroom
soup
1 teaspoon Italian seasoning
¼ teaspoon garlic powder
¼ teaspoon dried parsley

Cook spaghetti according to package directions. Sauté onion, zucchini, squash, mushrooms, and carrots in oil until onions are softened. Add tomatoes, tomato paste, soup, and seasonings and simmer until vegetables a tender, about 20 to 30 minutes. Serve over spaghetti.

4 SERVINGS

Each with: 383 Calories (7% from Fat, 17% from Protein, 77% from Carb); 18 g Protein; 3 g Total Fat; 1 g Unsaturated Fat; 1 g Monounsaturated Fat; 1 g Polyunsaturated Fat; 81 g Carb; 13 g Fiber; 19 g Sugar; 387 mg Phosphorus; 135 mg Calcium; 406 mg Sodium; 2124 mg Potassium; 3639 IU Vitamin A; 1 mg ATE Vitamin E; 60 mg Vitamin C; 4 mg Cholesterol

Eggplant Lasagna

Eggplant takes the place of noodles in this vegetarian lasagna, providing increased nutrition and decreased calories. But the flavor is still great and a generous helping will fill you up and keep you that way.

½ pound (225 g) plum tomatoes, halved and seeded

½ teaspoon garlic, minced

4 tablespoons (60 ml) olive oil

1 teaspoon black pepper, divided

3 pounds (1⅓ kg) eggplant, sliced lengthwise ¼-inch (6 mm) thick

1 cup (250 g) ricotta

¼ cup (60 ml) egg substitute

½ cup (20 g) fresh basil, chopped

¼ cup (25 g) Parmesan, grated

4 cups (228 g) mixed greens

2 tablespoons (28 ml) balsamic vinegar

Heat broiler. In a food processor, puree the tomatoes, garlic, 1 tablespoon (15 ml) of the oil, and ¼ teaspoon black pepper. In 2 batches, arrange the eggplant slices on a broiler pan or baking sheet, brush with 2 tablespoons (28 ml) of the oil, and season with ¼ teaspoon black pepper. Broil until charred and tender, 3 to 4 minutes per side. Meanwhile, in a small bowl, combine the ricotta, egg substitute, basil, and ¼ teaspoon black pepper. Spread half the tomato sauce in the bottom of an 8-inch (20 cm) square baking dish. On top of it, layer a third of the eggplant slices and half the ricotta mixture. Repeat with another layer of eggplant and ricotta. Top with the remaining eggplant and tomato sauce. Sprinkle with the cheese. Reduce oven to 400°F (200°C, or gas mark 6). Bake the lasagna until bubbling, 15 to 20 minutes. Let rest for 10 minutes before serving. Divide the greens among plates and drizzle with the remaining tablespoon (15 ml) of oil, vinegar, and ¼ teaspoon of black pepper. Serve with the lasagna.

4 SERVINGS

Each with: 357 Calories (51% from Fat, 17% from Protein, 32% from Carb); 16 g Protein; 22 g Total Fat; 6 g Unsaturated Fat; 12 g Monounsaturated Fat; 2 g Polyunsaturated Fat; 30 g Carb; 15 g Fiber; 10 g Sugar; 311 mg Phosphorus; 382 mg Calcium; 219 mg Sodium; 1288 mg Potassium; 1338 IU Vitamin A; 72 mg ATE Vitamin E; 27 mg Vitamin C; 25 mg Cholesterol

Better Than It Sounds Pasta with Tofu

OK, it sounds funny, but it works. Tofu is crumbled and stir-fried with vegetables and then added to pasta sauce to produce a meal that is incredibly nutritious, but it's also even lower in calories than most of the meals here.

8 ounces (225 g) whole wheat pasta

1 tablespoon (15 ml) olive oil

1 cup (160 g) onion, chopped

½ teaspoon garlic, minced

14 ounces (390 g) firm tofu

2 teaspoons dried basil

8 ounces (225 g) mushrooms, sliced

2 cups (240 g) zucchini, sliced

25 ounces (700 g) low sodium spaghetti sauce

Cook pasta according to package directions. Heat the oil in a pan and add the chopped onion and garlic. When they get golden in color, add an entire block of firm tofu. Don't chop it but crumble it finely instead. Add the basil. Turn the heat down and let the tofu cook with the onion and spices for about 5 minutes. Meanwhile, chop the mushrooms and slice the zucchini. Stir them into the tofu mixture. Cook until mushrooms and zucchini are softened. Add the tomato sauce. Stir well. Heat through. Serve over the pasta.

4 SERVINGS

Each with: 301 Calories (26% from Fat, 20% from Protein, 54% from Carb); 16 g Protein; 9 g Total Fat; 1 g Unsaturated Fat; 4 g Monounsaturated Fat; 3 g Polyunsaturated Fat; 43 g Carb; 7 g Fiber; 6 g Sugar; 290 mg Phosphorus; 112 mg Calcium; 845 mg Sodium; 1308 mg Potassium; 868 IU Vitamin A; 4 mg ATE Vitamin E; 31 mg Vitamin C; 0 mg Cholesterol

A Pizza Full of Vegetables

There is nothing like hot pizza, fresh from the oven. The problem with most pizza is that it's loaded with calories and fat from large quantities of cheese and high fat meats like sausage and pepperoni. We've cut back on the amount of cheese, eliminated the meat, and used fresh tomatoes instead of sauce, which often has added oil and sugar. In their place is a layer of fresh tomatoes and a mound of other vegetables. And you can still eat ¼ of this pizza and stay within your 400 calories.

Whole wheat pizza crust

1 cup (120 g) whole wheat flour

1 teaspoon yeast

½ cup (120 ml) hot water

2 tablespoons (28 ml) olive oil, divided

Pizza Topping

1 cup (160 g) onion, minced

8 ounces (225 g) mushrooms, coarsely chopped

1 cup (150 g) green bell pepper, sliced

1 cup (120 g) zucchini, thinly sliced

1 cup (71 g) broccoli florets

¼ teaspoon black pepper

½ teaspoon dried oregano

4 ounces (115 g) mozzarella, shredded

2 cups (360 g) tomatoes, sliced

2 ounces (55 g) Parmesan cheese, grated

In a small bowl, mix flour and yeast. With fork, stir in water and 1 tablespoon (15 ml) olive oil to form a soft dough. Cover lightly with plastic wrap. Let rise in warm place for about 30 minutes. Fit into a greased 12-inch (30 cm) pizza pan, building up edges slightly. Bake at 425°F (220°C, or gas mark 7) for 10 minutes. Sauté onion, mushrooms, and green bell pepper in oil in small skillet for 10 minutes or until mushroom liquid is evaporated. Add zucchini and broccoli. Sprinkle with black pepper and oregano. Distribute onion mixture evenly over partially baked crust. Sprinkle with mozzarella. Top with sliced tomatoes. Sprinkle with Parmesan cheese. Bake at 425°F (220°C, or gas mark 7) for 10 minutes or until hot and bubbly and crust is browned.

4 SERVINGS

Each with: 373 Calories (42% from Fat, 21% from Protein, 37% from Carb); 20 g Protein; 18 g Total Fat; 7 g Saturated Fat; 8 g Monounsaturated Fat; 2 g Polyunsaturated Fat; 37 g Carb; 7 g Fiber; 5 g Sugar; 429 mg Phosphorus; 346 mg Calcium; 417 mg Sodium; 790 mg Potassium; 1463 IU Vitamin A; 66 mg ATE Vitamin E; 75 mg Vitamin C; 35 mg Cholesterol

Chinese Restaurant Tofu Stir-Fry

Full of vegetables plus the protein of tofu, this stir-fry is sure to please, both in terms of taste and the ability to fill you up and keep you satisfied.

1 tablespoon (15 ml) olive oil

1 cup (160 g) onion, cut in wedges

1 cup (100 g) celery, cut on the diagonal

2 cups (140 g) bok choy, shredded

½ cup (75 g) green bell pepper, sliced

½ cup (75 g) red bell pepper, sliced

8 ounces (225 g) mushrooms, sliced

12 ounces (340 g) tofu, cubed

1 tablespoon (15 ml) low sodium soy sauce

1 cup (195 g) brown rice, cooked

Heat oil in wok and stir-fry ingredients gently, being careful not to overcook.

2 SERVINGS

Each with: 383 Calories (29% from Fat, 17% from Protein, 54% from Carb); 17 g Protein; 13 g Total Fat; 2 g Unsaturated Fat; 6 g Monounsaturated Fat; 4 g Polyunsaturated Fat; 54 g Carb; 8 g Fiber; 11 g Sugar; 357 mg Phosphorus; 146 mg Calcium; 588 mg Sodium; 1259 mg Potassium; 1623 IU Vitamin A; 0 mg ATE Vitamin E; 115 mg Vitamin C; 0 mg Cholesterol

Top of the List Vegetarian Fried Rice

When you have fried rice that tastes this good, you won't even miss the meat. Eggs add protein, and a whole lot of vegetables contribute to the nutrient levels. And the taste is superb.

¼ cup (60 ml) olive oil

1 teaspoon garlic, minced or mashed

¼ cup (25 g) green onion, diagonally sliced

¾ cup (120 g) onion, sliced

1 cup (70 g) bok choy, coarsely shredded

4 ounces (115 g) mushrooms, julienned

1 cup (145 g) snow pea pods

½ cup (120 ml) egg substitute

3 cups (585 g) brown rice, cooked and cooled

3 tablespoons (45 ml) low sodium soy sauce, or to taste

Heat wok. Add 1 tablespoon oil (15 ml) and heat. Add garlic, green onion, and regular onion and stir-fry until onions are tender. Add bok choy, mushrooms, and snow peas. Sauté 2 minutes. Remove vegetables. Add 1 tablespoon oil (15 ml) and heat. Add egg substitute. Stir until set. Remove eggs and break into very small pieces. Add remaining 2 tablespoons (28 ml) oil and add rice. Cook, stirring, until heated through. Season with soy sauce. Add vegetables and eggs and toss to mix well.

4 SERVINGS

Each with: 356 Calories (40% from Fat, 11% from Protein, 49% from Carb); 10 g Protein; 16 g Total Fat; 2 g Unsaturated Fat; 11 g Monounsaturated Fat; 2 g Polyunsaturated Fat; 44 g Carb; 5 g Fiber; 3 g Sugar; 217 mg Phosphorus; 65 mg Calcium; 524 mg Sodium; 465 mg Potassium; 454 IU Vitamin A; 0 mg ATE Vitamin E; 20 mg Vitamin C; 0 mg Cholesterol

Full Meal Vegetarian Curry

This is a moderately spicy vegetarian curry meal. Adjust the amount of cayenne pepper to your taste. It's full of vegetables, with the extra protein of beans and hard boiled eggs.

1 tablespoon (15 ml) olive oil

1 cup (160 g) onion, thinly sliced

¾ teaspoon garlic, crushed

1 apple, peeled, cored and chopped

1½ teaspoons curry powder

1½ teaspoons lemon peel, grated

1 teaspoon ground ginger

1 teaspoon coriander

⅛ teaspoon turmeric

⅛ teaspoon cayenne pepper

2 cups (342 g) black eyed peas, cooked and drained

2 cups (512 g) cooked kidney beans

⅓ cup (50 g) raisins

1 cup (230 g) plain fat-free yogurt

3 eggs, hard boiled and halved

6 radishes, thinly sliced

¼ cup (25 g) green onion, sliced

½ cup (8 g) fresh cilantro, chopped

¼ cup (35 g) peanuts, chopped

3 cups (585 g) brown rice, cooked

Heat oil in skillet. Sauté onion, garlic, and apple until soft. Combine curry powder, lemon peel, ginger, coriander, turmeric, and cayenne pepper. Stir into onion mixture. Add black-eyed peas, kidney beans, and raisins. Cover; simmer 5 minutes. Remove from heat, stir in yogurt. Place egg halves in bowl. Spoon curry over. Top with radishes, green onion, cilantro, and peanuts. Serve with rice.

6 SERVINGS

Each with: 400 Calories (15% from Fat, 19% from Protein, 66% from Carb); 19 g Protein; 7 g Total Fat; 2 g Saturated Fat; 3 g Monounsaturated Fat; 1 g Polyunsaturated Fat; 67 g Carb; 10 g Fiber; 15 g Sugar; 340 mg Phosphorus; 173 mg Calcium; 107 mg Sodium; 831 mg Potassium; 499 IU Vitamin A; 41 mg ATE Vitamin E; 10 mg Vitamin C; 123 mg Cholesterol

Curried Eggplant with Tomatoes and Basil

This creamy vegetarian curry featuring eggplant and cherry tomatoes offers great nutrition and low calories.

1 cup (185 g) brown basmati rice,
  uncooked
1 tablespoon (15 ml) olive oil
1 cup (160 g) onion, chopped
32 cherry tomatoes, halved
1 pound (455 g) eggplant, cut
  into ½-inch (1.3 cm) pieces
1½ teaspoons curry powder
¼ teaspoons black pepper
2 cups (475 ml) water
2 cups (480 g) chickpeas, drained
½ cup (20 g) fresh basil
¼ cup (60 g) plain low fat yogurt

Cook the rice according to package directions. Meanwhile, heat the oil in a saucepan over medium-high heat. Add the onion and cook, stirring occasionally, until softened, 4 to 6 minutes. Stir in the tomatoes, eggplant, curry powder, and black pepper. Cook, stirring, until fragrant, about 2 minutes. Add 2 cups water (475 ml) and bring to a boil. Reduce heat and simmer, partially covered, until eggplant is tender, 12 to 15 minutes. Stir in the chickpeas and cook just until heated through, about 3 minutes. Remove the vegetables from heat and stir in the basil. Fluff the rice with a fork. Serve the vegetables over the rice with yogurt.

4 SERVINGS

Each with: 429 Calories (14% from Fat, 13% from Protein, 73% from Carb); 15 g Protein; 7 g Total Fat; 1 g Unsaturated Fat; 3 g Monounsaturated Fat; 2 g Polyunsaturated Fat; 80 g Carb; 15 g Fiber; 10 g Sugar; 276 mg Phosphorus; 200 mg Calcium; 24 mg Sodium; 1106 mg Potassium; 1311 IU Vitamin A; 2 mg ATE Vitamin E; 35 mg Vitamin C; 1 mg Cholesterol

On The Road to Marrakesh Stew

This spicy Moroccan stew of vegetables and dried fruit is sure to be a hit.
It contains an amazing amount of flavor and great nutrition.

1 tablespoon (15 ml) olive oil

1½ cups (240 g) onion, chopped

2 garlic cloves, minced

1 teaspoon cinnamon, ground

½ teaspoon ginger, ground

½ teaspoon turmeric, ground

¼ teaspoon nutmeg, ground

¼ teaspoon red pepper, ground

2 cups (475 ml) water

3 cloves, whole

2 cups (244 g) carrot, sliced

2 cups (280 g) butternut squash, cubed

2 cups (480 g) chickpeas, cooked or canned, drained

1½ cups (200 g) sweet potatoes, cubed

½ cup (75 g) raisins

⅓ cup (43 g) dried apricots, diced

3 tablespoons (3 g) brown sugar substitute, such as Splenda

In a 4-quart (3.8 L) saucepan, heat the oil over medium-high heat. Add the onion and garlic and cook, stirring, until softened. Add the cinnamon, ginger, turmeric, nutmeg, and red pepper, stirring until absorbed. Add the water and cloves; bring to a boil. Add the carrot, squash, chickpeas, sweet potato, raisins, apricots, and brown sugar substitute and return to a boil. Reduce the heat and simmer uncovered, stirring occasionally, 40 to 45 minutes or until the sweet potato is tender.

4 SERVINGS

Each with: 416 Calories (13% from Fat, 11% from Protein, 77% from Carb); 12 g Protein; 6 g Total Fat; 1 g Saturated Fat; 3 g Monounsaturated Fat; 2 g Polyunsaturated Fat; 84 g Carb; 15 g Fiber; 32 g Sugar; 266 mg Phosphorus; 164 mg Calcium; 94 mg Sodium; 1261 mg Potassium; 34 916 IU Vitamin A; 0 mg ATE Vitamin E; 41 mg Vitamin C; 0 mg Cholesterol

Dinners: Soups, Stews, and Chilis

Sometimes you just want a simple meal, one bowl full of goodness to satisfy both your taste and your hunger without a lot of fuss. That's when we often turn to soups and stews. Just as salads seem to be warm weather meals, soups are what I crave when the weather turns cooler. And they are a great deal nutritionally. You can fill them with all kinds of vegetables and they never seem out of place. You can add such nutrient boosters as dark green leafy vegetables. And you can, as in many of these recipes, cook them in the slow cooker and end up with tender, flavorful meals using less fatty and less expensive cuts of meat. All in all there is just a lot to like about soups, stews, and chilis.

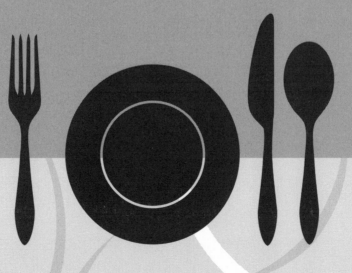

Beef Stew with Fall Veggies and Fruits

Apple cider gives this stew its unique flavor. Generous amounts of vegetables
give it its nutrition and filling qualities.

3 tablespoons (24 g) all purpose
  flour
¼ teaspoon black pepper
¼ teaspoon dried thyme
2 pound (900 g) beef round steak,
  cut in 1-inch (2.5 cm) cubes
2 tablespoons (28 ml) olive oil
2 cups (475 ml) apple cider
2 tablespoons (28 ml) cider
  vinegar
3 medium potatoes, peeled and
  quartered
1½ cups (183 g) carrot, sliced
1 cup (160 g) onion, quartered
1 cup (100 g) celery, sliced
1½ cups (210 g) butternut
  squash, peeled and cubed
1 apple, peeled and chopped

Combine flour, black pepper, and thyme. Dredge meat in flour
mixture. Heat oil in Dutch oven. Brown half the meat at a time
in the oil. Return all meat to pan. Stir in cider and vinegar.
Cook and stir until mixture boils. Reduce heat, cover, and
simmer about 1¼ hours until meat is tender. Stir in vegetables
and apple. Cover and cook until vegetables and apples are
done, about 30 minutes more.

8 SERVINGS

Each with: 428 Calories (20% from Fat, 42% from Protein, 38% from Carb);
45 g Protein; 9 g Total Fat; 2 g Saturated Fat; 5 g Monounsaturated Fat; 1 g
Polyunsaturated Fat; 40 g Carb; 4 g Fiber; 11 g Sugar; 371 mg Phosphorus; 51 mg
Calcium; 92 mg Sodium; 1308 mg Potassium; 5760 IU Vitamin A; 0 mg ATE Vitamin
E; 23 mg Vitamin C; 102 mg Cholesterol

Classic Beef Vegetable Soup (with Added Veggies)

There's nothing fancy here, just a flavorful soup Campbell's wishes they could put in a can. The addition of a few nonclassic vegetables pushes up the nutrition without adding significantly to the calories.

1½ pound (680 g) round steak, cut in ½-inch (1.3 cm) pieces

1 cup (160 g) onion, coarsely chopped

1 cup (100 g) celery, sliced

4 medium potatoes, cubed

4 cups (950 ml) low sodium beef broth

1 cup (90 g) cabbage, coarsely chopped

4 cups (652 g) frozen mixed vegetables

1 cup (71 g) broccoli florets

1 cup (100 g) cauliflower florets

2 cups (360 g) no-salt-added tomatoes

Brown meat in a skillet and transfer to slow cooker. Add onion, celery, and potatoes. Pour broth over. Cook on low for 8 to 10 hours. Add cabbage, mixed vegetables, broccoli, cauliflower, and tomatoes. Turn to high and cook until vegetables are done, about ½ hour to an hour.

8 SERVINGS

Each with: 399 Calories (16% from Fat, 35% from Protein, 49% from Carb); 35 g Protein; 7 g Total Fat; 2 g Saturated Fat; 3 g Monounsaturated Fat; 0 g Polyunsaturated Fat; 49 g Carb; 8 g Fiber; 7 g Sugar; 386 mg Phosphorus; 85 mg Calcium; 178 mg Sodium; 1248 mg Potassium; 4322 IU Vitamin A; 0 mg ATE Vitamin E; 44 mg Vitamin C; 82 mg Cholesterol

Filling Soup for a Winter's Night

This old-fashioned soup is quick and easy to make. The warm broth and homey vegetables are perfect for a cold day, filling and warming your entire body.

3 cups (700 ml) low sodium beef broth

1 cup (100 g) celery, chopped

2 cups (360 g) no-salt-added tomatoes

10 ounces (280 g) frozen mixed vegetables

1 cup (160 g) onion, chopped

1 cup (122 g) carrot, sliced

1 cup (90 g) cabbage, shredded

1 teaspoon black pepper

1¾ pounds (795 g) extra lean ground beef

2 tablespoons (16 g) cornstarch

½ cup (120 ml) water

Brown ground beef in skillet until barely cooked. Put all ingredients, except cornstarch and water, in large stew pot. Cover and simmer for 45 minutes. Add cornstarch to water and stir until smooth. Pour into pot and stir. Cook until thickened.

6 SERVINGS

Each with: 401 Calories (52% from Fat, 29% from Protein, 18% from Carb); 29 g Protein; 23 g Total Fat; 9 g Saturated Fat; 10 g Monounsaturated Fat; 1 g Polyunsaturated Fat; 18 g Carb; 5 g Fiber; 7 g Sugar; 265 mg Phosphorus; 81 mg Calcium; 217 mg Sodium; 898 mg Potassium; 4825 IU Vitamin A; 0 mg ATE Vitamin E; 22 mg Vitamin C; 91 mg Cholesterol

Full of Fall Minestrone

When the weather gets cooler, our slow cooker gets more use. This is a different variation on the traditional Italian soup, with fall or winter vegetables predominating.

1 cup (184 g) dried kidney beans

1 pound (455 g) extra lean ground beef

2½ cups (350 g) butternut squash, peeled and cubed

2 medium potatoes, peeled and cubed

2 bulbs fennel bulbs, cut in 1-inch (2.5 cm) pieces

1½ cups (240 g) onion, coarsely chopped

4 cups (120 g) spinach, chopped

2 cloves garlic, minced

1 tablespoon (6 g) Italian seasoning

4 cups (950 ml) low sodium chicken broth

1 cup (235 ml) white wine

Cook beans according to package directions until almost done. In a skillet, brown beef, breaking up into coarse chunks. Drain. In a large slow cooker, place vegetables on the bottom. Sprinkle seasoning over top. Add beans and beef. Pour broth and wine over all. Cook on low for 8 to 10 hours.

8 SERVINGS

Each with: 374 Calories (25% from Fat, 24% from Protein, 51% from Carb); 22 g Protein; 10 g Total Fat; 4 g Saturated Fat; 4 g Monounsaturated Fat; 1 g Polyunsaturated Fat; 47 g Carb; 12 g Fiber; 3 g Sugar; 317 mg Phosphorus; 159 mg Calcium; 399 mg Sodium; 1612 mg Potassium; 6238 IU Vitamin A; 0 mg ATE Vitamin E; 36 mg Vitamin C; 39 mg Cholesterol

Have a Beer with Your Stew

This recipe proves that you can have your beer and eat it too. Beer flavors this stew, but it is really the great variety of vegetables that carries it.

2 pound (900 g) beef round steak

2 teaspoons black pepper, fresh ground

2 bay leaves

1 tablespoon (4 g) dried thyme

1 tablespoon (3 g) dried rosemary

2 tablespoons (28 ml) olive oil

1 cup (160 g) onion, peeled and diced

¼ cup (31 g) all purpose flour

12 ounces (355 ml) dark beer

4 cups (950 ml) low sodium beef broth

½ cup (90 g) tomatoes, crushed

1 cup (130 g) carrot, peeled and diced

1 cup (100 g) celery, diced

1 cup (150 g) rutabaga, peeled and diced,

1 cup (110 g) parsnips, peeled and diced

1 cup (150 g) turnip

1 large potato

Season the beef with black pepper. Tie the bay leaves, thyme, and rosemary into cheesecloth. In a Dutch oven, brown the beef well on all sides in the oil. Remove the beef, set aside, and add the onion and cook until softened. Sprinkle the onion with the flour and stir to combine well. Return the beef to the pan. Add the beer, broth, herbs, and tomatoes. Bring to a boil and reduce the heat to a slow simmer. Cover and cook for ¾ hour. Add the vegetables and continue to cook for 1 additional hour.

6 SERVINGS

Each with: 377 Calories (28% from Fat, 49% from Protein, 23% from Carb); 42 g Protein; 11 g Total Fat; 3 g Saturated Fat; 6 g Monounsaturated Fat; 1 g Polyunsaturated Fat; 20 g Carb; 4 g Fiber; 5 g Sugar; 463 mg Phosphorus; 82 mg Calcium; 299 mg Sodium; 1160 mg Potassium; 2766 IU Vitamin A; 0 mg ATE Vitamin E; 21 mg Vitamin C; 97 mg Cholesterol

Easy Meatball Soup

This is a nontraditional soup with Mexican flavors, with ham adding flavor to meatballs and a minimum of seasonings. But we've found that we like its simple warming goodness.

½ pound (225 g) extra lean ground beef

¼ pound (115 g) ham, chopped

8 cups (1.9 L) low sodium chicken broth

4 tablespoons (32 g) all purpose flour

¼ cup (60 ml) egg substitute

4 ounces (115 g) green chilies, chopped

1 cup (110 g) carrot, grated

⅓ cup (32 g) instant brown rice, uncooked

½ pound (225 g) fresh spinach

½ teaspoon dried oregano

1 teaspoon ground cumin

2½ tablespoons (10 g) fresh parsley

Mix beef, ½ cup (120 ml) broth, flour, and egg substitute. Form into small balls. Set aside. Put remaining broth, green chilies, carrot, and rice in slow cooker on high and allow to simmer. When simmering, add meatballs, cover, and cook for ½ hour. Then turn heat on low and cook for another 3 hours. Add other ingredients and cover and cook for 20 more minutes.

4 SERVINGS

Each with: 391 Calories (37% from Fat, 32% from Protein, 31% from Carb); 32 g Protein; 16 g Total Fat; 6 g Unsaturated Fat; 7 g Monounsaturated Fat; 2 g Polyunsaturated Fat; 31 g Carb; 4 g Fiber; 2 g Sugar; 402 mg Phosphorus; 127 mg Calcium; 694 mg Sodium; 1251 mg Potassium; 9473 IU Vitamin A; 0 mg ATE Vitamin E; 31 mg Vitamin C; 51 mg Cholesterol

Just Like Grandma's Beef Vegetable Soup

This provides not only classic beef vegetable soup flavor, but even better than classic nutrition with the addition of the spinach, one of the most nutrient dense foods around.

1½ pounds (680 g) extra lean ground beef

1½ cups (183 g) carrot, sliced

1 cup (100 g) celery, sliced

1 tablespoon (15 ml) Worcestershire sauce

4 cups (720 g) no-salt-added tomatoes, chopped

2 cups (475 ml) low sodium tomato juice

3 cups (700 ml) low sodium beef broth

1 teaspoon onion powder

½ teaspoon black pepper

½ cup (100 g) pearl barley

2 medium potatoes, diced

6 ounces (170 g) mushrooms

6 ounces (170 g) spinach, torn into bite-sized pieces

In a Dutch oven, brown beef. Drain and return to pot. Add next 8 ingredients. Bring to a boil. Reduce heat and simmer 1 hour. Add barley and remaining vegetables. Simmer until barley is tender, about another hour.

8 SERVINGS

Each with: 373 Calories (37% from Fat, 25% from Protein, 38% from Carb); 23 g Protein; 16 g Total Fat; 6 g Saturated Fat; 6 g Monounsaturated Fat; 1 g Polyunsaturated Fat; 36 g Carb; 7 g Fiber; 9 g Sugar; 293 mg Phosphorus; 113 mg Calcium; 360 mg Sodium; 1405 mg Potassium; 6633 IU Vitamin A; 0 mg ATE Vitamin E; 50 mg Vitamin C; 59 mg Cholesterol

Steak and Potato Soup

Here's a thick and hearty stew full of beef and vegetables, with a flavor that is sure to please.

2 pound (900 g) beef round steak

2 tablespoons (28 ml) olive oil

1½ cups (240 g) onion, coarsely chopped

1 teaspoon garlic cloves, minced

2 large red potatoes, cut into ¾-inch (1.9 cm) pieces

3 cups (366 g) carrot, sliced

16 ounces (455 g) frozen green beans

2 tablespoons (5 g) fresh basil, chopped

½ teaspoon black pepper, freshly ground

8 cups (1.9 L) low sodium beef broth

3 tablespoons (45 g) steak sauce

Cut beef into ½-inch (1.3 cm) thick strips; cut each strip into 1-inch (2.5 cm) pieces. Heat oil in 8-quart (7.6 L) stockpot or Dutch oven over medium-high heat until hot. Add beef. Cook and stir 4 to 5 minutes or until browned. Add onion and garlic. Cook and stir 2 minutes. Add all remaining ingredients and mix well. Bring to a boil over medium-high heat. Reduce heat. Cover and simmer 12 to 15 minutes or until vegetables are tender, stirring occasionally.

10 SERVINGS

Each with: 259 Calories (23% from Fat, 40% from Protein, 37% from Carb); 26 g Protein; 7 g Total Fat; 2 g Unsaturated Fat; 3 g Monounsaturated Fat; 1 g Polyunsaturated Fat; 24 g Carb; 5 g Fiber; 6 g Sugar; 313 mg Phosphorus; 84 mg Calcium; 250 mg Sodium; 1048 mg Potassium; 4981 IU Vitamin A; 0 mg ATE Vitamin E; 26 mg Vitamin C; 42 mg Cholesterol

Northern Italian Beef and Barley Stew

This is a hearty beef stew, full of beans and veggies and featuring great Italian flavor. The white Italian kidney beans called cannellini beans are preferred, but if you can't find them, great northern or navy beans will work just as well.

1 cup (200 g) white beans
1½ pound (680 g) beef round steak
¼ cup (32 g) all purpose flour
1 tablespoon (15 ml) olive oil
1 cup (160 g) onion, chopped
½ teaspoon garlic, crushed
3 cups (700 ml) low sodium beef broth
½ teaspoon dried oregano
1 tablespoon (6 g) Italian seasoning
2 cups (244 g) carrot, sliced
½ cup (50 g) celery, chopped
½ teaspoon black pepper
¼ cup (25 g) Parmesan cheese, shredded

Soak beans according to package directions. Trim fat from meat and cut into bite-sized cubes. Dust beef with flour. Using a heavy pot, brown beef in hot oil, browning all sides. Remove meat and set aside. Add onion and garlic to drippings and cook until onion is transparent. Return the meat to pot. Add broth, oregano, Italian seasoning, and drained beans. Cover and simmer for 45 minutes. Add carrot and celery and simmer until meat is tender and beans are soft, about 40 minutes. Add additional water as needed. Season with black pepper to taste. Sprinkle with cheese to serve.

6 SERVINGS

Each with: 416 Calories (19% from Fat, 50% from Protein, 31% from Carb); 51 g Protein; 9 g Total Fat; 3 g Saturated Fat; 4 g Monounsaturated Fat; 1 g Polyunsaturated Fat; 32 g Carb; 7 g Fiber; 4 g Sugar; 403 mg Phosphorus; 124 mg Calcium; 157 mg Sodium; 1241 mg Potassium; 5177 IU Vitamin A; 0 mg ATE Vitamin E; 5 mg Vitamin C; 102 mg Cholesterol

More Than You Expect Tortilla Soup

Traditional Mexican tortilla soup is usually just broth with chicken and onion, not enough for a full meal. So we've bulked it up while keeping it low in calories with additional vegetables and beans. I think you'll like the result, and it will surely fill you and keep you that way.

1 pound (455 g) boneless skinless chicken breast

2 poblano chilies, fresh

1 cup (160 g) onion, chopped

8 cups (1.9 L) low sodium chicken broth

2 cups (240 g) zucchini, sliced and quartered

½ cup (75 g) green bell pepper, cut in 1-inch (2.5 cm) cubes

10 ounces (280 g) frozen corn

1 cup (256 g) kidney beans, drained

6 corn tortillas

lime juice, to taste

Rinse chicken and cut into 1-inch (2.5 cm) chunks. Rinse poblano chilies and trim and discard stems, seeds, and veins. Cut chilies lengthwise into ⅛- to ¼-inch (4 to 6 mm) strips. In a 4- or 5-quart (3.8 to 4.7 L) pan over high heat, bring chilies, onion, and broth to a boil. Reduce heat, cover, and simmer for 5 minutes. Add chicken, zucchini, green bell pepper, corn, and beans. Cover and simmer until meat is no longer pink and vegetables are tender, about 15 minutes. Cut tortillas into 1-inch (2.5 cm) squares and divide equally among soup bowls. Ladle soup over the tortillas. Add lime juice to taste.

4 SERVINGS

Each with: 419 Calories (13% from Fat, 41% from Protein, 46% from Carb); 45 g Protein; 6 g Total Fat; 2 g Saturated Fat; 2 g Monounsaturated Fat; 2 g Polyunsaturated Fat; 51 g Carb; 8 g Fiber; 7 g Sugar; 622 mg Phosphorus; 120 mg Calcium; 710 mg Sodium; 1436 mg Potassium; 628 IU Vitamin A; 7 mg ATE Vitamin E; 60 mg Vitamin C; 66 mg Cholesterol

Southwestern Pork and Vegetable Stew

Filling and flavorful, this pork stew, filled with vegetables and hominy is a family favorite of ours. I think it may become one of yours too. The lean pork loin holds down the fat and calories, while the vegetables provide nutrients and the hominy fiber. It's a perfect meal.

1 tablespoon (15 ml) olive oil

1 pound (455 g) boneless pork loin, cut into ½-inch (1.3 cm) pieces

1 cup (160 g) onion, coarsely chopped

½ teaspoon garlic, minced

1 large red potato, cut into ½-inch (1.3 cm) pieces

10 ounces (280 g) frozen corn

½ cup (75 g) green bell pepper, coarsely chopped

½ cup (75 g) red bell pepper, coarsely chopped

2 cups (475 ml) low sodium chicken broth

14 ounces (390 g) hominy, drained, rinsed

4 ounces (115 g) green chilies, chopped

3 teaspoons (8 g) chili powder

1 teaspoon dried oregano

1 teaspoon ground cumin

Heat oil in large saucepan or Dutch oven over medium-high heat until hot. Add pork. Cook and stir 3 to 4 minutes or until browned. Add onion and garlic. Cook and stir 1 to 2 minutes or until onion is crisp-tender. Add all remaining ingredients and mix well. Bring to a boil. Reduce heat. Cover and simmer 18 to 20 minutes, stirring occasionally, until potatoes are tender and pork is no longer pink in the center.

5 SERVINGS

Each with: 410 Calories (36% from Fat, 24% from Protein, 40% from Carb); 25 g Protein; 17 g Total Fat; 5 g Unsaturated Fat; 8 g Monounsaturated Fat; 2 g Polyunsaturated Fat; 42 g Carb; 7 g Fiber; 7 g Sugar; 358 mg Phosphorus; 59 mg Calcium; 538 mg Sodium; 1088 mg Potassium; 1162 IU Vitamin A; 2 mg ATE Vitamin E; 78 mg Vitamin C; 57 mg Cholesterol

Creamy Pork Stew

This creamy stew is full of lean pork and vegetables, yet it's low enough in calories to allow you to have potatoes with it.

1 tablespoon (15 ml) olive oil

1½ teaspoons garlic, finely chopped

8 ounces (225 g) fresh mushrooms, sliced

1½ pound (680 g) pork loin roast, cut into 1-inch (2.5 cm) pieces

2½ cups (570 ml) low sodium chicken broth

1 cup (235 ml) white wine

½ cup (80 g) onion, chopped

1 carrot, cut lengthwise in half, then cut into strips

¼ teaspoon black pepper

1 cup (235 ml) fat-free evaporated milk

⅓ cup (42 g) all purpose flour

2 tablespoons (8 g) fresh parsley

3 cups (675 g) mashed potatoes, prepared according to package directions

Heat oil in large 6-quart (5.7 L) Dutch oven over medium-high heat. Cook garlic and mushrooms in oil mixture 5 to 6 minutes, stirring frequently, until mushrooms are softened. Stir in pork. Cook 6 to 7 minutes, stirring frequently, until pork is lightly browned. Stir in broth, wine, onion, carrot, and black pepper. Heat to boiling; reduce heat to medium low. Cover and cook 25 to 30 minutes, stirring occasionally, until pork is tender and no longer pink in the center. Beat in evaporated milk and flour with wire whisk. Cook 5 to 6 minutes, stirring constantly, until hot and slightly thickened. Sprinkle with parsley. Serve with mashed potatoes.

6 SERVINGS

Each with: 377 Calories (22% from Fat, 39% from Protein, 39% from Carb); 33 g Protein; 9 g Total Fat; 3 g Unsaturated Fat; 4 g Monounsaturated Fat; 1 g Polyunsaturated Fat; 34 g Carb; 3 g Fiber; 9 g Sugar; 466 mg Phosphorus; 183 mg Calcium; 761 mg Sodium; 1206 mg Potassium; 2767 IU Vitamin A; 57 mg ATE Vitamin E; 12 mg Vitamin C; 75 mg Cholesterol

Zucchini Sausage Soup

This Italian soup is flavored with sausage, but only enough to give it that authentic taste, not enough to blow your diet. Considering that a normal sized serving of Italian sausage contains more calories than a helping of this soup, it seems like a good trade off to me.

2 tablespoons (28 ml) olive oil

1½ cups (180 g) zucchini, sliced

½ cup (80 g) chopped onion, chopped

¼ cup (22 g) fennel, chopped

½ teaspoon garlic, minced

2 cups (475 ml) low sodium tomato juice

1 cup (245 g) no-salt-added tomato sauce

1 cup (235 ml) low sodium chicken broth

1 cup (255 g) no-salt-added stewed tomatoes

1 bay leaf

1 tablespoon (3 g) chopped fresh basil

¼ teaspoon black pepper

½ pound (225 g) Italian sausage, cooked

1 cup (140 g) whole wheat pasta, cooked

In 4-quart (3.8 L) saucepan, heat oil; add zucchini, onion, fennel, and garlic and sauté until vegetables are clear. Add tomato juice, tomato sauce, broth, stewed tomatoes, bay leaf, basil, and black pepper and mix well. Reduce heat to low and cover. Cook, stirring frequently, until flavors are blended, about 30 minutes. Add sausage and pasta and cook 5 to 10 minutes longer. Remove bay leaf before serving.

4 SERVINGS

Each with: 390 Calories (57% from Fat, 14% from Protein, 29% from Carb); 14 g Protein; 26 g Total Fat; 8 g Unsaturated Fat; 13 g Monounsaturated Fat; 3 g Polyunsaturated Fat; 29 g Carb; 5 g Fiber; 11 g Sugar; 211 mg Phosphorus; 87 mg Calcium; 916 mg Sodium; 995 mg Potassium; 2359 IU Vitamin A; 0 mg ATE Vitamin E; 58 mg Vitamin C; 43 mg Cholesterol

Slow Cooker Sort of Minestrone

This soup will remind you of minestrone but with some differences like the use of ham. Picking a lean meat and using lots of vegetables gives you a soup that is hearty and filling while remaining low in calories.

1 cup (150 g) ham, diced
16 ounces (455 g) chickpeas
1 cup (160 g) onion, minced
½ teaspoon garlic, minced
1 cup (130 g) carrot, diced
1 cup (100 g) celery, diced
10 ounces (280 g) frozen spinach
15 ounces (425 g) no-salt-added tomatoes
2 medium potatoes, diced
2 tablespoons (8 g) fresh parsley
1 quart (950 ml) low sodium chicken broth
½ cup (53 g) whole wheat pasta, uncooked
6 tablespoons (30 g) Parmesan cheese, grated

Combine all ingredients except pasta and cheese in slow cooker. Cook on low 8 to 10 hours. One half hour before serving, add pasta. Serve soup sprinkled with cheese.

6 SERVINGS

Each with: 371 Calories (17% from Fat, 24% from Protein, 59% from Carb); 23 g Protein; 7 g Total Fat; 2 g Unsaturated Fat; 2 g Monounsaturated Fat; 2 g Polyunsaturated Fat; 57 g Carb; 12 g Fiber; 10 g Sugar; 412 mg Phosphorus; 242 mg Calcium; 492 mg Sodium; 1466 mg Potassium; 8613 IU Vitamin A; 7 mg ATE Vitamin E; 30 mg Vitamin C; 15 mg Cholesterol

Hearty Minestrone Soup

Full of all kinds of vegetables plus two kinds of beans, this soup is a great example of what we mean by nutrient density.

2 tablespoons (28 ml) olive oil

1½ cups (240 g) onion, coarsely chopped

1 cup (122 g) carrot, thinly sliced

1 cup (100 g) celery, thinly sliced

2 teaspoons garlic, minced

4 cups (480 g) zucchini, cubed

28 (785 g) ounces no-salt-added tomatoes, undrained

4 cups (950 ml) low sodium chicken broth

2 teaspoons dried basil

½ teaspoon dried oregano

3 cups (270 g) cabbage, thinly sliced

2 cups (480 g) chickpeas, drained

2 cups (512 g) kidney beans, drained

2 cups (200 g) green beans, cut into 1-inch (2.5 cm) pieces

½ cup (53 g) whole wheat pasta, uncooked

¼ teaspoon black pepper

¼ cup (25 g) Parmesan cheese, grated

In 8-quart (7.6 L) pot, heat oil over moderate heat. Add onion, carrot, celery, and garlic and cook 3 to 5 minutes, stirring occasionally. Stir in zucchini, tomatoes, broth, basil, and oregano. Cover, reduce heat to low, and simmer about 40 minutes, stirring occasionally. Add cabbage, chickpeas, kidney beans, green beans, and macaroni. Simmer about 15 minutes until cabbage and pasta are tender. Season with black pepper. Serve with grated cheese.

6 SERVINGS

Each with: 352 Calories (21% from Fat, 21% from Protein, 58% from Carb); 20 g Protein; 9 g Total Fat; 2 g Unsaturated Fat; 5 g Monounsaturated Fat; 2 g Polyunsaturated Fat; 54 g Carb; 16 g Fiber; 13 g Sugar; 368 mg Phosphorus; 239 mg Calcium; 182 mg Sodium; 1449 mg Potassium; 3389 IU Vitamin A; 5 mg ATE Vitamin E; 60 mg Vitamin C; 4 mg Cholesterol

King's Gold Cream of Potato Soup

Rich and creamy and full of vegetables and cheese, this potato soup tastes like anything but diet fare.

3 medium potatoes, finely
  chopped
1 cup (100 g) celery, chopped
1 cup (122 g) carrot, chopped
1 tablespoon (1 g) dried parsley
¼ cup (40 g) onion, chopped
⅛ teaspoon black pepper
1½ cups (355 ml) skim milk
2 tablespoons (16 g) all purpose
  flour
1 cup (115 g) low fat cheddar
  cheese, cubed

Combine first 7 ingredients. Simmer 20 to 30 minutes or until potatoes are soft. Mix flour and skim milk and add to broth. Cook until thickened and then add cheese and stir until melted.

4 SERVINGS

Each with: 352 Calories (8% from Fat, 21% from Protein, 71% from Carb); 19 g Protein; 3 g Total Fat; 2 g Unsaturated Fat; 1 g Monounsaturated Fat; 0 g Polyunsaturated Fat; 62 g Carb; 7 g Fiber; 3 g Sugar; 452 mg Phosphorus; 354 mg Calcium; 327 mg Sodium; 1671 mg Potassium; 4400 IU Vitamin A; 76 mg ATE Vitamin E; 35 mg Vitamin C; 9 mg Cholesterol

Way Low Vegetarian Noodle Soup

So full of vegetables, with a rich tasty broth and a generous helping of noodles, you won't believe this soup only contains about 300 calories per serving. And you certainly won't go away hungry.

2 cups (326 g) frozen mixed
  vegetables
9 ounces (255 g) frozen lima
  beans
1 cup (160 g) onion, chopped
½ cup (50 g) celery, sliced
2 cups (142 g) broccoli florets
2 cups (240 g) yellow squash
2 cups (360 g) no-salt-added
  tomatoes, diced
5 cups (1.2 L) low sodium
  vegetable broth
½ teaspoon dried basil
⅛ teaspoon dried thyme
⅛ teaspoon black pepper
5 ounces (140 g) egg noodles

In large saucepan, combine all ingredients except noodles. Bring to a boil. Add noodles. Return to a boil. Reduce heat. Cover and simmer 8 to 10 minutes or until vegetables and noodles are tender, stirring occasionally.

5 SERVINGS

Each with: 308 Calories (19% from Fat, 15% from Protein, 66% from Carb); 12 g Protein; 7 g Total Fat; 2 g Unsaturated Fat; 3 g Monounsaturated Fat; 2 g Polyunsaturated Fat; 53 g Carb; 9 g Fiber; 8 g Sugar; 230 mg Phosphorus; 134 mg Calcium; 223 mg Sodium; 967 mg Potassium; 4351 IU Vitamin A; 2 mg ATE Vitamin E; 61 mg Vitamin C; 9 mg Cholesterol

Welcome to Winter Soup

This rich soup is full of good things like squash and apples. And it has at least one unexpected thing, bananas. But by the time the banana has been pureed and topped with cheese, it just tastes sweet and good, not strange.

3 cups (420 g) butternut squash, peeled and cubed

2 apples, peeled and cubed

4 cups (950 ml) low sodium chicken broth

1 quart (950 ml) water

1 cup (160 g) onion, chopped

1 cup (100 g) celery, diced

¼ teaspoon dried rosemary, crumbled

¼ teaspoon marjoram, crumbled

2 bananas, peeled and chunked

½ teaspoon black pepper

½ cup (30 g) fresh parsley, chopped

1 cup (110 g) Swiss cheese, shredded

½ cup (15 g) croutons

Combine squash and apple with chicken broth, water, onion, celery, rosemary, and marjoram. Cover and simmer 30 minutes until squash is tender. Cool 10 minutes. Remove squash to blender along with ¼ cup (60 ml) pan broth. Blend until smooth. Pour back into pan. Spoon apples into blender along with ¼ cup (60 ml) pan broth. Blend until smooth. Add bananas to blender. Blend until smooth. Pour back into pan, stirring until mixture is smooth. Add black pepper and parsley. Simmer 15 minutes longer. Top serving with cheese and croutons.

4 SERVINGS

Each with: 354 Calories (27% from Fat, 19% from Protein, 54% from Carb); 18 g Protein; 11 g Total Fat; 7 g Unsaturated Fat; 3 g Monounsaturated Fat; 1 g Polyunsaturated Fat; 51 g Carb; 7 g Fiber; 22 g Sugar; 364 mg Phosphorus; 427 mg Calcium; 143 mg Sodium; 1186 mg Potassium; 12 413 IU Vitamin A; 70 mg ATE Vitamin E; 75 mg Vitamin C; 30 mg Cholesterol

Cajun Stew to Warm You Two Ways

Actually this stew isn't as spicy as the name might imply, but if you want it hotter you can always add more cayenne pepper. What it is, however, is filling. With the bulk of beans, barley, and brown rice (not to mention 14 grams of fiber), plus lots of vegetables, you can count on not going away hungry.

2 tablespoons (28 ml) olive oil
1 cup (160 g) onion, chopped
1 cup (122 g) carrot, sliced
1½ cups (105 g) mushrooms, sliced
6 cups (1 kg) pinto beans, drained
2 cups (360 g) no-salt-added tomatoes
¼ teaspoon Cajun seasoning
¼ teaspoon dried basil
¼ teaspoon dried tarragon
¼ teaspoon dried oregano
¼ teaspoon celery seed
¼ teaspoon dried thyme
¼ teaspoon marjoram
¼ teaspoon dried sage
¼ teaspoon black pepper
¼ teaspoon cayenne pepper
½ cup (95 g) brown rice, uncooked
⅓ cup (67 g) pearl barley, uncooked
6 cups (1.4 L) low sodium vegetable broth

Heat oil in a large kettle: Add onion, carrot, and mushrooms and sauté until softened, about 5 minutes. Add remaining ingredients. Bring to a boil. Reduce heat. Simmer 1 to 2 hours until grains are tender.

8 SERVINGS

Each with: 392 Calories (21% from Fat, 16% from Protein, 63% from Carb); 16 g Protein; 9 g Total Fat; 2 g Saturated Fat; 5 g Monounsaturated Fat; 2 g Polyunsaturated Fat; 63 g Carb; 14 g Fiber; 4 g Sugar; 304 mg Phosphorus; 114 mg Calcium; 912 mg Sodium; 755 mg Potassium; 2041 IU Vitamin A; 0 mg ATE Vitamin E; 15 mg Vitamin C; 0 mg Cholesterol

Ragin' Cajun Catfish Stew

This stew is the kind of warming meal that tastes great at the end of a cold day. You can vary the heat from mild to hot based on the amount of Tabasco sauce you add. The fish and vegetables are low in calories, so you get a generous portion and tons of nutrition.

2 pounds (900 g) catfish
1 cup (160 g) onion, diced
1 cup (150 g) red bell pepper, diced
1 cup (150 g) green bell pepper, diced
½ cup (50 g) celery, sliced
8 ounces (225 g) no-salt-added tomato sauce
2 cups (360 g) no-salt-added tomatoes, diced
½ teaspoon Worcestershire sauce
2 slices low sodium bacon, diced
1 teaspoon garlic, minced
2 medium potatoes, diced
1 cup (130 g) carrot, diced
¼ teaspoon Tabasco sauce, or to taste
¼ cup (15 g) fresh parsley, chopped

Place fish in soup pot. Cover with water. Simmer until fish is just done (about 20 minutes). Strain, reserving liquid. Flake fish, removing any bones, and set aside. Lightly sauté onion and garlic with bacon until lightly browned. Add fish broth, red and green bell pepper, celery, carrot, potatoes, tomato sauce, tomatoes, and seasoning to taste. Simmer for at least one hour. Add fish and cook a few minutes longer. Serve in bowls. Sprinkle parsley on top.

6 SERVINGS

Each with: 377 Calories (31% from Fat, 31% from Protein, 38% from Carb); 29 g Protein; 13 g Total Fat; 3 g Saturated Fat; 6 g Monounsaturated Fat; 3 g Polyunsaturated Fat; 36 g Carb; 6 g Fiber; 8 g Sugar; 447 mg Phosphorus; 86 mg Calcium; 353 mg Sodium; 1570 mg Potassium; 4020 IU Vitamin A; 23 mg ATE Vitamin E; 102 mg Vitamin C; 74 mg Cholesterol

Tuna and Cauliflower Chowder

This chowder makes a nice warm meal on a cool evening, and it's the kind of thing you can throw together quickly when you haven't planned something for dinner. It's thick and creamy and tastes rich, but it is in fact low in calories and high in nutrition.

2 cups (475 ml) water

2 cups (475 ml) low sodium chicken broth

6 potatoes, diced

14 ounces (390 g) tuna, water packed

½ cup (61 g) carrot, sliced

½ cup (50 g) celery, sliced

½ cup (80 g) onion, diced

½ cup (82 g) frozen corn

1½ cups (150 g) cauliflower, finely chopped

½ teaspoon dried basil

½ teaspoon dill weed

1 tablespoon (1 g) dried parsley

½ cup (120 ml) skim milk

In a large saucepan, mix broth with water. Add potatoes and simmer 10 to 15 minutes until tender. Remove cooked potatoes from broth, reserving liquid. Puree cooked potatoes with ¼ cup (60 ml) broth. Add tuna, vegetables, seasonings, and pureed potatoes to remaining broth in saucepan. Simmer 8 to 10 minutes until vegetables are tender. Stir in skim milk and heat to serving temperature without boiling.

6 SERVINGS

Each with: 402 Calories (7% from Fat, 26% from Protein, 67% from Carb); 26 g Protein; 3 g Total Fat; 1 g Saturated Fat; 1 g Monounsaturated Fat; 1 g Polyunsaturated Fat; 68 g Carb; 8 g Fiber; 6 g Sugar; 444 mg Phosphorus; 100 mg Calcium; 115 mg Sodium; 2094 mg Potassium; 1476 IU Vitamin A; 16 mg ATE Vitamin E; 90 mg Vitamin C; 28 mg Cholesterol

Italian Clam Soup

This is a deliciously flavored clam soup, with an Italian orientation. Like much seafood, clams are naturally high in protein and low in fat and calories. This soup adds vegetables and pasta for a filling taste treat.

2 slices low sodium bacon, chopped
½ cup (80 g) onion, chopped
2 cups (475 ml) water
2 cups (240 g) zucchini, diced
2 cups (510 g) no-salt-added stewed tomatoes, undrained, cut up
8 ounces (225 ml) clam juice
8 ounces (225 g) whole wheat orzo, uncooked
½ teaspoon dried basil
12 ounces (340 g) minced clams, undrained

Cook bacon in large nonstick saucepan over medium heat until browned. Remove bacon from saucepan with slotted spoon. Drain on paper towels. Set aside. Add onion to bacon drippings. Cook and stir over medium heat for 1 to 2 minutes or until tender. Add water, zucchini, tomatoes, and clam juice. Bring to a boil. Add orzo and basil and mix well. Reduce heat. Simmer 10 to 15 minutes or until orzo is tender, stirring occasionally. Stir in clams. Cook about 3 minutes or until thoroughly heated, stirring occasionally. Sprinkle each serving with bacon.

4 SERVINGS

Each with: 414 Calories (10% from Fat, 31% from Protein, 59% from Carb); 33 g Protein; 5 g Total Fat; 1 g Unsaturated Fat; 1 g Monounsaturated Fat; 1 g Polyunsaturated Fat; 63 g Carb; 2 g Fiber; 6 g Sugar; 531 mg Phosphorus; 160 mg Calcium; 631 mg Sodium; 1025 mg Potassium; 839 IU Vitamin A; 146 mg ATE Vitamin E; 33 mg Vitamin C; 61 mg Cholesterol

Split Pea and Kielbasa Soup

Turkey kielbasa helps to hold down the calories and fat in this hearty soup. Extra vegetables like spinach up the nutrition even more. And the split peas provide over half your daily fiber in one bowl.

8 ounces (225 g) turkey kielbasa, cut in ½-inch (1.3 cm) slices, then halved

4 cups (950 ml) low sodium chicken broth

4 cups (950 ml) water

1 cup (225 g) split peas, picked over and rinsed

1 cup (200 g) pearl barley

¾ cup (120 g) onion, coarsely chopped

¾ cup (75 g) celery, chopped

¾ teaspoons dried thyme

1 pound (455 g) fresh spinach, rinsed, thick stems removed, leaves torn

Cook kielbasa in a 4- to 5-quart (3.8 to 4.7 L) pot over medium-high heat for 5 to 7 minutes, stirring often, until lightly browned. Remove to a small bowl. Add broth, water, split peas, barley, onion, celery, and thyme to pot. Bring to a boil. Reduce heat and simmer, uncovered 40 to 45 minutes until barley is tender. Stir in kielbasa and spinach and cook 3 to 4 minutes until spinach is wilted.

5 SERVINGS

Each with: 354 Calories (25% from Fat, 22% from Protein, 54% from Carb); 20 g Protein; 10 g Total Fat; 3 g Unsaturated Fat; 4 g Monounsaturated Fat; 2 g Polyunsaturated Fat; 50 g Carb; 12 g Fiber; 3 g Sugar; 240 mg Phosphorus; 134 mg Calcium; 697 mg Sodium; 1008 mg Potassium; 8605 IU Vitamin A; 0 mg ATE Vitamin E; 35 mg Vitamin C; 32 mg Cholesterol

Hearty Pea Soup

Here's something that's a little more than most split pea soups, with turnips and lots of other vegetables adding more than the usual substance and flavor.

1 cup (225 g) yellow split peas

1 cup (225 g) green split peas

7 cups (1.6 L) cold water

2 cups (244 g) carrot, sliced

2 cups (300 g) turnip, diced

2 cups (320 g) onion, chopped

1 cup (100 g) celery, chopped

½ cup (95 g) brown rice

¾ pound (340 g) ham

Sort and rinse peas. Add cold water and bring to boil. Cook for 1 hour. Add vegetables and rice and cook for 1 additional hour. Cut ham into small cubes and add for last 20 minutes of cooking.

6 SERVINGS

Each with: 390 Calories (13% from Fat, 30% from Protein, 57% from Carb); 30 g Protein; 6 g Total Fat; 2 g Saturated Fat; 3 g Monounsaturated Fat; 1 g Polyunsaturated Fat; 56 g Carb; 20 g Fiber; 12 g Sugar; 418 mg Phosphorus; 95 mg Calcium; 697 mg Sodium; 1197 mg Potassium; 5324 IU Vitamin A; 0 mg ATE Vitamin E; 17 mg Vitamin C; 23 mg Cholesterol

Jamaican Split Pea Soup

This is an island version of split pea soup, with curry powder kicking up the flavor.
Pork also adds flavor and vegetables make it healthier.

1½ pound (680 g) boneless pork
loin roast

1 cup (225 g) green split peas,
rinsed and drained

1½ cups (195 g) carrot, finely
chopped

1 cup (100 g) celery, finely
chopped

1½ cups (240 g) onion, finely
chopped

6 cups (1.4 L) low sodium
chicken broth

2 teaspoons curry powder

½ teaspoon paprika

½ teaspoon ground cumin

¼ teaspoon black pepper

4 cups (120 g) fresh spinach, torn

Trim fat from pork and cut pork into ½-inch (1.3 cm) pieces.
Combine split peas, carrot, celery, and onion in Dutch oven.
Stir in broth, curry powder, paprika, cumin, and black pepper.
Stir in pork. Cover. Cook and simmer until pork is tender and
peas are soft, about 1 hour. Stir in spinach and cook for 10
minutes more.

6 SERVINGS

Each with: 361 Calories (21% from Fat, 42% from Protein, 37% from Carb);
39 g Protein; 9 g Total Fat; 3 g Saturated Fat; 3 g Monounsaturated Fat; 1 g
Polyunsaturated Fat; 35 g Carb; 15 g Fiber; 7 g Sugar; 449 mg Phosphorus; 250 mg
Calcium; 219 mg Sodium; 1413 mg Potassium; 19 390 IU Vitamin A; 2 mg ATE
Vitamin E; 9 mg Vitamin C; 62 mg Cholesterol

Pasta e Fagioli (That's a Good Thing)

In Italian, that means pasta and beans. This traditional Italian soup is full of the kind of vegetables that Italians love. This version uses whole wheat pasta to up the nutrition even more.

1½ cups (323 g) dried navy beans
6 cups (1.4 L) water
½ pound (225 g) whole wheat pasta
3 tablespoons (45 ml) olive oil
1 cup (160 g) onion, chopped
1 cup (122 g) carrot, sliced
1 cup (100 g) celery, sliced
½ teaspoon garlic, crushed
2 cups (360 g) tomatoes, peeled and diced
1 teaspoon dried sage
½ teaspoon dried oregano
¼ teaspoon black pepper

In large bowl, combine beans with 6 cups (1.4 L) cold water. Refrigerate overnight. Next day, pour beans and water into 6-quart (5.7 L) kettle. Bring to a boil, reduce heat, and simmer covered, about 3 hours or until beans are tender. Stir several times during cooking. Drain, reserving about 2 cups (475 ml) of liquid. Cook pasta. Heat oil in a large skillet. Sauté onion, carrot, celery, and garlic until soft (about 20 minutes). Do not brown. Add tomato, sage, oregano, and black pepper. Cover and cook over medium heat, 15 minutes. In large saucepan or kettle, combine beans, pasta, and sautéed vegetables. Add 1½ cups (355 ml) of reserved bean liquid. Bring to a boil, cover, and simmer 35 to 40 minutes, stirring several times and adding more liquid if needed.

6 SERVINGS

Each with: 398 Calories (18% from Fat, 17% from Protein, 65% from Carb); 18 g Protein; 8 g Total Fat; 1 g Saturated Fat; 5 g Monounsaturated Fat; 1 g Polyunsaturated Fat; 67 g Carb; 18 g Fiber; 5 g Sugar; 360 mg Phosphorus; 126 mg Calcium; 45 mg Sodium; 955 mg Potassium; 3084 IU Vitamin A; 0 mg ATE Vitamin E; 12 mg Vitamin C; 0 mg Cholesterol

Harvest Moon Vegetable Soup

This soup is full of flavor from the garden, with a fiber and nutrition boost from canned beans. It cooks quickly, making it easy to prepare when you get home from work.

1 tablespoon (15 ml) olive oil

2 cups (320 g) onion, chopped

1½ cups (183 g) carrot, thinly sliced

1 cup (100 g) celery, thinly sliced

1 teaspoon garlic, minced

2 teaspoons Italian seasoning

6 cups (1.4 L) low sodium chicken broth

3 cups (700 ml) low sodium tomato juice

¼ pound (115 g) green beans

1 bay leaf

⅛ teaspoon black pepper

2 cups (512 g) kidney beans, drained

2 cups (524 g) navy beans, drained

2 cups (240 g) yellow squash, coarsely chopped

 Tip: If you have other fresh vegetables, such as tomatoes or zucchini, they make a great addition.

In 6-quart (5.7 L) Dutch oven over medium heat, cook onion, carrot, and celery with garlic and Italian seasoning in hot oil until vegetables are tender. Stir in remaining ingredients except kidney beans, navy beans, and squash. Heat to boiling. Reduce heat to low; simmer 30 minutes. Add beans and squash and cook 5 minutes more or until squash is tender. Remove bay leaf before serving.

8 SERVINGS

Each with: 427 Calories (8% from Fat, 25% from Protein, 67% from Carb); 28 g Protein; 4 g Total Fat; 1 g Saturated Fat; 2 g Monounsaturated Fat; 1 g Polyunsaturated Fat; 74 g Carb; 27 g Fiber; 9 g Sugar; 527 mg Phosphorus; 200 mg Calcium; 349 mg Sodium; 1852 mg Potassium; 4544 IU Vitamin A; 0 mg ATE Vitamin E; 41 mg Vitamin C; 0 mg Cholesterol

Italian Sausage and Bean Soup

This is a hearty Italian-style soup full of good things for you. It's the kind of thing I particularly like in cold weather.

½ pound (225 g) Italian sausage

½ teaspoon garlic, minced

1 cup (160 g) onion, chopped

⅓ cup (20 g) fresh parsley, chopped

¾ cup (92 g) carrot, sliced

1 cup (70 g) mushrooms, sliced

2 cups (480 g) garbanzo beans

3 cups (700 ml) low sodium beef broth

½ teaspoon dried sage

½ teaspoon black pepper

Crumble sausage and cook in 3-quart (2.8 L) saucepan over medium-high heat, stirring often, until browned. Add garlic, onion, parsley, carrot, and mushrooms. Cook until limp. Add beans and remaining ingredients. Bring to a boil and then lower heat and simmer covered, about 10 minutes. Skim off excess fat.

4 SERVINGS

Each with: 385 Calories (46% from Fat, 18% from Protein, 36% from Carb); 17 g Protein; 20 g Total Fat; 7 g Saturated Fat; 9 g Monounsaturated Fat; 3 g Polyunsaturated Fat; 35 g Carb; 7 g Fiber; 3 g Sugar; 250 mg Phosphorus; 87 mg Calcium; 900 mg Sodium; 670 mg Potassium; 3345 IU Vitamin A; 0 mg ATE Vitamin E; 17 mg Vitamin C; 43 mg Cholesterol

Hearty Turkey, Vegetable, and Bean Stew

This hearty soup will fill you up and warm you. Full of protein and other nutrients, high in fiber, and easy to fix by using packaged coleslaw mix, there is a lot to like here.

1 cup (160 g) onion, chopped

½ teaspoon garlic, minced

1¼ pounds (570 g) lean ground turkey

2 tablespoons (9 g) poultry seasoning

16 ounces (455 g) coleslaw mix

28 ounces (785 g) no-salt-added stewed tomatoes

40 ounces (1.1 kg) no-salt-added tomatoes

4 ounces (115 g) green chilies, chopped

15 ounces (425 g) black beans, drained

15 ounces (425 g) red kidney beans, drained

46 ounces (1.4 L) tomato juice, low sodium

 Tip: This is also great made with leftover roast turkey.

Sauté onion and garlic until tender in a large stock pot. Add fresh ground turkey and brown. Add remaining ingredients to the large stock pot. Simmer for 1 hour, stirring frequently.

6 SERVINGS

Each with: 410 Calories (7% from Fat, 36% from Protein, 58% from Carb); 38 g Protein; 3 g Total Fat; 1 g Unsaturated Fat; 0 g Monounsaturated Fat; 1 g Polyunsaturated Fat; 62 g Carb; 16 g Fiber; 26 g Sugar; 530 mg Phosphorus; 264 mg Calcium; 1166 mg Sodium; 2360 mg Potassium; 1653 IU Vitamin A; 0 mg ATE Vitamin E; 112 mg Vitamin C; 57 mg Cholesterol

Nicely Spiced Black Bean and Pork Stew

Cumin and cilantro give this stew a Southwestern flavor, while beans and squash provide a contrast in tastes and textures. This recipe gives you a great value in flavor, nutrition, and volume for being less than 400 calories.

4 cups (950 ml) water

¾ cup (188 g) black beans, dried

2 ancho chilies

1 pound (455 g) boneless pork loin

1½ cups (270 g) tomatoes, chopped

½ cup (80 g) onion, chopped

½ cup (120 ml) dry red wine

1 teaspoon dried sage

1 teaspoon marjoram

½ teaspoon ground cumin

¼ teaspoon cinnamon

½ teaspoon garlic, minced

2 cups (280 g) butternut squash, peeled and cubed

1 cup (150 g) red bell pepper, diced

2 tablespoons (2 g) fresh cilantro, chopped

Heat water, beans, and chilies to boiling in Dutch oven. Boil uncovered 2 minutes. Remove from heat. Cover and let stand 1 hour. Remove chilies; reserve. Heat beans to boiling; reduce heat. Simmer covered for 1 hour. Seed and coarsely chop chilies. Trim any fat from pork. Cut pork into 1-inch (2.5 cm) cubes. Stir pork, chilies, and remaining ingredients except squash, red bell pepper, and cilantro into beans. Heat to boiling; reduce heat. Cover and simmer 30 minutes, stirring occasionally. Stir in squash. Cover and simmer 30 minutes, stirring occasionally, until squash is tender. Stir in red bell pepper and cilantro. Cover and simmer about 5 minutes or until red bell pepper is crisp-tender.

4 SERVINGS

Each with: 377 Calories (38% from Fat, 31% from Protein, 31% from Carb); 28 g Protein; 16 g Total Fat; 5 g Saturated Fat; 7 g Monounsaturated Fat; 2 g Polyunsaturated Fat; 28 g Carb; 8 g Fiber; 4 g Sugar; 345 mg Phosphorus; 96 mg Calcium; 77 mg Sodium; 1252 mg Potassium; 10 816 IU Vitamin A; 2 mg ATE Vitamin E; 103 mg Vitamin C; 71 mg Cholesterol

Spicy Mexican Bean Soup

This is bean soup with a Mexican kick. Start with our healthier refried beans, add some Mexican flavor and a nice sprinkling of toppings, and you'll get not only most of your day's fiber needs in one bowl, but a filling soup that may become the new standard for bean soup in your house.

2 cups (476 g) refried beans, see recipe in chapter 14
4 ounces (115 g) green chilies, chopped
1 teaspoon ground cumin
½ teaspoon garlic powder
1 cup (235 ml) water
1 cup (63 g) tortilla chips, coarsely crushed
2 teaspoons green onion, sliced
1 teaspoon jalapeño pepper, finely chopped

In medium saucepan, combine refried beans, green chilies, cumin, garlic powder, and water. Mix well. Cook over medium heat until mixture just comes to a boil, stirring frequently. Sprinkle each serving with crushed tortilla chips, green onion, and chopped jalapeno pepper.

2 SERVINGS

Each with: 365 Calories (18% from Fat, 17% from Protein, 65% from Carb); 17 g Protein; 8 g Total Fat; 2 g Unsaturated Fat; 4 g Monounsaturated Fat; 2 g Polyunsaturated Fat; 66 g Carb; 16 g Fiber; 3 g Sugar; 335 mg Phosphorus; 156 mg Calcium; 1046 mg Sodium; 898 mg Potassium; 475 IU Vitamin A; 0 mg ATE Vitamin E; 55 mg Vitamin C; 21 mg Cholesterol

Warm and Filling Barley and Lentil Soup

This meatless soup contains so many other good things that you won't even miss the meat. It is truly a meal in a bowl, full of taste, nutrition, and the kind of ingredients that will satisfy you without a lot of calories.

2 tablespoons (28 ml) olive oil

2 cups (320 g) onion, chopped

1 teaspoon garlic, minced

1½ cups (183 g) carrot, sliced

1 cup (100 g) celery, sliced

1½ cups (225 g) red bell pepper, sliced

¼ cup (14 g) sun-dried tomatoes, drained and chopped

2 teaspoons dried basil

1 teaspoon dried oregano

6 cups (1.4 L) low sodium beef broth

2 cups (360 g) no-salt-added tomatoes, whole

2 tablespoons (32 g) no-salt-added tomato paste

1½ cups (300 g) pearl barley

1½ cups (288 g) lentils

½ teaspoon black pepper

Heat oil in a large Dutch oven over medium-high heat. Add onion and sauté until translucent. Add next 7 ingredients and cook until red bell pepper just softens, about 5 minutes. Mix in the broth, tomatoes, and tomato paste. Bring to a boil. Stir in barley and lentils. Reduce heat and simmer until barley and lentils are tender, stirring occasionally, about 1½ hours. Season to taste with black pepper.

6 SERVINGS

Each with: 357 Calories (18% from Fat, 17% from Protein, 66% from Carb); 16 g Protein; 7 g Total Fat; 1 g Saturated Fat; 4 g Monounsaturated Fat; 1 g Polyunsaturated Fat; 61 g Carb; 16 g Fiber; 10 g Sugar; 310 mg Phosphorus; 109 mg Calcium; 213 mg Sodium; 1154 mg Potassium; 5404 IU Vitamin A; 0 mg ATE Vitamin E; 95 mg Vitamin C; 0 mg Cholesterol

Winter's Night Lentil Barley Soup

Warm and filling, this is true comfort food. Easy to fix and hearty,
it will become a favorite.

¾ cup (120 g) onion, chopped
¾ cup (75 g) celery, chopped
½ teaspoon garlic, minced
2 tablespoons (28 ml) olive oil
28 ounces (785 g) no-salt-added
  tomatoes, cut up, undrained
¾ cup (144 g) lentils, rinsed and
  drained
¾ cup (150 g) pearl barley
6 cups (1.4 L) low sodium
  vegetable broth
½ teaspoon dried rosemary
½ teaspoon dried oregano
¼ teaspoon black pepper
1 cup (122 g) carrot, sliced

In 4-quart (3.8 L) Dutch oven, cook onion, celery, and garlic in oil until tender. Add tomatoes, lentils, barley, broth, rosemary, oregano, and black pepper. Bring to boil; reduce heat. Cover and simmer 45 minutes. Add carrot and simmer for 15 minute or more until carrots are tender.

5 SERVINGS

Each with: 370 Calories (31% from Fat, 10% from Protein, 59% from Carb); 10 g Protein; 13 g Total Fat; 3 g Unsaturated Fat; 7 g Monounsaturated Fat; 3 g Polyunsaturated Fat; 57 g Carb; 11 g Fiber; 8 g Sugar; 236 mg Phosphorus; 123 mg Calcium; 220 mg Sodium; 836 mg Potassium; 3396 IU Vitamin A; 0 mg ATE Vitamin E; 32 mg Vitamin C; 0 mg Cholesterol

Lentil and Brown Rice Soup

You can't get a more hardy soup than this for less than 400 calories. Full of chicken, lentils,
brown rice, and lots of veggies, it will warm you up and keep you full.

⅓ cup (64 g) lentils
⅔ cup (127 g) brown rice, uncooked
1 potato, peeled and diced
½ cup (50 g) celery, diced
1 cup (122 g) carrot, sliced thin
8 ounces (225 g) mushrooms, sliced
½ cup (80 g) onion, diced
1 pound (455 g) boneless skinless
  chicken breast, uncooked, diced
4 cups (950 ml) low sodium
  chicken broth
¼ teaspoon black pepper

Mix all ingredients together in slow cooker and cook on low for 8 to 10 hours.

4 SERVINGS

Each with: 399 Calories (9% from Fat, 39% from Protein, 52% from Carb); 39 g Protein; 4 g Total Fat; 1 g Unsaturated Fat; 1 g Monounsaturated Fat; 1 g Polyunsaturated Fat; 52 g Carb; 6 g Fiber; 5 g Sugar; 549 mg Phosphorus; 62 mg Calcium; 191 mg Sodium; 1382 mg Potassium; 3951 IU Vitamin A; 7 mg ATE Vitamin E; 16 mg Vitamin C; 66 mg Cholesterol

A Taste of North Africa Soup

With flavors of the cuisine of Morocco or other countries in northwest Africa, this hearty soup full of beef and vegetables is sure to please. But the use of a lean cut of beef and vegetables with high nutrient density keeps the calorie count low.

2 tablespoons (28 ml) extra virgin olive oil

1 cup (160 g) onion, finely diced

2 teaspoons turmeric

1 pound (455 g) beef round steak, cut into ½-inch (1.3 cm) cubes

6 cups (1.4 L) low sodium beef broth, or water

2 cups (360 g) no-salt-added tomatoes, diced

2 small turnips, peeled and diced

½ cup (65 g) carrot, diced

½ cup (50 g) celery, leaves included, thinly sliced

¼ cup (15 g) fresh parsley, whole sprigs

¼ cup (4 g) fresh cilantro, whole sprigs

1½ cups (180 g) zucchini, peeled and cut into ¼-inch (6 mm) dice

4 ounces (115 g) whole wheat spaghetti, broken into small pieces

½ teaspoon black pepper, fresh ground

additional fresh parsley and/or cilantro for garnish, if desired

Heat oil in a Dutch oven over medium-high heat. Add onion and turmeric; stir to coat. Add meat and cook, stirring occasionally, until the onion is tender, 4 to 5 minutes. Add broth, tomatoes and their juice, turnips, carrot, and celery. Tie parsley and cilantro sprigs together with kitchen string and add to the pot. Bring the soup to a boil. Cover and reduce to a simmer. Cook until the meat is tender, 45 to 50 minutes. Stir in zucchini and cook, covered, until soft, 8 to 10 minutes. Add pasta and cook until soft, 4 to 10 minutes, depending on the type of pasta. Discard the parsley and cilantro sprigs. Season with black pepper. Serve sprinkled with fresh parsley and/or cilantro leaves, if desired.

4 SERVINGS

Each with: 418 Calories (26% from Fat, 35% from Protein, 39% from Carb); 38 g Protein; 12 g Total Fat; 3 g Unsaturated Fat; 7 g Monounsaturated Fat; 1 g Polyunsaturated Fat; 41 g Carb; 8 g Fiber; 11 g Sugar; 466 mg Phosphorus; 159 mg Calcium; 391 mg Sodium; 1463 mg Potassium; 2737 IU Vitamin A; 0 mg ATE Vitamin E; 54 mg Vitamin C; 52 mg Cholesterol

African Style Groundnut Stew

Groundnut means peanut, a typical North African ingredient. The other key point about North African cooking is it tends to be quite spicy. I didn't add as much red pepper as would have been needed to make it authentic, but feel free to add either more or less depending on your taste.

1½ cups (355 ml) low sodium chicken broth

1 cup (100 g) celery, thinly sliced

1 cup (160 g) onion, thinly sliced

1 cup (150 g) red bell pepper, sliced

1 cup (150 g) green bell pepper, sliced

4 boneless skinless chicken breast, skinned

½ cup (130 g) chunky peanut butter

¼ teaspoon red pepper flakes

2 sweet potatoes, peeled and cubed

Combine broth, celery, onion, red and green bell pepper, and sweet potatoes in slow cooker. Spread peanut butter over both sides of chicken pieces. Sprinkle with red pepper flakes. Place on top of ingredients in slow cooker. Cover. Cook on low for 5 to 6 hours.

4 SERVINGS

Each with: 377 Calories (41% from Fat, 28% from Protein, 31% from Carb); 26 g Protein; 17 g Total Fat; 3 g Saturated Fat; 8 g Monounsaturated Fat; 5 g Polyunsaturated Fat; 29 g Carb; 6 g Fiber; 12 g Sugar; 300 mg Phosphorus; 69 mg Calcium; 159 mg Sodium; 875 mg Potassium; 13 406 IU Vitamin A; 4 mg ATE Vitamin E; 115 mg Vitamin C; 41 mg Cholesterol

Back to the Islands Caribbean Fish Stew

This is a fairly spicy stew if you use the habañero pepper. I use a jalapeño instead, which still gives you some heat but in moderation.

½ cup (61 g) carrot, sliced

1 cup (160 g) onion, sliced

1 cup (150 g) red bell pepper, sliced

½ teaspoon garlic, minced

1 teaspoon ground ginger

½ teaspoon ground cloves

½ teaspoon allspice

½ teaspoon cardamom

⅓ teaspoon turmeric

2 teaspoons coriander

4 cups (720 g) no-salt-added tomatoes

12 ounces (355 ml) beer

1 habañero pepper, whole

2 medium potatoes, diced

1 pound (455 g) tilapia fillets, cut into 2-inch (5 cm) pieces

1 tablespoon (1 g) fresh cilantro, chopped

½ cup (120 ml) lime juice

Sauté the carrot, onion, and red bell pepper until slightly soft and then add in the ginger and garlic. When it's nice and soft, add the spices and sauté about 1 minute longer. Then add the tomatoes and beer. Bring to a boil. Add the habañero pepper. Reduce the heat, let it simmer for 20 minutes, and then add the potatoes. When the potatoes are tender, add the fish. Cook about another 5 minutes. Then add the cilantro and lime juice. Stir and serve.

4 SERVINGS

Each with: 395 Calories (9% from Fat, 34% from Protein, 58% from Carb); 31 g Protein; 4 g Total Fat; 1 g Saturated Fat; 1 g Monounsaturated Fat; 1 g Polyunsaturated Fat; 53 g Carb; 7 g Fiber; 14 g Sugar; 449 mg Phosphorus; 173 mg Calcium; 115 mg Sodium; 2151 mg Potassium; 3709 IU Vitamin A; 53 mg ATE Vitamin E; 140 mg Vitamin C; 36 mg Cholesterol

A Healthier Kind of Chili

This is a healthier version of chili that doesn't suffer at all in the taste department. It's low in fat, high in fiber, but still just as tasty and full of nutrition. It also cooks a lot quicker than most chili recipes, letting you fix it when you get home from work.

---

1 pound (455 g) ground turkey

4 cups (684 g) pinto beans, undrained

18 ounces (510 g) no-salt-added tomato sauce

6 ounces (170 g) no-salt-added tomato paste

2 cups (475 ml) low sodium tomato juice

2 tablespoons (16 g) chili powder

1 teaspoon ground cumin

1 teaspoon cinnamon

½ cup (50 g) bulgur

Brown turkey and drain. Add remaining ingredients. Simmer ½ hour. Stir often.

6 SERVINGS

Each with: 408 Calories (12% from Fat, 36% from Protein, 52% from Carb); 37 g Protein; 6 g Total Fat; 2 g Saturated Fat; 1 g Monounsaturated Fat; 2 g Polyunsaturated Fat; 54 g Carb; 16 g Fiber; 10 g Sugar; 423 mg Phosphorus; 117 mg Calcium; 348 mg Sodium; 1417 mg Potassium; 2732 IU Vitamin A; 0 mg ATE Vitamin E; 42 mg Vitamin C; 58 mg Cholesterol

Warm and Filling White Chili

White chili is made with chicken and white beans and without the typical tomatoes. This tends to give it a more subtle flavor than tomato chili, which many people seem to prefer once they've tried it. Our version here has added vegetables to make it a more filling meal.

1 pound (455 g) navy beans

6 boneless skinless chicken breast

1 tablespoon (15 ml) olive oil

1½ cups (240 g) onion, chopped

1 teaspoon garlic cloves, minced

¼ cup (36 g) green chili peppers, chopped

1½ cups (225 g) green bell pepper, chopped

1½ cups (183 g) carrot, sliced

2 teaspoons ground cumin

1½ teaspoons dried oregano

¼ teaspoon ground cloves

¼ teaspoon cayenne pepper

6 cups (1.4 L) low sodium chicken broth

2 cups (230 g) low fat Monterey Jack cheese, grated

½ cup (115 g) fat-free sour cream

½ cup (130 g) salsa

¼ cup (4 g) fresh cilantro, chopped

Place beans in a heavy large pot. Add enough cold water to cover by at least 3 inches (7.5 cm) and soak overnight. Place chicken in heavy large saucepan. Add cold water to cover and bring to simmer. Cook until just tender, about 15 minutes. Drain and cool. Cut chicken into cubes. Drain beans. Heat oil in same pot over medium-high heat. Add onion and sauté until translucent, about 10 minutes. Stir in garlic, green chilies, green bell pepper, carrot, cumin, oregano, cloves, and cayenne pepper and sauté 2 minutes. Add beans and broth and bring to boil. Reduce heat and simmer until beans are very tender, stirring occasionally, about 2 hours. Add chicken and 1 cup (115 g) cheese to chili and stir until cheese melts. Serve with remaining cheese, sour cream, salsa, and cilantro.

6 SERVINGS

Each with: 391 Calories (25% from Fat, 41% from Protein, 35% from Carb); 40 g Protein; 11 g Total Fat; 5 g Saturated Fat; 4 g Monounsaturated Fat; 1 g Polyunsaturated Fat; 34 g Carb; 7 g Fiber; 4 g Sugar; 598 mg Phosphorus; 312 mg Calcium; 446 mg Sodium; 983 mg Potassium; 4354 IU Vitamin A; 51 mg ATE Vitamin E; 39 mg Vitamin C; 58 mg Cholesterol

Chili for a Chilly Night

This is a great low fat chili featuring ground turkey and black beans.
It makes a mild chili, but you can easily add more chili powder or
some red pepper flakes to spice it up.

1 pound (455 g) ground turkey

1 tablespoon (15 ml) olive oil

½ onion, chopped

½ green bell pepper, seeded and chopped

2 cloves garlic, minced

4 cups (688 g) black beans, no-salt-added, rinsed and drained

1 can (14½ ounces, or 410 g) no-salt-added stewed tomatoes

1 can (8 ounces, or 225 g) no-salt-added tomato sauce

1 cup (235 ml) dark beer, or low sodium beef broth

1 tablespoon (8 g) chili powder

1 tablespoon (7 g) ground cumin

1 teaspoon ground coriander

1 teaspoon dried oregano

Heat large heavy saucepan or Dutch oven to medium high. Brown the meat until done. Drain meat and set aside. In the skillet, add the oil and bring to medium heat. Add the onion, green bell pepper, and garlic and cook until vegetables are tender, about 5 to 6 minutes. Return meat to pan. Add remaining ingredients. Bring chili to a boil; then reduce heat and simmer for 30 to 45 minutes or until thickened, stirring occasionally. Taste and adjust seasonings if necessary.

6 SERVINGS

Each with: 394 Calories (17% from Fat, 37% from Protein, 46% from Carb); 36 g Protein; 7 g Total Fat; 2 g Saturated Fat; 3 g Monounsaturated Fat; 2 g Polyunsaturated Fat; 44 g Carb; 15 g Fiber; 7 g Sugar; 392 mg Phosphorus; 123 mg Calcium; 109 mg Sodium; 1354 mg Potassium; 1100 IU Vitamin A; 0 mg ATE Vitamin E; 17 mg Vitamin C; 60 mg Cholesterol

Chock Full of Vegetables Chili

The flavor definitely says chili, but the ingredients are not what you would usually expect.
A wide assortment of vegetables join the beans for a warming, filling, flavorful bowl.

1 cup (184 g) kidney beans, dried
4 cups (950 ml) water
½ cup (50 g) bulgur
¼ cup (60 ml) olive oil
1 cup (160 g) red onion, diced
1 cup (160 g) onion, diced
1½ tablespoons (15 g) garlic, minced
1 cup (100 g) celery, sliced
1 cup (122 g) carrot, sliced
2 tablespoons chili powder
2 tablespoons (14 g) ground cumin
½ teaspoon cayenne pepper
1 tablespoon (3 g) fresh basil
1 tablespoon (4 g) fresh oregano
1 cup (120 g) yellow squash, cubed
1 cup (120 g) zucchini, cubed
1 cup (150 g) green bell pepper, cubed
1 cup (150 g) red bell pepper, cubed
8 ounces (225 g) mushrooms, sliced
4 cups (720 g) no-salt-added tomatoes, diced
½ (130 g) cup no-salt-added tomato paste
¾ cup (175 ml) white wine, dry
black pepper, to taste

Soak beans in cold water to cover overnight. Drain off water. Add 3 cups (700 ml) fresh water to beans and cook over medium heat until tender, about 45 minutes. Drain beans, reserving cooking liquid. Bring 1 cup (235 ml) water to boil. Pour over bulgur in bowl. Let stand 30 minutes to soften wheat (the water will be absorbed). Heat olive oil in large saucepan. Add red and white onion and sauté until tender. Add garlic, celery, and carrot. Sauté until softened. Add chili powder, cumin, cayenne pepper, basil, and oregano. Cook over low heat until carrots are almost tender. Add squash, zucchini, red and green bell pepper, and mushrooms and cook 4 minutes. Stir in bulgur, kidney beans, tomatoes, and reserved cooking liquid from beans. Cook 30 minutes or until vegetables are tender. Mix tomato paste with white wine until smooth and then stir into vegetable mixture. Season with black pepper to taste.

6 SERVINGS

Each with: 371 Calories (26% from Fat, 16% from Protein, 58% from Carb); 15 g Protein; 11 g Total Fat; 2 g Saturated Fat; 7 g Monounsaturated Fat; 2 g Polyunsaturated Fat; 55 g Carb; 17 g Fiber; 15 g Sugar; 322 mg Phosphorus; 190 mg Calcium; 115 mg Sodium; 1718 mg Potassium; 5046 IU Vitamin A; 0 mg ATE Vitamin E; 112 mg Vitamin C; 0 mg Cholesterol

It May Sound Funny Zucchini Chili

This is an unusual chili, with vegetables such as zucchini and mushrooms providing the bulk and taking the place of the meat. But have no fear, the flavor is true to form with a spicy tomato base.

6 cups (720 g) zucchini, shredded
1 cup (100 g) celery, sliced
1 cup (160 g) onion, chopped
3 tablespoons (45 ml) olive oil
15 ounces (425 g) no-salt-added
  tomato sauce
8 ounces (225 g) water
28 ounces (785 g) no-salt-added
  tomatoes
2 tablespoons (16 g) chili powder
1 teaspoon garlic powder
1 teaspoon black pepper
½ teaspoon cayenne pepper
½ cup (70 g) ripe olives, sliced
15 ounces (425 g) kidney beans
4 ounces (115 g) mushrooms,
  sliced

Sauté zucchini, celery, and onion in hot oil in large kettle or saucepan until celery is tender but not browned, about 6 minutes. Add tomato sauce, water, tomatoes and juice, chili powder, garlic powder, and black pepper. Simmer slowly, uncovered, 1 to 1½ hours. Add olives, kidney beans, and mushrooms. Simmer another 10 to 15 minutes.

4 SERVINGS

Each with: 391 Calories (29% from Fat, 17% from Protein, 54% from Carb); 17 g Protein; 14 g Total Fat; 2 g Unsaturated Fat; 9 g Monounsaturated Fat; 2 g Polyunsaturated Fat; 57 g Carb; 19 g Fiber; 17 g Sugar; 347 mg Phosphorus; 224 mg Calcium; 267 mg Sodium; 2094 mg Potassium; 2413 IU Vitamin A; 0 mg ATE Vitamin E; 82 mg Vitamin C; 0 mg Cholesterol

Beef and Bean Chili

Mildly spicy and full of nutrition, this chili has an extra amount of beans, increasing the fiber content.

2 tablespoons (28 ml) olive oil

1 cup (160 g) onion, coarsely
chopped

2 teaspoons garlic, finely chopped

2 tablespoons (16 g) chili powder

1 tablespoon (7 g) ground cumin

¼ teaspoon black pepper

1¼ pound (570 g) beef round
steak, cut into 1-inch (2.5 cm)
cubes

4 cups (720 g) no-salt-added
tomatoes, undrained

4 cups (688 g) black beans,
rinsed and drained

4 ounces (115 g) green chilies,
chopped

½ cup (120 ml) water

Heat oil in 12-inch (30 cm) skillet over medium-high heat. Cook onion and garlic in oil 4 to 5 minutes, stirring frequently, until onions are softened. Stir in chili powder, cumin, black pepper, and beef. Cook 6 to 8 minutes, stirring occasionally, until beef is lightly browned. Place beef mixture in 3- to 4-quart (2.8 to 3.8 L) slow cooker. Stir in tomatoes, black beans, green chilies, and water. Cover and cook on low heat setting 8 to 10 hours. Stir well before serving.

5 SERVINGS

Each with: 385 Calories (26% from Fat, 33% from Protein, 42% from Carb); 32 g Protein; 11 g Total Fat; 2 g Unsaturated Fat; 6 g Monounsaturated Fat; 2 g Polyunsaturated Fat; 41 g Carb; 10 g Fiber; 14 g Sugar; 506 mg Phosphorus; 162 mg Calcium; 1303 mg Sodium; 1621 mg Potassium; 1209 IU Vitamin A; 0 mg ATE Vitamin E; 42 mg Vitamin C; 43 mg Cholesterol

Two Bean Turkey Chili

This makes a big batch of very good chili, so it's a great recipe if you are having guests for dinner. But it also freezes well, so it's good even for a small family. It's a white chili, without tomatoes, featuring low fat ground turkey, lots of vegetables, and two kinds of beans. In other words, it's low in fat and high in fiber and other nutrients.

2 tablespoons (28 ml) olive oil

2 pounds (900 g) ground turkey

1½ cups (240 g) onion, coarsely chopped

1½ cups (150 g) celery, chopped

1 teaspoon garlic, minced

3 teaspoons (7 g) ground cumin

1½ teaspoons dried oregano

4 cups (750 ml) low sodium chicken broth

4 cups (708 g) great northern beans, drained and rinsed

4 cups (684 g) black eyed peas, drained and rinsed

10 ounces (280 g) frozen corn

8 ounces (225 g) green chilies, chopped

2 tablespoons (28 ml) lime juice

Heat oil in 6-quart (5.6 L) saucepan or Dutch oven over medium-high heat until hot. Add turkey, onion, celery, garlic, cumin, and oregano. Mix well. Cook 5 to 6 minutes or until turkey is browned and no longer pink, stirring frequently. Add broth, beans, peas, corn, and chilies. Mix well. Bring to a boil. Reduce heat and simmer 25 to 30 minutes to blend flavors, stirring occasionally. Stir in lime juice.

10 SERVINGS

Each with: 398 Calories (14% from Fat, 38% from Protein, 49% from Carb); 38 g Protein; 6 g Total Fat; 1 g Unsaturated Fat; 3 g Monounsaturated Fat; 1 g Polyunsaturated Fat; 50 g Carb; 11 g Fiber; 6 g Sugar; 483 mg Phosphorus; 109 mg Calcium; 380 mg Sodium; 1200 mg Potassium; 317 IU Vitamin A; 0 mg ATE Vitamin E; 24 mg Vitamin C; 54 mg Cholesterol

Mix and Match Meals

In the recipes so far, you've seen a complete meal in each recipe. In some cases, this has included side dishes and extras that make it a complete meal, one that gives you maximum nutrition while holding the calories around 400. This is the easiest way to get started on a mega meal diet. All of the work of finding the right combination of dishes and ingredients to reach that final product has been done for you.

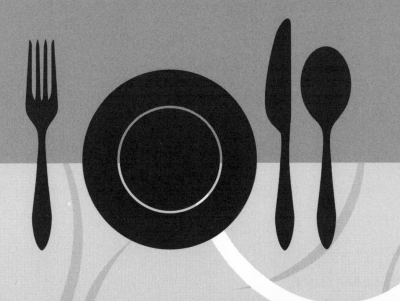

But what if you decide that you really aren't in the mood for that exact combination? That is where the next few chapters come into play. It's sort of like the old choose *one from column A and one from column B*. There are four chapters of recipes, one of main dishes, one of appetizers and side dishes, one of desserts, and one of bread. To get your perfect meal, both in nutrition and calories and in satisfying what you feel like eating, you simply choose. The goal is twofold. First, to help you select a combination of dishes that is exactly what you *like*. But just as important, as we talked about in chapter 1, is to get you thinking about the way 400-calorie mega meals are constructed so that you can be successful in sticking to your diet when you don't have this book and the stove in front of you, for instance when you go out to eat or are at a friend's house. These recipes will help you to understand what you can combine and still stay on your mega diet.

To build your perfect meal, start with chapter 13 and pick a main dish (no, it's not acceptable to just pick four different desserts). Once you've got your main dish take note of how many calories it contains. Most are around 200 calories, give or take a little. But there are some that have fewer and a few that are closer to 300. That figure will guide you in picking things to go with your main dish. The idea is to end up with something close to 400 calories total. Depending on what you pick, that could be a main dish, a couple of side dishes, and a dessert. Or it might be a main dish and some cornbread or a biscuit. Or it could be a main dish, salad, and dessert. There are a lot of possible combinations, and the choice is up to you.

So go take a look and see what appeals to you.

Mix and Match:
Main Dishes

The recipes in this chapter are a starting point for your mix and match 400-calorie meal. There are a variety of dishes with different meats, fish, seafood, and vegetarian options. Use these as a starting point for building your meal, then add things out of chapters 14 through 16 until you are close to 400 calories.

Of course, you don't have to start with a recipe at all. You can also start with just a plain piece of meat. Then you can grill it, broil it, or bake it. Without extras, it will be even lower in calories than many of the recipes in this chapter. Approximate calorie values for different options are below. But keep in mind that if you add oil to cook it in, sauces, and extras other than simple herbs and spices, the calorie count will go up.

Fish: 4 ounce (115 g) serving

Haddock	99 calories
Flounder	103 calories
Tilapia	125 calories
Tuna (water packed)	145 calories
Catfish	153 calories
Tuna steaks	163 calories
Salmon fillets	208 calories

Seafood: 4 ounce (115 g) serving

Crab meat	99 calories
Scallops	100 calories
Shrimp	120 calories
Clams	168 calories

Meat: 4 ounce (115 g) serving

Chicken breast	125 calories
Turkey breast	130 calories
Ground turkey	135 calories
Beef round steak	144 calories
Pork loin chop	145 calories
Pork loin roast	145 calories
Extra lean ground beef	265 calories

Creamy, Dreamy Chicken Breasts

To taste these chicken breasts in their creamy sauce you would think they have to be full
of calories. But the use of boneless skinless breasts and low fat dairy products allows
all that decadence for less than 150 calories.

4 boneless skinless chicken
  breasts
1 cup (230 g) plain low-fat yogurt
¼ cup (60 g) fat-free sour cream
½ teaspoon lime peel, grated
½ teaspoon dried oregano
¼ teaspoon celery seed
¼ teaspoon garlic powder
¼ teaspoon coriander
¼ teaspoon dried parsley
¼ teaspoon dried thyme
3 tablespoons (45 ml) lime juice

Preheat oven to 375°F (190°C, or gas mark 5). Spray roasting
pan with nonstick vegetable oil spray, place chicken breasts in
it, and set aside. Combine all other ingredients. Baste chicken
breasts with mixture and bake for 20 minutes. Remove from
oven. Turn chicken breasts, baste with sauce, and bake 15
minutes longer until meat is tender. Turn off oven. Cover
chicken with foil and let stand in oven 10 minutes. Remove
aluminum foil, arrange chicken breasts on serving dish, and
serve hot with any remaining sauce.

4 SERVINGS

Each with: 142 Calories (24% from Fat, 58% from Protein, 18% from Carb);
20 g Protein; 4 g Total Fat; 2 g Unsaturated Fat; 1 g Monounsaturated Fat; 0 g
Polyunsaturated Fat; 6 g Carb; 0 g Fiber; 5 g Sugar; 245 mg Phosphorus; 143 mg
Calcium; 96 mg Sodium; 366 mg Potassium; 128 IU Vitamin A; 28 mg ATE Vitamin E;
6 mg Vitamin C; 51 mg Cholesterol

Carry Me Away to Hawaii Chicken

This was thrown together the first night we made it when we didn't know what to have for dinner. But now
it gets a regular turn on the menu. It's low in fat and high in nutrition, a great start for a mega meal.

8 ounces (225 g) pineapple
  chunks, drained
¼ cup (85 g) honey
¼ cup (60 ml) red wine vinegar
4 boneless skinless chicken breast
1 cup (150 g) red bell pepper,
  chopped
1 cup (160 g) onion, coarsely
  chopped

Drain pineapple, reserving juice. Combine juice, honey, and
vinegar. Place chicken in an 8 × 13-inch (20 × 33 cm) baking
pan. Sprinkle pineapple and vegetables over top. Pour juice
mixture over chicken. Bake at 350°F (180°C, or gas mark 4)
until chicken is done, about 45 minutes.

4 SERVINGS

Each with: 189 Calories (5% from Fat, 35% from Protein, 60% from Carb);
17 g Protein; 1 g Total Fat; 0 g Saturated Fat; 0 g Monounsaturated Fat; 0 g
Polyunsaturated Fat; 29 g Carb; 2 g Fiber; 26 g Sugar; 164 mg Phosphorus; 30 mg
Calcium; 50 mg Sodium; 415 mg Potassium; 1203 IU Vitamin A; 4 mg ATE Vitamin E;
79 mg Vitamin C; 41 mg Cholesterol

Chicken Florentine

These chicken breasts, cooked with spinach and then covered with a creamy mushroom sauce, make a great company meal. But the easy preparation and great taste make them the kind of thing you can have regularly just for the family too. Add a salad and a slice of bread for a great meal.

4 boneless skinless chicken breast
1 cup (160 g) onion, chopped
1½ pounds (680 g) spinach, torn into bite-sized pieces
2 tablespoons (14 g) Swiss cheese, shredded
⅛ teaspoon nutmeg
8 ounces (225 g) mushrooms, sliced
1 cup (235 ml) skim milk
1 cup (235 ml) low sodium chicken broth
1 tablespoon (14 g) unsalted butter, melted

Flatten chicken to ¼-inch (6 mm). Set aside. Sauté onion in large skillet with coated nonstick vegetable oil spray. Remove from heat and stir in spinach, cheese, and nutmeg. Divide mixture in fourths and shape into mounds. Transfer mounds to a 10 × 6 × 2-inch (25 × 15 × 5 cm) dish coated with cooking spray. Top each portion with a chicken breast half. Bake at 350°F (180°C, or gas mark 4) for 25 minutes or until chicken is done. Place mushrooms in skillet. Stir in skim milk and remaining ingredients and bring to a boil. Simmer 6 minutes, stirring frequently, until liquid is reduce and thickened. Spoon over chicken.

4 SERVINGS

Each with: 223 Calories (24% from Fat, 48% from Protein, 27% from Carb); 28 g Protein; 6 g Total Fat; 3 g Saturated Fat; 1 g Monounsaturated Fat; 1 g Polyunsaturated Fat; 16 g Carb; 5 g Fiber; 4 g Sugar; 394 mg Phosphorus; 318 mg Calcium; 412 mg Sodium; 1535 mg Potassium; 16 213 IU Vitamin A; 74 mg ATE Vitamin E; 53 mg Vitamin C; 54 mg Cholesterol

How Low Can You Go Italian Chicken Breasts

This is a variation on an oven baked chicken recipes, this one with an Italian flavor. It's great with pasta and a salad for dinner and low enough in calories that you can afford to do that.

4 boneless chicken breasts

¼ cup (60 ml) egg substitute

12 saltines, crushed

1 teaspoon brown sugar substitute, such as Splenda

½ teaspoon sesame seeds

1 tablespoon (7 g) wheat germ

½ teaspoon dried oregano

¼ teaspoon celery seed

¼ teaspoon garlic powder

1 teaspoon onion, minced

½ teaspoon dried parsley

1 teaspoon Italian seasoning

Combine all ingredients except chicken and egg substitute. Dip the chicken in the egg substitute and then in the crumb mixture, turning to cover on all sides. Place in a baking dish sprayed with nonstick vegetable oil spray. Spray chicken with same spray until crumbs are moistened. Bake at 350°F (180°C, or gas mark 4) until done, about 30 to 40 minutes.

4 SERVINGS

Each with: 160 Calories (11% from Fat, 53% from Protein, 36% from Carb); 20 g Protein; 2 g Total Fat; 0 g Saturated Fat; 0 g Monounsaturated Fat; 1 g Polyunsaturated Fat; 14 g Carb; 1 g Fiber; 0 g Sugar; 198 mg Phosphorus; 29 mg Calcium; 170 mg Sodium; 279 mg Potassium; 112 IU Vitamin A; 4 mg ATE Vitamin E; 1 mg Vitamin C; 41 mg Cholesterol

Buffalo Chicken Rolls

Made lower in fat by using skinless breasts instead of wings and baking instead of frying, this will still give you the full flavor of Buffalo chicken. It makes a nice flavorful start to a healthy meal.

---

4 boneless skinless chicken breast, boned and skinned
2 tablespoons (28 g) unsalted butter, melted
¼ cup (60 ml) Tabasco sauce
4 tablespoons (32 g) blue cheese, crumbled
½ cup (50 g) celery sticks

 Tip: These chicken rolls can be sliced to be used as appetizers.

Pound the chicken breasts down to a ¼-inch (6 mm) thickness. In a large glass bowl, make the marinade by mixing together the butter and Tabasco sauce. Add the chicken into the marinade, turning to coat; cover and refrigerate 15 to 30 minutes. Preheat the oven to 400°F (200°C, or gas mark 6). Remove the chicken from the marinade and spoon 1 tablespoon (8 g) of the blue cheese onto the center of each chicken breast. Lay a celery stick over the blue cheese. Fold in the sides, rolling the chicken around the filling. Secure with wooden picks. Place the chicken rolls in a baking pan. Bake at 400°F (200°C, or gas mark 6) for 30 minutes or until chicken is fork-tender. Set the temperature control to broil. Cook the chicken for about 5 minutes longer or until brown. Remove the wooden picks from the chicken before serving.

4 SERVINGS

Each with: 133 Calories (47% from Fat, 51% from Protein, 2% from Carb); 17 g Protein; 7 g Total Fat; 4 g Unsaturated Fat; 2 g Monounsaturated Fat; 0 g Polyunsaturated Fat; 1 g Carb; 0 g Fiber; 0 g Sugar; 148 mg Phosphorus; 17 mg Calcium; 148 mg Sodium; 240 mg Potassium; 490 IU Vitamin A; 52 mg ATE Vitamin E; 2 mg Vitamin C; 56 mg Cholesterol

Mexican Drunken Chicken

A generous helping of tequila ensures that this chicken will be both tender and flavorful.
The use of boneless skinless breasts ensures that it will be low in calories.

4 boneless skinless chicken
  breasts
1 cup (235 ml) low sodium
  chicken broth
1 teaspoon garlic, minced
1 tablespoon (15 ml) olive oil
1 cup (180 g) no-salt-added
  tomatoes, undrained
½ cup (120 ml) tequila
¼ cup (60 ml) lime juice
dash cayenne pepper
1 teaspoon chili powder
1 teaspoon ground cumin
½ teaspoon coriander

 *Tip: Serve this over noodles or
rice and with a salad for a
complete meal.*

Simmer the chicken breasts in the broth until tender. Remove
and cube. Set aside, reserving stock. Sauté the garlic in olive
oil. Add tomatoes (breaking them up) and the remaining
ingredients; simmer, covered, for ½ hour. Add chicken and
reheat. If sauce becomes too thick, add the reserved stock.

4 SERVINGS

Each with: 202 Calories (32% from Fat, 53% from Protein, 16% from Carb);
18 g Protein; 5 g Total Fat; 1 g Unsaturated Fat; 3 g Monounsaturated Fat; 1 g
Polyunsaturated Fat; 6 g Carb; 1 g Fiber; 2 g Sugar; 177 mg Phosphorus; 38 mg
Calcium; 78 mg Sodium; 413 mg Potassium; 297 IU Vitamin A; 4 mg ATE Vitamin E;
15 mg Vitamin C; 41 mg Cholesterol

Just Peachy Chicken

Sweet and juicy, this chicken is sure to be popular with kids as well as adults. And because it used skinless chicken breasts, it is almost fat free.

4 boneless chicken breasts
16 ounces (455 g) peaches, in juice
2 tablespoons (28 ml) lemon juice
⅛ teaspoon black pepper

 Tip: Serve with ½ cup (98 g) brown rice and green beans for a complete meal.

Drain peach juice into a cup; add lemon juice. Place chicken into a baking pan. Sprinkle chicken with black pepper. Pour peach juice over chicken. Bake at 350°F (180°C, or gas mark 4) about 35 to 40 minutes. Remove and add peach slices or peach halves. Return to oven and bake for another 10 to 15 minutes.

4 SERVINGS

Each with: 130 Calories (6% from Fat, 52% from Protein, 42% from Carb); 17 g Protein; 1 g Total Fat; 0 g Unsaturated Fat; 0 g Monounsaturated Fat; 0 g Polyunsaturated Fat; 14 g Carb; 2 g Fiber; 12 g Sugar; 159 mg Phosphorus; 15 mg Calcium; 51 mg Sodium; 336 mg Potassium; 448 IU Vitamin A; 4 mg ATE Vitamin E; 8 mg Vitamin C; 41 mg Cholesterol

Easy Low Calorie Grilled Blackened Chicken

This gives you a nice Cajun flavor off the grill. It's low in calories and fat, giving you a number of choices to make it a complete meal. We like it with a big plate of grilled vegetables such as zucchini, onion, bell peppers, and tomato slices.

4 boneless skinless chicken breasts
2 tablespoons (28 g) unsalted butter, melted
5 teaspoons (15 g) Cajun blackening spice mix

Trim excess fat from the chicken. Cut slashes through the skin and ½-inch (1.3 cm) deep to allow spices to penetrate the meat. Brush the chicken breasts with the melted butter and then rub the spices in. Cook on a medium grill for about 25 minutes.

4 SERVINGS

Each with: 129 Calories (48% from Fat, 52% from Protein, 0% from Carb); 16 g Protein; 7 g Total Fat; 4 g Unsaturated Fat; 2 g Monounsaturated Fat; 0 g Polyunsaturated Fat; 0 g Carb; 0 g Fiber; 0 g Sugar; 141 mg Phosphorus; 10 mg Calcium; 47 mg Sodium; 183 mg Potassium; 191 IU Vitamin A; 52 mg ATE Vitamin E; 1 mg Vitamin C; 56 mg Cholesterol

Indian Chicken Meal Starter

This is a slightly tangy but not overly hot chicken flavored like the classic Tandori chicken. It's a real bargain in terms of flavor for calories. Try it with the *So Easy and Tasty Curried Fresh Vegetables* or *Spice Up Your Dinner with Indian Spinach and Carrots* in chapter 14. Or have it with both and still be under your calorie limit.

1 cup (260 g) plain fat free yogurt
½ teaspoon cardamom
½ teaspoon ground cumin
½ teaspoon turmeric
⅛ teaspoon cayenne pepper
1 teaspoon bay leaf, crushed
½ teaspoon garlic powder
¾ teaspoon ground ginger
¼ cup (40 g) onion, minced
¼ cup (60 ml) lime juice
¼ teaspoon black pepper
1 teaspoon cinnamon
1 teaspoon coriander
8 boneless chicken breasts

Combine yogurt with all other spice, mixing well. Prick chicken with a fork. In a plastic food bag or glass pan large enough to hold chicken, cover chicken with yogurt marinade, making sure all surfaces of chicken are coated. Cover and refrigerate minimum of 3 hours but overnight is best. Turn at least once while marinating. Grill over medium coals until done or place chicken in a greased roasting pan with marinade and cook at 375°F (190°C, or gas mark 5) for 45 minutes to 1 hour or until chicken is tender.

8 SERVINGS

Each with: 103 Calories (9% from Fat, 73% from Protein, 18% from Carb); 18 g Protein; 1 g Total Fat; 0 g Saturated Fat; 0 g Monounsaturated Fat; 0 g Polyunsaturated Fat; 4 g Carb; 0 g Fiber; 3 g Sugar; 192 mg Phosphorus; 78 mg Calcium; 71 mg Sodium; 293 mg Potassium; 44 IU Vitamin A; 5 mg ATE Vitamin E; 4 mg Vitamin C; 42 mg Cholesterol

Come Home to the Islands Coconut Chicken

With the natural sweetness of coconut and fresh fruit, these chicken breasts are sure to be a hit with young and old alike. And that's not even to mention the nutrients they contain.

⅓ cup (28 g) flaked coconut

2 tablespoons (28 g) unsalted butter

8 boneless skinless chicken breasts

1 tablespoon (6 g) fresh ginger, finely chopped or ¾ teaspoon ground ginger

1 cup (235 ml) fat-free evaporated milk

2 cups bananas, sliced

1 papaya, peeled, seeded, halved, and sliced

1 lime, cut into 8 sections

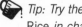 *Tip: Try these with* Tropical Rice *in chapter 14.*

Toast coconut in a 300°F (150°C, or gas mark 3) oven for 10 minutes. Set aside. In a large frying pan, brown chicken breasts in butter. Sprinkle ginger and 3 tablespoons (15 g) coconut over chicken. Add evaporated milk, cover, and cook over medium heat for 10 minutes or until done. Remove chicken and arrange with fruit on a large platter. Spoon sauce over chicken and sprinkle with remaining toasted coconut. Garnish with limes to be squeezed over chicken and fruit. Serve with brown rice, if desired.

8 SERVINGS

Each with: 204 Calories (22% from Fat, 38% from Protein, 40% from Carb); 20 g Protein; 5 g Total Fat; 3 g Unsaturated Fat; 1 g Monounsaturated Fat; 0 g Polyunsaturated Fat; 21 g Carb; 2 g Fiber; 12 g Sugar; 221 mg Phosphorus; 110 mg Calcium; 85 mg Sodium; 562 mg Potassium; 461 IU Vitamin A; 66 mg ATE Vitamin E; 19 mg Vitamin C; 50 mg Cholesterol

Chicken with Spinach and Mushrooms

Tasty pan fried chicken breasts are paired with super healthy spinach, which has been stir-fried with mushrooms, for this filling main dish that still leaves you over 150 mix and match calories to spend.

2 tablespoons (28 ml) olive oil

4 boneless skinless chicken breasts

¼ teaspoon black pepper

1 pound (455 g) mushrooms, quartered

1 cup (150 g) red bell pepper, cut into ½-inch (1.3 cm) pieces

½ teaspoon garlic, minced

½ cup (120 ml) dry white wine

1½ pounds (680 g) spinach, thick stems removed

Heat 1 tablespoon (15 ml) of the oil in a large skillet over medium-high heat. Season the chicken with black pepper. Cook the chicken until browned and cooked through, 5 to 7 minutes per side. Transfer to a plate. Return the skillet to medium-high heat and heat the remaining tablespoon (15 ml) of oil. Cook the mushrooms and red bell pepper, tossing, for 3 minutes. Add the garlic and wine and cook until the mushrooms are tender and the wine is nearly evaporated, 2 to 3 minutes. Toss in the spinach and cook until wilted. Serve the spinach with the chicken.

4 SERVINGS

Each with: 232 Calories (34% from Fat, 44% from Protein, 22% from Carb); 25 g Protein; 9 g Total Fat; 1 g Unsaturated Fat; 5 g Monounsaturated Fat; 1 g Polyunsaturated Fat; 13 g Carb; 6 g Fiber; 4 g Sugar; 333 mg Phosphorus; 186 mg Calcium; 188 mg Sodium; 1592 mg Potassium; 17 131 IU Vitamin A; 4 mg ATE Vitamin E; 122 mg Vitamin C; 41 mg Cholesterol

Spinach Stuffed Chicken Breasts

These chicken breasts, stuffed with a spinach dressing, make a great start to just about any meal. They are naturally low in fat and calories and high in nutrient density.

8 slices low sodium bacon

1 cup (160 g) onion, finely chopped

½ pound (225 g) fresh spinach, washed and chopped

¼ cup (60 ml) egg substitute

½ cup (15 g) croutons, lightly crushed

¼ teaspoon garlic powder

8 boneless skinless chicken breasts

black pepper to taste

 Tip: These are great on a grill. Try them on medium for about 20 minutes.

Fry bacon; drain and crumble. Reserve 2 tablespoons (28 ml) drippings. Sauté onion in bacon drippings until soft. Remove from heat and stir in spinach, egg substitute, croutons, garlic, and crumbled bacon. Cut pocket in thick side of each chicken breast. Stuff with spinach mixture and close with wooden pick. Sprinkle with black pepper. Place breast in 9 × 12-inch (23 × 30 cm) baking dish and cook in preheated 350°F (180°C, or gas mark 4) oven until done, about ½ hour. Remove the wooden picks before serving.

8 SERVINGS

Each with: 151 Calories (29% from Fat, 58% from Protein, 13% from Carb); 22 g Protein; 5 g Total Fat; 1 g Unsaturated Fat; 2 g Monounsaturated Fat; 1 g Polyunsaturated Fat; 5 g Carb; 1 g Fiber; 1 g Sugar; 213 mg Phosphorus; 47 mg Calcium; 179 mg Sodium; 443 mg Potassium; 2704 IU Vitamin A; 5 mg ATE Vitamin E; 10 mg Vitamin C; 50 mg Cholesterol

Chicken Breasts with Balsamic Vinegar Sauce

I'm a big fan of balsamic vinegar. It adds so much flavor for so few calories and goes well with just about any meat or vegetable. Here it helps produce a juicy flavorful chicken with very few calories.

4 boneless skinless chicken breasts

¼ teaspoon black pepper

2 tablespoons (28 ml) olive oil

1 tablespoon (10 g) shallots, finely chopped

3 tablespoons (45 ml) balsamic vinegar

1½ cups (355 ml) low sodium chicken broth

2 teaspoons fresh marjoram, finely chopped

Sprinkle chicken with black pepper. Heat oil in large heavy frying pan over high heat. Add chicken and cook on both sides until browned. Reduce heat to medium low and cook until chicken is no longer pink inside, about 12 minutes. Transfer chicken to heated platter and keep warm in oven. Add shallots and cook over medium-low heat for 3 minutes or until translucent, scraping up any browned bits. Add vinegar and bring to a boil. Boil for 3 minutes or until reduced to a glaze, stirring constantly. Add broth and boil until reduced to ½ cup (120 ml), stirring occasionally. Remove sauce from heat and whisk in marjoram and any juices from chicken. Spoon sauce over chicken and serve immediately.

4 SERVINGS

Each with: 157 Calories (47% from Fat, 47% from Protein, 6% from Carb); 18 g Protein; 8 g Total Fat; 1 g Unsaturated Fat; 5 g Monounsaturated Fat; 1 g Polyunsaturated Fat; 2 g Carb; 0 g Fiber; 1 g Sugar; 170 mg Phosphorus; 19 mg Calcium; 74 mg Sodium; 284 mg Potassium; 67 IU Vitamin A; 4 mg ATE Vitamin E; 1 mg Vitamin C; 41 mg Cholesterol

Bayou Creole Soup

This is a delightful soup of chicken and vegetables in a Creole-influenced broth. It provides lots of nutrition for not many calories, leaving you plenty of room left for a slice of bread and a dessert from the mix and match chapters.

4 slices low sodium bacon, cut in ½-inch (1.3 cm) pieces

¾ cup (75 g) green onion, sliced

1 cup (150 g) green bell pepper, cut into ½-inch (1.3 cm) pieces

1 teaspoon garlic, minced

14½ ounces (410 g) no-salt-added stewed tomatoes

4 cups (950 ml) low sodium chicken broth

1½ cups (355 ml) water

1 bay leaf

2 cups (280 g) cooked chicken breast, cut in bite-sized pieces

hot sauce to taste

In soup kettle, cook bacon until crisp over medium heat. Remove bacon and drain fat, leaving 2 tablespoons (28 ml) in pot. Add green onion, green bell pepper, and garlic; cook over medium heat until crisp-tender. Add tomatoes, broth, water, and bay leaf. Bring just to boil and then reduce heat. Simmer, uncovered, 10 minutes. Add chicken and bacon. Cover and heat gently for 5 more minutes. Remove bay leaf. Add hot sauce to taste and serve.

4 SERVINGS

Each with: 239 Calories (28% from Fat, 51% from Protein, 21% from Carb); 31 g Protein; 8 g Total Fat; 2 g Unsaturated Fat; 3 g Monounsaturated Fat; 1 g Polyunsaturated Fat; 13 g Carb; 2 g Fiber; 6 g Sugar; 310 mg Phosphorus; 76 mg Calcium; 440 mg Sodium; 763 mg Potassium; 521 IU Vitamin A; 5 mg ATE Vitamin E; 42 mg Vitamin C; 68 mg Cholesterol

Filling Chicken Rolls

These delicious chicken rolls will give you your protein and a starch all for under 200 calories. Add a couple of helping of vegetables and you'll still have enough calories left for dessert.

4 boneless skinless chicken breast
¼ cup (40 g) onion, chopped
1¼ cup (25 g) celery, chopped
1 teaspoon olive oil
⅔ cup (130 g) brown rice, cooked
¼ teaspoon poultry seasoning
¼ teaspoon black pepper
¼ teaspoon garlic powder
1⅓ cups (315 ml) low sodium
  chicken broth

Pound breasts with meat mallet until ¼-inch (6 mm) thick. Cook onion and celery in oil until tender. Mix in rice and seasonings. Place quarter of rice mixture on each breast half. Start with narrowest end and roll. Tie kitchen twice around each end of roll to hold it together. Leave the ends of the string long so they can be easily removed before serving. Brown chicken rolls on all sides in hot frying pan. Add broth and bring to a boil. Reduce heat, cover, and simmer until tender, about 15 minutes.

4 SERVINGS

Each with: 173 Calories (14% from Fat, 46% from Protein, 40% from Carb); 20 g Protein; 3 g Total Fat; 1 g Saturated Fat; 1 g Monounsaturated Fat; 0 g Polyunsaturated Fat; 17 g Carb; 1 g Fiber; 1 g Sugar; 188 mg Phosphorus; 38 mg Calcium; 105 mg Sodium; 383 mg Potassium; 215 IU Vitamin A; 4 mg ATE Vitamin E; 3 mg Vitamin C; 41 mg Cholesterol

What in the World Is Mulligatawny Soup?

The answer is that its soup brought back from India by the British, rich with a curry flavored broth and lots of vegetables and fruits. This makes a big batch, but it freezes well. You can serve it over brown rice or with a slice of dark bread.

2 pounds (900 g) boneless skinless chicken breast
1 quart (950 ml) water
1 tablespoon (1 g) dried parsley
1 bay leaf
2 teaspoons curry powder
⅛ teaspoon nutmeg
⅛ teaspoon ground cloves
2 tablespoons (28 ml) olive oil
1 cup (160 g) onion, chopped
1 cup (160 g) carrot, chopped
1 cup (150 g) green bell pepper, chopped
1 apple, pared, cored, and chopped
14 ounces (390 g) no-salt-added tomatoes
¼ teaspoon cayenne pepper

In large soup pot or kettle, combine first 7 ingredients; cover and simmer approximately 45 minutes (until chicken is tender). Cut meat into small chunks. In another large pot, heat oil over medium heat and add vegetables and apple; simmer until tender. Remove from heat and stir in flour. Stir in chicken, tomatoes (with juice), and cayenne pepper. Bring to boil and reduce heat. Cover and simmer about 1 hour.

8 SERVINGS

Each with: 193 Calories (24% from Fat, 57% from Protein, 19% from Carb); 27 g Protein; 5 g Total Fat; 1 g Unsaturated Fat; 3 g Monounsaturated Fat; 1 g Polyunsaturated Fat; 9 g Carb; 2 g Fiber; 5 g Sugar; 251 mg Phosphorus; 47 mg Calcium; 94 mg Sodium; 545 mg Potassium; 2159 IU Vitamin A; 7 mg ATE Vitamin E; 27 mg Vitamin C; 66 mg Cholesterol

Italian Steak in Sauce

This creates an Italian sauce that's beefy but low in fat and calories because of the lean cut of meat used. The slow cooker both makes the beef very tender and provides that long simmering that makes sauces even richer. It can be served over pasta or other starches or in building other Italian meals with vegetables.

1 pound (455 g) beef round steak, cubed

1 can (14½ ounces, or 410 g) low sodium tomatoes

2 tablespoons (28 ml) red wine

¼ teaspoon garlic powder

1 teaspoon Italian seasoning

1 cup (160 g) onion, coarsely chopped

4 ounces (115 g) mushrooms, sliced

6 ounces (170 g) low sodium tomato paste

Place meat in bottom of slow cooker. Stir together remaining ingredients except tomato paste. Pour over meat. Cover and cook on low 8 to 10 hours. Turn to high. Stir in tomato paste and cook until thickened, 10 to 15 minutes.

4 SERVINGS

Each with: 200 Calories (16% from Fat, 54% from Protein, 29% from Carb); 27 g Protein; 4 g Total Fat; 1 g Unsaturated Fat; 1 g Monounsaturated Fat; 0 g Polyunsaturated Fat; 15 g Carb; 3 g Fiber; 7 g Sugar; 229 mg Phosphorus; 36 mg Calcium; 77 mg Sodium; 877 mg Potassium; 817 IU Vitamin A; 0 mg ATE Vitamin E; 20 mg Vitamin C; 60 mg Cholesterol

A Meal's Worth of Curried Beef for Half the Calories

Beef is not a traditional ingredient for curried dishes. The generous helping of fruit and vegetables makes it a meal in itself, but the calories are low enough that you can add brown rice or whole wheat pasta or one of our mix and match desserts.

½ pound (225 g) extra lean ground beef
½ cup (80 g) onion, chopped
½ teaspoon garlic, minced
¾ cup (113 g) apple, chopped, unpeeled
¼ cup (15 g) fresh parsley, chopped
1½ teaspoons curry powder
½ teaspoon ground cumin
⅛ teaspoon cayenne pepper
¼ cup (60 ml) apple juice, unsweetened
16 ounces (455 g) no-salt-added tomatoes, undrained
2 cups (240 g) zucchini, chopped

Cook ground beef, onion, and garlic in 10-inch (25 cm) nonstick skillet over medium heat, stirring frequently, until no longer pink; drain. Stir in remaining ingredients. Break up the tomatoes. Heat to boiling and then reduce heat. Simmer uncovered about 5 minutes or until apple is tender, stirring occasionally.

4 SERVINGS

Each with: 195 Calories (46% from Fat, 26% from Protein, 29% from Carb); 13 g Protein; 10 g Total Fat; 4 g Unsaturated Fat; 4 g Monounsaturated Fat; 1 g Polyunsaturated Fat; 14 g Carb; 3 g Fiber; 9 g Sugar; 141 mg Phosphorus; 66 mg Calcium; 60 mg Sodium; 687 mg Potassium; 631 IU Vitamin A; 0 mg ATE Vitamin E; 34 mg Vitamin C; 39 mg Cholesterol

Really Low Calorie Beef and Tomato Curry

Beef, tomatoes, and other vegetables are simmered in a mild curry sauce to make this tasty dish. Using a lean cut of beef holds down the calories and fat, while vegetables provide nutrient density without adding to those totals.

1 pound (455 g) beef round steak
½ cup (120 ml) low sodium beef broth
1½ cups (270 g) tomatoes, coarsely chopped
1 cup (150 g) green bell pepper, cut in 1-inch (2.5 cm) pieces
1½ cups (80 g) onion, coarsely chopped
1 teaspoon curry powder
1 tablespoon (8 g) cornstarch
1 tablespoon (15 ml) water

Cut meat into 1 × 2-inch (2.5 to 5 cm) strips. Spray skillet with nonstick vegetable oil spray. Cook meat in broth until tender. Add tomatoes, peeled and cut up, green bell pepper, onion, and curry powder and heat to boiling. Cover and cook on medium for 3 to 5 minutes. Mix cornstarch and water. Stir into mixture and cook until thick and boiling.

4 SERVINGS

Each with: 202 Calories (19% from Fat, 56% from Protein, 25% from Carb); 28 g Protein; 4 g Total Fat; 1 g Unsaturated Fat; 2 g Monounsaturated Fat; 0 g Polyunsaturated Fat; 13 g Carb; 2 g Fiber; 3 g Sugar; 297 mg Phosphorus; 49 mg Calcium; 99 mg Sodium; 723 mg Potassium; 492 IU Vitamin A; 0 mg ATE Vitamin E; 48 mg Vitamin C; 52 mg Cholesterol

 Tip: Serve over noodles or rice.

Ginger Orange Pork Chops

These tasty and low calorie chops can be the start of a number of meals. These are good with Asian vegetables and brown rice or potatoes and vegetables.

4 boneless pork loin chops
1 tablespoon (15 ml) oil
¼ teaspoon black pepper
1 teaspoon ground ginger
¼ cup (60 ml) orange juice

 Tip: These are especially good with baked sweet potatoes.

Brown chops in oil on both sides. Sprinkle with spices and pour orange juice over. Cover and cook until done, 10 to 15 minutes.

4 SERVINGS

Each with: 168 Calories (43% from Fat, 53% from Protein, 5% from Carb); 21 g Protein; 8 g Total Fat; 2 g Unsaturated Fat; 3 g Monounsaturated Fat; 2 g Polyunsaturated Fat; 2 g Carb; 0 g Fiber; 0 g Sugar; 223 mg Phosphorus; 16 mg Calcium; 52 mg Sodium; 411 mg Potassium; 20 IU Vitamin A; 2 mg ATE Vitamin E; 6 mg Vitamin C; 64 mg Cholesterol

East and West Pork Chops

It's a little hard to categorize the marinade for these chops. The soy sauce and spices say Asian, but the mustard gives it a New World flavor. Whatever you call it and whatever you put with it, it's the start of a healthy low fat meal.

1 tablespoon (11 g) Dijon mustard

3 tablespoons (45 ml) low sodium soy sauce

⅛ teaspoon garlic powder

¼ cup (60 ml) dry white wine

2 teaspoons vegetable oil

2 teaspoons sherry extract

1 pound (455 g) boneless pork loin chops

Combine marinade ingredients and pour over chops. Marinate several hours or overnight. Broil or grill, turning occasionally and basting until done.

4 SERVINGS

Each with: 184 Calories (38% from Fat, 58% from Protein, 4% from Carb); 25 g Protein; 7 g Total Fat; 2 g Unsaturated Fat; 3 g Monounsaturated Fat; 2 g Polyunsaturated Fat; 2 g Carb; 0 g Fiber; 0 g Sugar; 266 mg Phosphorus; 21 mg Calcium; 501 mg Sodium; 460 mg Potassium; 13 IU Vitamin A; 2 mg ATE Vitamin E; 1 mg Vitamin C; 71 mg Cholesterol

Pineapple Stuffed Pork Chops

These chops have a sweet and sour flavor. They are low in calories because of the lean cut of pork used. We like them with brown rice, using the rest of the sauce to flavor it, and a large helping of steamed broccoli.

4 pork loin chops, 1-inch (2.5 cm) thick

8 ounces (225 g) pineapple slices

¼ cup (60 g) low sodium catsup

1 tablespoon (6 g) green onion, chopped

½ teaspoon dry mustard

Cut a pocket in each chop to make room for pineapple. Drain pineapple, reserving liquid. Cut two slices in half, cut up remaining pineapple, and set aside. Place a half pineapple slice in the pocket of each chop. Heat grill to medium and grill about 20 minutes, turning once. Meanwhile, in a small saucepan, combine catsup, green onion, mustard, and the reserved pineapple juice and pieces. Heat to boiling, reduce heat, and simmer 10 minutes. Grill chops 5 minutes more, brushing with sauce and turning several times.

4 SERVINGS

Each with: 190 Calories (21% from Fat, 46% from Protein, 33% from Carb); 22 g Protein; 4 g Total Fat; 1 g Unsaturated Fat; 2 g Monounsaturated Fat; 1 g Polyunsaturated Fat; 16 g Carb; 1 g Fiber; 13 g Sugar; 231 mg Phosphorus; 25 mg Calcium; 55 mg Sodium; 510 mg Potassium; 187 IU Vitamin A; 2 mg ATE Vitamin E; 8 mg Vitamin C; 64 mg Cholesterol

Asian Barbecued Pork Chops

An Asian flavored barbecue sauce is used first to marinate, then as a topping for these flavorful and lean chops.

4 pork loin chops
6 tablespoons (90 ml) low sodium
  soy sauce
½ teaspoon garlic powder
2 teaspoons sherry
½ cup (61 g) no-salt-added
  tomato sauce
¼ cup (60 ml) water

 Tip: If you prefer, you can also pan-fry or broil the chops instead of grilling.

Trim fat from pork chops. Mix soy sauce, garlic, sherry, and tomato sauce. Pour over meat in flat pan. Let stand, covered, in refrigerator for 3 hours. Drain off marinade and pour into small pan. Add water and heat to boiling. Reduce heat and simmer 5 minutes. Grill chops over medium heat until done, turning once. Serve sauce with meat.

4 SERVINGS

Each with: 158 Calories (26% from Fat, 61% from Protein, 13% from Carb); 23 g Protein; 4 g Total Fat; 1 g Unsaturated Fat; 2 g Monounsaturated Fat; 0 g Polyunsaturated Fat; 5 g Carb; 1 g Fiber; 2 g Sugar; 258 mg Phosphorus; 22 mg Calcium; 852 mg Sodium; 536 mg Potassium; 113 IU Vitamin A; 2 mg ATE Vitamin E; 5 mg Vitamin C; 64 mg Cholesterol

Asian Pork Chops with Mushrooms and Onion

Mushrooms and onions cook around these Asian-style chops, giving you a great start for your mix and match meal. You can combine these with either stir-fried vegetables and rice or in a more American type setting with pasta or potatoes and vegetables.

4 loin pork chops
1 tablespoon (15 ml) oil
8 ounces (225 g) mushrooms,
  sliced
1 cup (160 g) onion, sliced
¼ teaspoon black pepper
1 teaspoon ground ginger
¼ cup (60 ml) orange juice

Brown chops in oil on both sides in a large skillet. Place mushrooms and onion around chops. Sprinkle with spices and pour orange juice over. Cover and cook until done, 10 to 15 minutes.

4 SERVINGS

Each with: 197 Calories (36% from Fat, 48% from Protein, 16% from Carb); 24 g Protein; 8 g Total Fat; 2 g Saturated Fat; 3 g Monounsaturated Fat; 3 g Polyunsaturated Fat; 8 g Carb; 1 g Fiber; 3 g Sugar; 282 mg Phosphorus; 26 mg Calcium; 55 mg Sodium; 647 mg Potassium; 21 IU Vitamin A; 2 mg ATE Vitamin E; 10 mg Vitamin C; 64 mg Cholesterol

Balsamic Salmon

Fish is a great choice to start your 400 calorie meal. Here we add lots of flavor to a salmon fillet while holding down the calories. When we prepared this, we steamed broccoli over it while it cooked. The broccoli ended up with much more flavor than had it been cooked plain.

½ cup (120 ml) balsamic vinegar
¼ (60 ml) cup water
2 tablespoons (40 g) maple syrup
¼ teaspoon garlic powder
1 pound (455 g) salmon fillets

Heat all ingredients except salmon in a large skillet, stirring to combine. Add salmon fillets. Cover and cook until salmon is done, about 10 minutes, turning once.

4 SERVINGS

Each with: 239 Calories (47% from Fat, 38% from Protein, 15% from Carb); 23 g Protein; 12 g Total Fat; 2 g Saturated Fat; 4 g Monounsaturated Fat; 4 g Polyunsaturated Fat; 9 g Carb; 0 g Fiber; 8 g Sugar; 268 mg Phosphorus; 23 mg Calcium; 68 mg Sodium; 463 mg Potassium; 57 IU Vitamin A; 17 mg ATE Vitamin E; 4 mg Vitamin C; 67 mg Cholesterol

Crunchy Oven Fried Fish

This fish is baked in the oven and features a nice crunchy coating low in fat and calories. It's a great start for your mix and match meal, perhaps with some slaw.

¼ cup (60 ml) egg substitute
2 tablespoons (28 ml) skim milk
½ cup (30 g) potato flakes, mashed
¼ teaspoon black pepper
1 pound (455 g) catfish fillets

Mix egg substitute and skim milk together. Stir together potatoes and black pepper. Dip fish in egg mixture, then potato flakes. Repeat. Place on baking sheet. Spray with nonfat vegetable oil spray. Bake at 325°F (170°C, or gas mark 3) until fish flakes easily, about 15 minutes.

4 SERVINGS

Each with: 191 Calories (44% from Fat, 44% from Protein, 12% from Carb); 20 g Protein; 9 g Total Fat; 2 g Saturated Fat; 4 g Monounsaturated Fat; 2 g Polyunsaturated Fat; 5 g Carb; 0 g Fiber; 0 g Sugar; 266 mg Phosphorus; 32 mg Calcium; 99 mg Sodium; 472 mg Potassium; 130 IU Vitamin A; 22 mg ATE Vitamin E; 6 mg Vitamin C; 54 mg Cholesterol

Devilish Deviled Fish Broil

Fish is naturally low in calories and high is nutrients low omega-3 fatty acids,
but a spicy mustard sauce lifts these fish fillets out of the ordinary.

1 teaspoon onion flakes

¼ teaspoon hot pepper sauce

½ teaspoon Worcestershire sauce

½ teaspoon low sodium soy sauce

1 tablespoon (11 g) prepared
mustard

½ teaspoon fresh parsley, minced

8 ounces (225 g) tilapia fillets

Combine all ingredients except fish. Mix well. Brush on both
sides of fish. Broil until fish flakes easily with fork.

2 SERVINGS

Each with: 136 Calories (21% from Fat, 75% from Protein, 4% from Carb);
24 g Protein; 3 g Total Fat; 0 g Unsaturated Fat; 1 g Monounsaturated Fat; 1 g
Polyunsaturated Fat; 1 g Carb; 0 g Fiber; 0 g Sugar; 257 mg Phosphorus; 61 mg
Calcium; 122 mg Sodium; 553 mg Potassium; 221 IU Vitamin A; 53 mg ATE Vitamin
E; 3 mg Vitamin C; 36 mg Cholesterol

Fish Fillets Italian

These are great tasting fish rollups, flavored with Italian herbs and cooked in tomato sauce, topped
with bread crumbs. Fish is naturally low in calories and the herbs give this version a great flavor.
Serve with fresh steamed broccoli for a really heart healthy, low calorie meal.

1 pound (455 g) fish fillets, such
as cod, flounder, or perch

1 tablespoon (15 ml) olive oil

black pepper, to taste

1 tablespoon (4 g) fresh parsley,
chopped

1 teaspoon dried basil

¼ teaspoon dried oregano

1 cup (160 g) onion, sliced

8 ounces (225 g) no-salt-added
tomato sauce, sliced

¼ cup (30 g) bread crumbs, dry

¼ cup (25 g) Parmesan cheese

Brush fillets with oil. Season with black pepper to taste and
with parsley, basil, and oregano. Roll up fillets. Spray an
8 × 8-inch (20 × 20 cm) baking dish with nonstick vegetable
oil spray. Lay slices of onion on bottom of dish. Place rolled
fillets, seam side down, on top of onion. Pour tomato sauce
over fillets. Combine bread crumbs and cheese. Sprinkle on
fillets. Bake at 400°F (200°C, or gas mark 6) for 20 minutes or
until fish flakes easily with a fork.

4 SERVINGS

Each with: 122 Calories (42% from Fat, 14% from Protein, 44% from Carb);
4 g Protein; 6 g Total Fat; 2 g Unsaturated Fat; 3 g Monounsaturated Fat; 1 g
Polyunsaturated Fat; 14 g Carb; 2 g Fiber; 5 g Sugar; 87 mg Phosphorus; 104 mg
Calcium; 153 mg Sodium; 301 mg Potassium; 325 IU Vitamin A; 7 mg ATE Vitamin E;
11 mg Vitamin C; 6 mg Cholesterol

Honey Mustard Fish

Mustard with just a little honey can give a great flavor to just about any kind of fish. And this simple starter allows you to pick and choose several side dishes and still stay within your 400 calories.

2 tablespoons (22 g) Dijon mustard

1 tablespoon (11 g) grainy mustard

2 teaspoons ground cumin

1 tablespoon (20 g) honey

1 pound (455 g) catfish, or other firm white fish

Preheat oven to 400°F (200°C, or gas mark 6). Line a baking sheet with foil and lightly spray with nonstick cooking spray. In a small bowl, stir together the mustards, cumin, and honey. Rinse fish and pat dry. Spoon mustard coating on both sides of fish and place on prepared baking sheet. For fish 1½ inches (3.8 cm) thick, bake 20 minutes. Place fish on individual plates and pour pan juices over top.

4 SERVINGS

Each with: 181 Calories (46% from Fat, 41% from Protein, 13% from Carb); 18 g Protein; 9 g Total Fat; 2 g Saturated Fat; 4 g Monounsaturated Fat; 2 g Polyunsaturated Fat; 6 g Carb; 0 g Fiber; 5 g Sugar; 245 mg Phosphorus; 29 mg Calcium; 193 mg Sodium; 377 mg Potassium; 85 IU Vitamin A; 17 mg ATE Vitamin E; 1 mg Vitamin C; 53 mg Cholesterol

Chowder from the Sea

Grab a slice of bread from one of the recipes in chapter 14 and you have a filling, great tasting meal. This recipe came about on a weekend when I didn't want to spend my day cooking, and I knew everyone was going to be available for dinner at a different time. The answer . . . the slow cooker and a fish and shrimp soup that people could ladle up whenever they were ready.

½ pound (225 g) cod, or other white fish, cubed

½ pound (225 g) shrimp, peeled

3 medium potatoes, shredded

1 cup (110 g) carrot, shredded

1 cup (160 g) onion, finely chopped

1 cup (150 g) red bell pepper, finely chopped

1 cup (100 g) celery, finely chopped

2 cups (475 ml) low sodium chicken broth

1 cup (235 ml) skim milk

1 teaspoon seafood seasoning

Place fish and shrimp in slow cooker. Add vegetables. Pour broth over fish and vegetables. Add skim milk and seasoning. Stir to mix. Cook on low for 6 to 8 hours.

6 SERVINGS

Each with: 257 Calories (6% from Fat, 33% from Protein, 62% from Carb); 21 g Protein; 2 g Total Fat; 0 g Saturated Fat; 0 g Monounsaturated Fat; 1 g Polyunsaturated Fat; 40 g Carb; 5 g Fiber; 5 g Sugar; 285 mg Phosphorus; 119 mg Calcium; 193 mg Sodium; 1072 mg Potassium; 3629 IU Vitamin A; 55 mg ATE Vitamin E; 64 mg Vitamin C; 91 mg Cholesterol

Something's Fishy About This Stew

What's fishy is that this is a great fish stew, full of vegetables and delicious, but very low in calories. So you can afford to have dessert or a slice of freshly baked bread with it.

6 slices low sodium bacon, chopped

2 cups (320 g) onion, sliced

1½ pounds (680 g) haddock, cut in 2½-inch (6.4 cm) pieces

1 pound (455 g) potatoes, cut in ¾-inch (1.9 cm) cubes

1 cup (100 g) celery, sliced

1 cup (122 g) carrot, sliced

½ cup (75 g) green bell pepper, diced

½ teaspoon black pepper

3 cups (700 ml) water

28 ounces (785 g) no-salt-added crushed tomatoes

2 tablespoons (8 g) fresh parsley, chopped

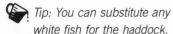 Tip: You can substitute any white fish for the haddock.

In a deep kettle or Dutch oven, sauté bacon until lightly browned; remove bacon, set aside. In same kettle, sauté onion until tender. Add fish, potatoes, celery, carrot, green bell pepper, black pepper, and water. Simmer, covered, until vegetables are tender, about 25 minutes. Add tomatoes; heat. Garnish with parsley and crumbled bacon bits.

6 SERVINGS

Each with: 261 Calories (17% from Fat, 42% from Protein, 41% from Carb); 28 g Protein; 5 g Total Fat; 1 g Saturated Fat; 2 g Monounsaturated Fat; 1 g Polyunsaturated Fat; 27 g Carb; 5 g Fiber; 5 g Sugar; 364 mg Phosphorus; 85 mg Calcium; 212 mg Sodium; 1262 mg Potassium; 3715 IU Vitamin A; 20 mg ATE Vitamin E; 67 mg Vitamin C; 73 mg Cholesterol

Low Calorie, High Bulk, Grilled Portobello Mushrooms

This is a fairly simple recipe for grilled portobello mushrooms, but one that still provides a flavorful meat alternative. If you start a mix and match meal with these, you have a lot of flexibility about what to add. While mushrooms are great at providing low calorie bulk to a meal, they aren't one of the higher things in nutrients, so make sure you add plenty of veggies or other nutrient dense side dishes.

4 portobello mushroom caps
¼ cup (60 ml) balsamic vinegar
1 tablespoon (15 ml) olive oil
1 teaspoon dried basil
1 teaspoon dried oregano
½ teaspoon garlic, minced
4 ounces (115 g) low fat
  provolone cheese, sliced

Place the mushroom caps smooth side up in a shallow dish. Mix together vinegar, oil, basil, oregano, and garlic. Pour over the mushrooms. Let stand at room temperature for 15 minutes or so, turning twice. Preheat grill for medium-high heat. Spray grate with nonstick vegetable oil spray. Place mushrooms on the grill, reserving marinade for basting. Grill for 5 to 8 minutes on each side or until tender. Brush with marinade frequently. Top with cheese during the last 2 minutes of grilling.

4 SERVINGS

Each with: 133 Calories (73% from Fat, 22% from Protein, 6% from Carb); 7 g Protein; 11 g Total Fat; 5 g Saturated Fat; 5 g Monounsaturated Fat; 1 g Polyunsaturated Fat; 2 g Carb; 0 g Fiber; 1 g Sugar; 144 mg Phosphorus; 224 mg Calcium; 249 mg Sodium; 66 mg Potassium; 283 IU Vitamin A; 65 mg ATE Vitamin E; 0 mg Vitamin C; 20 mg Cholesterol

Veggie Rich Pasta Toss

Kind of like a warm pasta salad, this version of pasta primavera has even more vegetables than usual. We like it with one of the Italian rolls from chapter 16.

2 cups (210 g) whole wheat pasta, uncooked
1 cup (71 g) broccoli florets
½ cup (61 g) carrot, sliced
½ cup (50 g) celery, sliced
½ cup (75 g) red bell pepper, cut into thin 2-inch (5 cm) long slices
½ cup (50 g) fresh green beans
¼ teaspoon black pepper
30 cherry tomatoes, halved
¼ cup (25 g) Parmesan, grated
2 tablespoons (3 g) fresh basil, chopped
2 tablespoons (28 ml) olive oil

Cook the pasta according to package directions. During the last 3 minutes of pasta cooking time, add the broccoli, carrot, celery, bell pepper, and green beans to the saucepan. Drain the pasta and vegetables. Sprinkle with black pepper and toss. Add the tomatoes, cheese, and basil, drizzle the olive oil, and toss well.

4 SERVINGS

Each with: 228 Calories (35% from Fat, 14% from Protein, 51% from Carb); 9 g Protein; 10 g Total Fat; 2 g Unsaturated Fat; 6 g Monounsaturated Fat; 1 g Polyunsaturated Fat; 31 g Carb; 6 g Fiber; 3 g Sugar; 147 mg Phosphorus; 137 mg Calcium; 130 mg Sodium; 587 mg Potassium; 3739 IU Vitamin A; 7 mg ATE Vitamin E; 84 mg Vitamin C; 6 mg Cholesterol

Take Me Away to the Islands Black Bean Soup

This is a wonderful, full flavored Caribean style soup that's low in fat. Serve it with a salad and a slice of dark bread, and you will have a meal that is fulfilling both in taste and volume.

1½ cups (375 g) black beans, dried
1 cup (160 g) onion, finely chopped
½ cup (75 g) green bell pepper, finely chopped
½ teaspoon garlic, minced
½ cup (55 g) carrot, finely chopped
½ cup (50 g) celery, finely chopped
1 tablespoon (15 ml) olive oil
1 teaspoon ground cumin
¼ teaspoon cayenne pepper
4 cups (950 ml) water
2 tablespoons (28 ml) lime juice
¼ cup (65 g) salsa

Soak beans in water overnight. In a large Dutch oven, sauté onion, green bell pepper, garlic, carrot, and celery in oil until almost soft. Add spices and sauté a few minutes more. Add beans, 4 cups (950 ml) water, lime juice, and salsa and simmer until beans are beginning to fall apart, 1½ to 2 hours. Add additional water if necessary.

6 SERVINGS

Each with: 102 Calories (23% from Fat, 17% from Protein, 60% from Carb); 5 g Protein; 3 g Total Fat; 0 g Saturated Fat; 2 g Monounsaturated Fat; 0 g Polyunsaturated Fat; 16 g Carb; 5 g Fiber; 3 g Sugar; 81 mg Phosphorus; 37 mg Calcium; 68 mg Sodium; 310 mg Potassium; 1488 IU Vitamin A; 0 mg ATE Vitamin E; 16 mg Vitamin C; 0 mg Cholesterol

You Won't Believe This Vegetable Soup

Look at all those vegetables, all that nutrition, and all that great taste. It's as filling as you could want. And it's all for about 100 calories. What's not to like? This is a great soup to experiment with if you have fresh vegetables. Just use them in place of the frozen ones.

4 cups (950 ml) low sodium vegetable broth
10 ounces (280 g) frozen corn
1 cup (130 g) carrot, chopped
10 ounces (280 g) frozen green beans
2 cups (240 g) zucchini, sliced
2 cup (360 g) tomatoes, chopped
1 cup (160 g) onion, chopped
½ teaspoon garlic, minced
½ teaspoon dried thyme
½ teaspoon dried basil
¼ teaspoon black pepper
1½ cups (107 g) broccoli, chopped
1 cup (130 g) frozen peas

Combine all ingredients in a large Dutch oven. Simmer until vegetables are tender, about 45 minutes.

8 SERVINGS

Each with: 109 Calories (10% from Fat, 22% from Protein, 68% from Carb); 7 g Protein; 1 g Total Fat; 0 g Saturated Fat; 0 g Monounsaturated Fat; 0 g Polyunsaturated Fat; 20 g Carb; 5 g Fiber; 4 g Sugar; 132 mg Phosphorus; 83 mg Calcium; 480 mg Sodium; 564 mg Potassium; 2720 IU Vitamin A; 1 mg ATE Vitamin E; 41 mg Vitamin C; 0 mg Cholesterol

Tortellini Soup

This quick and easy Italian soup is made in 15 minutes using one pan. There's lots of nutrition and only 217 calories, so you have lots to use on mix and match accompaniments.

½ teaspoon garlic, crushed
1 tablespoon (15 ml) olive oil
6 cups (1.4 L) low sodium chicken broth
8 ounces (225 g) cheese tortellini
10 ounces (280 g) frozen spinach, thawed
14½ ounces (410 g) no-salt-added stewed tomatoes, undrained and cut up
6 tablespoons (30 g) Parmesan cheese, grated

In large saucepan, over medium heat, cook garlic in oil for 2 to 3 minutes. Add broth and tortellini. Heat to boil. Reduce heat and simmer 10 minutes. Add spinach and tomatoes and simmer 5 minutes more. Serve with Parmesan cheese.

6 SERVINGS

Each with: 217 Calories (31% from Fat, 26% from Protein, 43% from Carb); 15 g Protein; 8 g Total Fat; 3 g Unsaturated Fat; 3 g Monounsaturated Fat; 2 g Polyunsaturated Fat; 24 g Carb; 3 g Fiber; 3 g Sugar; 155 mg Phosphorus; 192 mg Calcium; 502 mg Sodium; 621 mg Potassium; 4577 IU Vitamin A; 7 mg ATE Vitamin E; 19 mg Vitamin C; 31 mg Cholesterol

Summer Corn Chowder

Full of fresh vegetables in a rich, creamy stock, this soup will get your meal off to a great start, providing lots of filling nutrition for very few calories.

2 tablespoons (28 ml) olive oil

½ cup (80 g) onion, chopped

2 tablespoons (16 g) all purpose flour

2 cups (475 ml) low sodium chicken broth

2 cups (328 g) frozen corn, or fresh cut from cob

2 cups (360 g) tomatoes, peeled and chopped

½ cup (50 g) celery, chopped

½ cup (75 g) green bell pepper, chopped

½ teaspoon dried thyme

1 cup (235 ml) skim milk

¼ teaspoon black pepper

Heat oil in large saucepan. Add onion and flour; cook for 1 minute. Stir in broth. Heat to boiling. Add corn, tomatoes, celery, green bell pepper, and thyme. Heat to boiling. Cover and simmer soup over low heat for 20 minutes. Stir in skim milk and black pepper. Heat through.

6 SERVINGS

Each with: 143 Calories (34% from Fat, 15% from Protein, 51% from Carb); 6 g Protein; 6 g Total Fat; 1 g Unsaturated Fat; 4 g Monounsaturated Fat; 1 g Polyunsaturated Fat; 20 g Carb; 3 g Fiber; 3 g Sugar; 139 mg Phosphorus; 76 mg Calcium; 69 mg Sodium; 464 mg Potassium; 488 IU Vitamin A; 25 mg ATE Vitamin E; 28 mg Vitamin C; 1 mg Cholesterol

Fill Up on Vegetarian Chili Soup

This is really a combination of chili and vegetable soup, but whichever you call it,
the taste is great, the nutrition is great, and the calories are low.

1 cup (160 g) onion, chopped

1 teaspoon garlic, minced

1 tablespoon (15 ml) olive oil

1 cup (100 g) celery, chopped

2 cups (244 g) carrot, peeled and
thinly sliced

2 cups (300 g) green bell pepper,
chopped

10 ounces (280 g) frozen corn

1 cup (260 g) salsa

8 ounces (225 g) mushrooms,
sliced

1¼ cup (285 ml) water

14 ounces (390 g) kidney beans,
no-salt-added, drained

14 ounces (390 g) no-salt-added
tomatoes, undrained

1 teaspoon lemon juice

¼ teaspoon dried oregano

1 teaspoon ground cumin

1 teaspoon chili powder

1 teaspoon black pepper

Sauté onion and garlic in olive oil in a Dutch oven over
medium heat until tender. Add remaining fresh veggies. Sauté
2 to 3 minutes. Add remaining ingredients. Cover. Simmer until
flavors are blended and vegetables are tender, about ½ hour.

10 SERVINGS

Each with: 132 Calories (14% from Fat, 19% from Protein, 67% from Carb);
7 g Protein; 2 g Total Fat; 0 g Saturated Fat; 1 g Monounsaturated Fat; 1 g
Polyunsaturated Fat; 24 g Carb; 7 g Fiber; 6 g Sugar; 140 mg Phosphorus; 63 mg
Calcium; 156 mg Sodium; 645 mg Potassium; 3610 IU Vitamin A; 0 mg ATE Vitamin
E; 40 mg Vitamin C; 0 mg Cholesterol

Country Everything Soup

This soup really does have a little of everything: split peas, barley, lentils, brown rice, pasta, and a great assortment of vegetables. Yet with all that nutrition, fiber, and just plain fill you up goodness, it's low enough in calories that you can have a slice of bread from chapter 14 or a dessert from chapter 15 with it.

¾ cup (169 g) split green peas
¾ cup (150 g) barley
¾ cup (144 g) lentils
½ cup (95 g) brown rice, uncooked
2 tablespoons (8 g) fresh parsley, chopped
2 tablespoons (10 g) onion flakes
½ teaspoon lemon pepper
1½ cups (158 g) whole wheat pasta
3 quarts (2.8 L) low sodium vegetable broth
1 cup (100 g) celery, chopped
1 cup (122 g) carrot, sliced
2 cups (180 g) cabbage, shredded
2 cups (360 g) no-salt-added tomatoes

Combine all ingredients in a large soup pot and simmer until vegetables are tender, about 1 hour.

8 SERVINGS

Each with: 320 Calories (9% from Fat, 24% from Protein, 67% from Carb); 20 g Protein; 3 g Total Fat; 1 g Saturated Fat; 1 g Monounsaturated Fat; 1 g Polyunsaturated Fat; 55 g Carb; 13 g Fiber; 6 g Sugar; 342 mg Phosphorus; 181 mg Calcium; 1204 mg Sodium; 961 mg Potassium; 2221 IU Vitamin A; 4 mg ATE Vitamin E; 22 mg Vitamin C; 0 mg Cholesterol

Bean (and No Fat) Soup

Most large markets carry a bean mixture in their dried bean section. The one I happened to find had 16 varieties. This meatless soup contains only 200 calories per serving, but gives you large helpings of protein, potassium, and other good things. So you are free to pick another 200 calories from the other mix and match chapters. I'd suggest a big salad and a slice of freshly baked bread.

1 pound (455 g) dried bean
  mixture
1 onion, chopped
½ cup (50 g) celery, sliced
1 cup (122 g) carrot, sliced
1 tablespoon (6 g) low sodium
  chicken bouillon
2 cups (360 g) no-salt-added
  tomatoes, undrained
½ teaspoon black pepper
6 cups (1.4 L) water

Soak and drain beans according to package directions.
In a large saucepan or Dutch oven, combine all ingredients. Bring to a boil. Reduce heat, cover, and simmer until beans are tender, about 1½ hours.

8 SERVINGS

Each with: 216 Calories (3% from Fat, 25% from Protein, 72% from Carb); 14 g Protein; 1 g Total Fat; 0 g Saturated Fat; 0 g Monounsaturated Fat; 0 g Polyunsaturated Fat; 40 g Carb; 10 g Fiber; 5 g Sugar; 194 mg Phosphorus; 170 mg Calcium; 67 mg Sodium; 1257 mg Potassium; 2059 IU Vitamin A; 0 mg ATE Vitamin E; 11 mg Vitamin C; 0 mg Cholesterol

Mix and Match: Starters and Side Dishes

This chapter contains mainly side dishes for your mix and match pleasure, but there are also a couple of appetizers included. The idea was to come up with some dishes that were interesting and maybe a little out of the ordinary in taste. But when it comes to side dishes, you have lots of choices. Most fresh vegetables are very low in calories and high in nutrition. Along with the dishes in this chapter, you can also pick and choose from the following list. Keep in mind that fresh veggies will have more nutrition than frozen or canned ones, raw veggies more than cooked, and those minimally cooked by steaming more than those that are boiled.

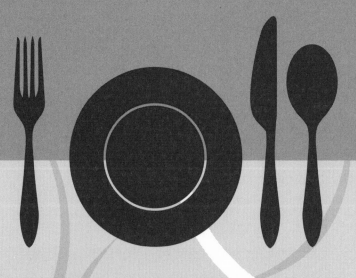

Fresh vegetables, 1 cup (225 g) serving

Mushrooms	13 calories
Yellow squash	18 calories
Zucchini	20 calories
Cauliflower	29 calories
Broccoli	30 calories
Green bell pepper	30 calories
Green beans	34 calories
Red bell pepper	39 calories
Onion	67 calories
Peas	125 calories
Corn	132 calories

How About Some Chicken Wings Honey?

Sweet, with a hint of Asian barbecue flavor, these wings are always popular, especially with those who don't like the heat of Buffalo wings. The honey ups the calories count of these a little, so be aware when you are picking mix and match dishes to go with them.

1¼ pounds (570 g) chicken wings
2 tablespoons (40 g) honey
½ cup (120 ml) low sodium soy sauce
2 tablespoons (28 ml) olive oil
2 tablespoons (30 g) catsup
½ teaspoon garlic, minced

Rinse chicken wings; pat dry. Cut off and discard wing tips and then cut each wing at the joint to make two sections. Place wings on a broiler pan spayed with nonstick vegetable oil spray. Broil about 4 inches (10 cm) from the heat for 5 minutes on each side or until chicken wings are nicely browned. Transfer chicken wings to baking dish. In a bowl, combine remaining ingredients. Pour sauce over chicken wings. Cover and cook at 350°F (180°C, or gas mark 4) until chicken is done, about 20 minutes.

8 SERVINGS

Each with: 148 Calories (36% from Fat, 45% from Protein, 19% from Carb); 16 g Protein; 6 g Total Fat; 1 g Saturated Fat; 3 g Monounsaturated Fat; 1 g Polyunsaturated Fat; 7 g Carb; 0 g Fiber; 5 g Sugar; 129 mg Phosphorus; 13 mg Calcium; 590 mg Sodium; 188 mg Potassium; 81 IU Vitamin A; 13 mg ATE Vitamin E; 1 mg Vitamin C; 40 mg Cholesterol

Asian Chicken Wing Starters

Chicken wings are usually fairly high in fat since they can't easily have their skin removed. We hold down the calorie count of these Asian flavored wings down by using sugar substitute and limiting the portion size. Served as an appetizer, each person will get 2 to 3 wing sections.

1¼ pounds (570 g) chicken wings
½ cup (80 g) onion, chopped
¼ cup (60 ml) low sodium soy sauce
½ cup (8 g) brown sugar substitute, such as Splenda
1 teaspoon ground ginger
½ teaspoon garlic, minced
¼ cup (60 ml) sherry

 Tip: If you want to use them as a main dish, double the portion size and pick another 200 mix and match calories, choosing items that contain significant bulk like salads or vegetables.

Rinse chicken wings; pat dry. Cut off and discard wing tips then cut each wing at the joint to make two sections. Place wings on a broiler pan spayed with nonstick vegetable oil spray. Broil about 4 inches (10 cm) from the heat for 5 minutes on each side or until chicken wings are nicely browned. Transfer chicken wings to baking dish. In a bowl, combine chopped onion, soy sauce, brown sugar, ginger, garlic, and sherry. Pour sauce over chicken wings. Cover and cook at 350°F (180°C, or gas mark 4) until chicken is done, about 20 minutes.

8 SERVINGS

Each with: 111 Calories (23% from Fat, 65% from Protein, 12% from Carb); 16 g Protein; 3 g Total Fat; 1 g Saturated Fat; 1 g Monounsaturated Fat; 1 g Polyunsaturated Fat; 3 g Carb; 0 g Fiber; 1 g Sugar; 123 mg Phosphorus; 14 mg Calcium; 324 mg Sodium; 177 mg Potassium; 42 IU Vitamin A; 13 mg ATE Vitamin E; 2 mg Vitamin C; 40 mg Cholesterol

Fresh Salsa PLUS

This salsa is for those people who like both salsa and guacamole. It's a tasty, healthy, low calorie combination of the two.

1 cup (180 g) plum tomatoes, seeded and finely chopped
¼ cup (40 g) red onion, diced
1 jalapeño pepper, seeded and chopped
1 avocado, diced
2 tablespoons (28 ml) lime juice
1 tablespoon (1 g) cilantro

Put all the ingredients in to a bowl. Stir to mix.

8 SERVINGS

Each with: 43 Calories (64% from Fat, 6% from Protein, 30% from Carb); 1 g Protein; 3 g Total Fat; 0 g Saturated Fat; 2 g Monounsaturated Fat; 0 g Polyunsaturated Fat; 4 g Carb; 2 g Fiber; 1 g Sugar; 19 mg Phosphorus; 7 mg Calcium; 3 mg Sodium; 171 mg Potassium; 225 IU Vitamin A; 0 mg ATE Vitamin E; 7 mg Vitamin C; 0 mg Cholesterol

Mega Starter Side Salad

What we have here is mix and match within mix and match. Pick and choose the vegetables you like from the various categories and end up with a starter that gets any meal off to a good start, providing lots of food and very few calories. Choosing from the items below as specified will give you a salad containing between 30 and 40 calories. The nutritional analysis below shows what you would get if you picked everything. Pick a low calorie dressing from chapter 2 and be sure to add those calories or just drizzle it with balsamic vinegar.

Choose one of the following as a base:

1 cup (47 g) romaine lettuce, torn into bite-sized pieces

1½ cups (45 g) spinach, torn into bite-sized pieces

1½ cups (108 g) iceberg lettuce, torn into bite-sized pieces

Add two of the following:

2 tablespoons (14 g) carrot, shredded

⅓ cup (33 g) celery, sliced

⅓ cup (40 g) zucchini, sliced

¼ cup (18 g) mushrooms, sliced

Add 1 one the following:

4 cherry tomatoes, halved

¼ cup (40 g) red onion, thinly sliced

Pick and choose and eat!!

1 SERVING

Each with: 82 Calories (8% from Fat, 21% from Protein, 71% from Carb); 5 g Protein; 1 g Total Fat; 0 g Saturated Fat; 0 g Monounsaturated Fat; 0 g Polyunsaturated Fat; 17 g Carb; 6 g Fiber; 7 g Sugar; 114 mg Phosphorus; 120 mg Calcium; 97 mg Sodium; 1042 mg Potassium; 10 350 IU Vitamin A; 0 mg ATE Vitamin E; 54 mg Vitamin C; 0 mg Cholesterol

Super Asian Side Salad

Like our *Mega Starter Side Salad*, this salad lets you pick and choose, including Asian ingredients. Depending on what you pick, you'll end up with a salad that contains between 35 and 45 calories. Try it with the *Creamy Asian Salad Dressing* in chapter 2 for a total of 56 calories or less.

Choose one of the following as a base:

1 cup (47 g) romaine lettuce, torn into bite-sized pieces

1½ cups (45 g) spinach, torn into bite-sized pieces

1½ cups (108 g) iceberg lettuce, torn into bite-sized pieces

Add two of the following:

¼ cup (26 g) fresh bean spouts

2 tablespoons (16 g) water chestnuts, sliced

¼ cup (38 g) red bell pepper, sliced

4 cherry tomatoes, halved

Add both of the following if desired:

¼ cup (18 g) mushrooms, sliced

¼ cup (30 g) cucumber, thinly sliced

Pick and choose and eat!!

1 SERVING

Each with: 70 Calories (9% from Fat, 25% from Protein, 66% from Carb); 5 g Protein; 1 g Total Fat; 0 g Saturated Fat; 0 g Monounsaturated Fat; 0 g Polyunsaturated Fat; 14 g Carb; 4 g Fiber; 5 g Sugar; 100 mg Phosphorus; 96 mg Calcium; 54 mg Sodium; 808 mg Potassium; 8932 IU Vitamin A; 0 mg ATE Vitamin E; 119 mg Vitamin C; 0 mg Cholesterol

MaxiFruit Salad

Here's one more Mix and Match salad builder for you, this one with the added flavor of fruit. This one has a few more calories, but you can still build yourself a great salad for around 50 and add a helping of the *Fruity Orange Yogurt Dressing* for a total of around 75 calories. This can also make a good dessert or addition to a breakfast by leaving out the greens. The nutrition below is for all the ingredients.

Choose one of the following as a base:

1 cup (47 g) romaine lettuce, torn into bite-sized pieces

1½ cups (45 g) spinach, torn into bite-sized pieces

1½ cups (108 g) iceberg lettuce, torn into bite-sized pieces

Add two of the following:

½ cup (73 g) strawberries, sliced

¼ cup (36 g) blueberries

¼ cup (46 g) orange sections

Add 1 one the following:

¼ cup (18 g) mushrooms, sliced

2 tablespoons (14 g) carrot, shredded

Pick and choose and eat!!

1 SERVING

Each with: 105 Calories (7% from Fat, 15% from Protein, 78% from Carb); 5 g Protein; 1 g Total Fat; 0 g Saturated Fat; 0 g Monounsaturated Fat; 0 g Polyunsaturated Fat; 24 g Carb; 7 g Fiber; 15 g Sugar; 106 mg Phosphorus; 118 mg Calcium; 60 mg Sodium; 847 mg Potassium; 9793 IU Vitamin A; 0 mg ATE Vitamin E; 103 mg Vitamin C; 0 mg Cholesterol

Pretty as It Is Good for You Broccoli and Tomato Salad

This salad is great with a piece of grilled meat or an egg dish like quiche. It can provide all the vegetables you need to make a filling, nutritious meal.

Salad

1 pound (455 g) broccoli

¼ pound (115 g) mushrooms

¾ cup (105 g) olives, drained

8 ounces (225 g) cherry tomatoes

Dressing

¼ cup (60 ml) olive oil

1 tablespoon (15 ml) white wine vinegar

1 tablespoon (15 ml) lemon juice

2 tablespoons (8 g) fresh parsley, chopped

¼ cup (25 g) green onion, minced

¼ teaspoon garlic, minced

¼ teaspoon black pepper, fresh ground

 Tip: This is a colorful salad that looks very impressive served in a glass bowl.

Trim florets from broccoli. You should have about 1 quart (1.1 kg). Reserve stems for another use. Drop broccoli florets into boiling water for 1 minute or just until they turn bright green; drain. Trim mushroom stems to ½ inch (1.3 cm). Combine broccoli, mushrooms, olives, and cherry tomatoes in bowl. Measure oil, vinegar, lemon juice, parsley, onion, garlic, and black pepper into small bowl. Whisk until blended. Pour dressing over vegetable mixture. Turn gently to coat vegetables. Cover and refrigerate 3 hours or more until ready to serve.

4 SERVINGS

Each with: 209 Calories (67% from Fat, 9% from Protein, 24% from Carb); 5 g Protein; 17 g Total Fat; 2 g Saturated Fat; 12 g Monounsaturated Fat; 2 g Polyunsaturated Fat; 14 g Carb; 5 g Fiber; 3 g Sugar; 104 mg Phosphorus; 88 mg Calcium; 261 mg Sodium; 603 mg Potassium; 1393 IU Vitamin A; 0 mg ATE Vitamin E; 117 mg Vitamin C; 0 mg Cholesterol

Good Luck (and Good Nutrition) Salad

This recipe has its roots in the southern United States. Black-eyed peas are supposed to be good luck when eaten on New Year's Day. This has become a traditional New Year's recipe in our house because it gets you the good luck peas in a side dish that can be paired with any meat.

1½ cups (257 g) dried black eyed peas, cooked

½ cup (75 g) green bell pepper, chopped

½ cup (75 g) red bell pepper, chopped

1 teaspoon garlic, minced

1 cup (160 g) onion, minced

3 tablespoons (45 ml) red wine vinegar

2 tablespoons (28 ml) olive oil

½ teaspoon dried thyme

Pour the drained black-eyed peas into a medium-sized bowl and add the red and green bell pepper, garlic, and onion. In another bowl, combine the vinegar, olive oil, and thyme to form the marinade. Pour the marinade over the black-eyed pea mixture, cover with plastic wrap, and refrigerate overnight so that the flavors blend, stirring occasionally.

4 SERVINGS

Each with: 171 Calories (37% from Fat, 14% from Protein, 49% from Carb); 6 g Protein; 7 g Total Fat; 1 g Saturated Fat; 5 g Monounsaturated Fat; 1 g Polyunsaturated Fat; 21 g Carb; 5 g Fiber; 6 g Sugar; 98 mg Phosphorus; 30 mg Calcium; 6 mg Sodium; 372 mg Potassium; 705 IU Vitamin A; 0 mg ATE Vitamin E; 55 mg Vitamin C; 0 mg Cholesterol

Garbanzo and Pasta Salad

Garbanzo beans can be purchased dried or canned. If using dried beans,
cook according to package directions.

4 ounces (115 g) whole wheat
pasta, uncooked

2 cups (480 g) garbanzo beans,
drained and rinsed

½ cup (75 g) red bell pepper,
chopped

⅓ cup (33 g) celery, sliced

⅓ cup (41 g) carrot, sliced

¼ cup (25 g) green onion,
chopped

3 tablespoons (45 ml) balsamic
vinegar

2 tablespoons (28 g) low fat
mayonnaise

2 teaspoons mustard

½ teaspoon black pepper

¼ teaspoon dried Italian seasoning

4 cup (188 g) leaf lettuce, torn
into bite-sized pieces

 Tip: This recipe can also be
used as a vegetarian main
dish, yielding 4 servings.

Cook pasta according to directions, omitting salt. Drain and
rinse well under cold water until pasta is cool; drain well.
Combine pasta, garbanzo beans, red bell pepper, celery, carrot,
and green onion in medium bowl. Whisk together vinegar,
mayonnaise, mustard, black pepper, and Italian seasoning in
small bowl until blended. Pour over salad; toss to coat evenly.
Cover and refrigerate up to 8 hours. Arrange lettuce on
individual plates. Spoon salad over lettuce.

8 SERVINGS

Each with: 151 Calories (16% from Fat, 15% from Protein, 69% from Carb);
6 g Protein; 3 g Total Fat; 0 g Saturated Fat; 0 g Monounsaturated Fat; 1 g
Polyunsaturated Fat; 27 g Carb; 4 g Fiber; 2 g Sugar; 102 mg Phosphorus; 43 mg
Calcium; 229 mg Sodium; 261 mg Potassium; F3094 IU Vitamin A; 2 mg ATE Vitamin
E; 26 mg Vitamin C; 15 mg Cholesterol

Grilled Vegetable Orzo Salad

This is colorful, tasty, and full of nutrition. Although it's a side dish, it's a good starting place for a meal. We had it with a grilled chicken breast, thinking we might as well put the rest of the grill to use while it was on.

1 cup (120 g) zucchini, cut into 1-inch (2.5 cm) pieces

½ cup (75 g) red bell pepper, cut into 1-inch (2.5 cm) pieces

½ cup (75 g) yellow bell pepper, cut into 1-inch (2.5 cm) pieces

½ cup (80 g) red onion, cut into 1-inch (2.5 cm) pieces

½ teaspoon garlic, minced

1 tablespoon (15 ml) olive oil

8 ounces (225 g) whole wheat orzo

⅓ cup (80 ml) lemon juice

1 teaspoon black pepper, fresh ground, divided

¼ cup (35 g) pine nuts, toasted

Prepare the grill. Toss zucchini, red and yellow bell pepper, onion, and garlic with the olive oil and ½ teaspoon black pepper in a large bowl. Transfer to a grill basket. Grill for 15 to 20 minutes, until browned, stirring occasionally. Meanwhile, cook the orzo in boiling water according to package directions. Drain and transfer to a large serving bowl. Add the roasted vegetables to the pasta. Combine the lemon juice and black pepper and pour on the pasta and vegetables. Let cool to room temperature. Stir in the pine nuts and serve.

8 SERVINGS

Each with: 161 Calories (28% from Fat, 11% from Protein, 61% from Carb); 5 g Protein; 5 g Total Fat; 1 g Saturated Fat; 2 g Monounsaturated Fat; 2 g Polyunsaturated Fat; 25 g Carb; 1 g Fiber; 2 g Sugar; 79 mg Phosphorus; 13 mg Calcium; 4 mg Sodium; 162 mg Potassium; 327 IU Vitamin A; 0 mg ATE Vitamin E; 26 mg Vitamin C; 0 mg Cholesterol

Low Calorie Mexican Bean Salad

This is a simple and tasty south of the border bean salad. Unlike much Mexican food, this salad is full of nutrition and very low in fat and calories.

1½ cups (384 g) no-salt-added kidney beans, drained

1½ cups (360 g) no-salt-added garbanzo beans, drained

1 cup (180 g) tomatoes, chopped

¾ cup (89 g) cucumber, peeled and chopped

2 tablespoons (20 g) onion, diced

½ cup (118 g) guacamole

½ cup (115 g) low fat plain yogurt

4 cups (288 g) iceberg lettuce, shredded

 Tip: Eden Organic and some other companies make no-salt-added beans if you are watching your sodium.

In a large bowl, toss together the kidney beans, garbanzo beans, tomatoes, cucumber, and onion. In a small bowl, mix the guacamole and yogurt. If dressing seems thick, stir in a little skim milk. Stir into the bean mixture and chill. Serve on top of shredded lettuce.

8 SERVINGS

Each with: 126 Calories (18% from Fat, 22% from Protein, 60% from Carb); 7 g Protein; 3 g Total Fat; 0 g Saturated Fat; 1 g Monounsaturated Fat; 1 g Polyunsaturated Fat; 20 g Carb; 6 g Fiber; 4 g Sugar; 139 mg Phosphorus; 63 mg Calcium; 18 mg Sodium; 408 mg Potassium; 284 IU Vitamin A; 2 mg ATE Vitamin E; 6 mg Vitamin C; 1 mg Cholesterol

Pasta and Kidney Bean Salad

This is really an easy salad to put together, especially if you're like me and tend to cook a whole pound of kidney beans while you are doing it, then wonder what to do with the leftovers. It goes well with just about any kind of meat and has a lot of nutrition on its own.

4 ounces (115 g) whole wheat rotini, or other small pasta
2 cups (512 g) red kidney beans, cooked
1 cup (120 g) zucchini, diced
1 cup (150 g) green bell pepper, diced
1 cup (180 g) tomato, chopped
⅓ cup (47 g) green olives, chopped
½ cup (115 g) low fat mayonnaise
½ teaspoon chili powder
½ teaspoon coriander
½ teaspoon paprika
¼ teaspoon dried sage

Cook pasta until al dente. Rinse and drain. Put in large bowl and add rest of the ingredients. Mix thoroughly and serve chilled or at room temperature.

6 SERVINGS

Each with: 190 Calories (9% from Fat, 19% from Protein, 72% from Carb); 9 g Protein; 2 g Total Fat; 0 g Saturated Fat; 1 g Monounsaturated Fat; 0 g Polyunsaturated Fat; 34 g Carb; 8 g Fiber; 3 g Sugar; 136 mg Phosphorus; 60 mg Calcium; 374 mg Sodium; 457 mg Potassium; 560 IU Vitamin A; 0 mg ATE Vitamin E; 28 mg Vitamin C; 2 mg Cholesterol

Fall Slaw

This is a different kind of coleslaw. The apples provide sweetness, great nutrition, and a sense that you've had more food than the calorie count shows.

Dressing

2 tablespoons (28 g) low fat mayonnaise, low sodium

¼ cup (60 g) low fat plain yogurt

½ tablespoon lemon juice

1 tablespoon (20 g) honey

¼ teaspoon celery seed

⅛ teaspoon black pepper

Slaw

2 cups (180 g) cabbage, shredded

2 cups (300 g) apple, chopped

Mix together all dressing ingredients and toss with cabbage and apples.

8 SERVINGS

Each with: 43 Calories (28% from Fat, 6% from Protein, 66% from Carb); 1 g Protein; 1 g Total Fat; 0 g Saturated Fat; 0 g Monounsaturated Fat; 0 g Polyunsaturated Fat; 8 g Carb; 1 g Fiber; 6 g Sugar; 21 mg Phosphorus; 25 mg Calcium; 39 mg Sodium; 92 mg Potassium; 44 IU Vitamin A; 1 mg ATE Vitamin E; 11 mg Vitamin C; 2 mg Cholesterol

Tip: This is good with pork or chicken.

Sweet and Low Pineapple Slaw

It's not named for the sweetener but for the taste and the calories. This fruity slaw is perfect with spiced or barbecued meats can has only 26 calories per serving.

2 tablespoons (19 g) green bell pepper, chopped

½ cup (75 g) apple, diced

1 teaspoon sugar substitute

¼ cup (60 ml) cider vinegar

3 cups (270 g) cabbage, shredded

1 cup (110 g) carrot, shredded

½ cup (120 g) crushed pineapple, drained

Combine green bell pepper, apple, sugar substitute, and vinegar. Pour over vegetables and pineapple and stir to combine.

8 SERVINGS

Each with: 26 Calories (4% from Fat, 8% from Protein, 89% from Carb); 1 g Protein; 0 g Total Fat; 0 g Saturated Fat; 0 g Monounsaturated Fat; 0 g Polyunsaturated Fat; 6 g Carb; 1 g Fiber; 4 g Sugar; 15 mg Phosphorus; 21 mg Calcium; 16 mg Sodium; 150 mg Potassium; 1976 IU Vitamin A; 0 mg ATE Vitamin E; 18 mg Vitamin C; 0 mg Cholesterol

Better Than the Original Deviled Eggs

A healthier alternative to the usual deviled eggs, these have no cholesterol, less fat, and 2 grams of fiber. And you won't miss the flavor of the yolks at all. These are a perfect addition to any picnic.

7 eggs, hard boiled, peeled
1 cup (240 g) garbanzo beans, drained
2 tablespoons (30 g) plain fat-free yogurt
1 teaspoon Dijon mustard
½ teaspoon garlic, minced

Slice eggs in half and discard yolks. In food processor, add beans and next 3 ingredients. Spoon mixture into egg cavities.

14 SERVINGS

Each with: 65 Calories (44% from Fat, 29% from Protein, 27% from Carb); 5 g Protein; 3 g Total Fat; 1 g Saturated Fat; 1 g Monounsaturated Fat; 0 g Polyunsaturated Fat; 4 g Carb; 1 g Fiber; 0 g Sugar; 75 mg Phosphorus; 26 mg Calcium; 98 mg Sodium; 75 mg Potassium; 146 IU Vitamin A; 40 mg ATE Vitamin E; 1 mg Vitamin C; 123 mg Cholesterol

Almost Calorie Free Fresh Veggie Medley

Come on, where else can you get this much taste and filling power for so few calories?
A big serving is less than 20 calories. For those of you looking for comparison,
that the same as 4 Jelly Belly jelly beans.

4 tomatoes, chopped
1 zucchini, cubed
½ pound (225 g) green beans
¼ teaspoon garlic powder
1 teaspoon dried basil

Wash, trim, and cook beans until almost tender. Drain. Return to pan with other ingredients and cook to desired doneness.

4 SERVINGS

Each with: 19 Calories (3% from Fat, 20% from Protein, 77% from Carb); 1 g Protein; 0 g Total Fat; 0 g Saturated Fat; 0 g Monounsaturated Fat; 0 g Polyunsaturated Fat; 4 g Carb; 2 g Fiber; 1 g Sugar; 23 mg Phosphorus; 25 mg Calcium; 4 mg Sodium; 126 mg Potassium; 408 IU Vitamin A; 0 mg ATE Vitamin E; 9 mg Vitamin C; 0 mg Cholesterol

Spinach and Bean Thread Casserole

This is a delicious mixture of ingredients that is surprisingly easy to make.

2 cups (475 ml) low sodium
   chicken broth
4 ounces (115 g) bean threads,
   also called cellophane noodles
10 ounces (280 g) frozen spinach
1 tablespoon (14 g) unsalted
   butter

 Tip: Beans threads are
available at most grocery
stores in the ethnic foods
section and at Asian markets.

Soak bean threads in warm water 5 minutes. If desired, bean threads can be cut in shorter lengths with kitchen scissors or knives after soaking. Put chicken broth in pan. Add drained bean threads. Boil until most of the liquid is absorbed by bean threads. Mix butter into bean threads. Thaw spinach until pieces can be broken apart. Mix spinach pieces into the noodle mixture. Pour into casserole dish and bake 30 minutes at 350°F (180°C, or gas mark 4).

4 SERVINGS

Each with: 160 Calories (21% from Fat, 11% from Protein, 68% from Carb); 5 g Protein; 4 g Total Fat; 2 g Unsaturated Fat; 1 g Monounsaturated Fat; 0 g Polyunsaturated Fat; 28 g Carb; 2 g Fiber; 0 g Sugar; 81 mg Phosphorus; 83 mg Calcium; 95 mg Sodium; 502 mg Potassium; 6735 IU Vitamin A; 24 mg ATE Vitamin E; 20 mg Vitamin C; 8 mg Cholesterol

Corn and Spinach Casserole

Spinach is a great nutrition value. Here it is paired with corn, which by itself tends to be higher in calories than many vegetables, holding down the overall calorie count in a dish reminiscent of corn pudding.

¼ cup (40 g) chopped onion
3 cups (492 g) frozen corn
½ cup (120 ml) egg substitute
½ cup (120 ml) skim milk
1 tablespoon (15 ml) white wine
  vinegar
¼ teaspoon black pepper, freshly
  ground
½ pound (225 g) spinach,
  coarsely chopped
2 tablespoons (10 g) Parmesan
  cheese, grated
¼ cup (30 g) bread crumbs

 Tip: This unusual combination is excellent served with roast pork or chicken.

Spray an 8-inch (20 cm) square pan or 1½-quart (1.4 L) casserole with nonstick vegetable oil spray. Sprinkle chopped onion in the pan. Add corn. Mix egg substitute with skim milk and pour over the corn. In a bowl, add vinegar and black pepper to chopped spinach and toss until well seasoned. Place spinach mixture on top of corn. Sprinkle with cheese. Top with bread crumbs and bake in a preheated oven at 375°F (190°C, or gas mark 5) for 45 minutes.

6 SERVINGS

Each with: 134 Calories (13% from Fat, 23% from Protein, 64% from Carb); 9 g Protein; 2 g Total Fat; 1 g Unsaturated Fat; 1 g Monounsaturated Fat; 1 g Polyunsaturated Fat; 23 g Carb; 4 g Fiber; 4 g Sugar; 139 mg Phosphorus; 135 mg Calcium; 155 mg Sodium; 366 mg Potassium; 4688 IU Vitamin A; 15 mg ATE Vitamin E; 4 mg Vitamin C; 2 mg Cholesterol

Full of Flavor Sautéed Spinach

A little bit of garlic takes this spinach over the top. It's perfect with almost any kind of meat and one of the most nutrient dense vegetables you can find.

1 pound (455 g) spinach
2 tablespoons (28 ml) olive oil
1 clove garlic, minced

Sauté spinach and garlic in hot oil in a heavy skillet until wilted.

6 SERVINGS

Each with: 57 Calories (69% from Fat, 14% from Protein, 17% from Carb); 2 g Protein; 5 g Total Fat; 1 g Unsaturated Fat; 3 g Monounsaturated Fat; 1 g Polyunsaturated Fat; 3 g Carb; 2 g Fiber; 0 g Sugar; 37 mg Phosphorus; 75 mg Calcium; 60 mg Sodium; 422 mg Potassium; 7089 IU Vitamin A; 0 mg ATE Vitamin E; 21 mg Vitamin C; 0 mg Cholesterol

Greens the Real Southern Way

This is a traditional long cooked Southern recipe for greens. Collards and kale are at the very top of the ANDI scale in nutrient density and are naturally low in calories, so eating more is a good thing. The long slow cooking here and the bacon and sugar ensure that they will not be bitter. I like them with a little vinegar drizzled over and a few drops of hot pepper sauce. If everyone you're cooking for likes them hotter, you could just add ¼ to ½ teaspoon of red pepper flakes.

2 pounds (900 g) collard greens, or kale
3 slices low sodium bacon
¼ cup (40 g) onion, chopped
½ teaspoon black pepper
1 tablespoon (13 g) sugar

Rinse greens thoroughly. Cut off stems and chop coarsely. Brown bacon in the bottom of a stew pot or Dutch oven. Remove. Place greens, onion, and spices in pot. Add enough water to cover. Cover and cook until tender, about 45 minutes to an hour. Drain. Crumble bacon over.

6 SERVINGS

Each with: 78 Calories (24% from Fat, 24% from Protein, 52% from Carb); 5 g Protein; 2 g Total Fat; 1 g Saturated Fat; 1 g Monounsaturated Fat; 0 g Polyunsaturated Fat; 12 g Carb; 6 g Fiber; 3 g Sugar; 39 mg Phosphorus; 222 mg Calcium; 72 mg Sodium; 290 mg Potassium; 10 084 IU Vitamin A; 0 mg ATE Vitamin E; 54 mg Vitamin C; 4 mg Cholesterol

So Easy and Tasty Curried Fresh Vegetables

Nothing could be easier than this curried vegetable dish. It could be served as is for a side dish or over brown rice or pasta as an accompaniment to a meat course. And it's very low in calories.

3 cup (540 g) tomatoes, chopped
1 cup (160 g) onion, coarsely chopped
1½ cups (180 g) zucchini, cubed
1 cup (150 g) green bell pepper, chopped
¼ teaspoon garlic powder
1 tablespoon (6 g) curry powder

Combine all ingredients in a saucepan. Cook and stir until vegetables are softened.

4 SERVINGS

Each with: 61 Calories (10% from Fat, 14% from Protein, 77% from Carb); 2 g Protein; 1 g Total Fat; 0 g Saturated Fat; 0 g Monounsaturated Fat; 0 g Polyunsaturated Fat; 14 g Carb; 3 g Fiber; 3 g Sugar; 69 mg Phosphorus; 33 mg Calcium; 18 mg Sodium; 519 mg Potassium; 943 IU Vitamin A; 0 mg ATE Vitamin E; 70 mg Vitamin C; 0 mg Cholesterol

Spice Up Your Dinner with Indian Carrots and Spinach

Whenever I'm looking for a little different flavor combination for a side dish, I often look at Indian recipes. This one isn't curry per se, but it is very flavorful and packed about as full of nutrition as you can for less than 100 calories.

½ cup (50 g) green onion, sliced

2 cloves garlic, minced

½ teaspoon turmeric

1 tablespoon (15 ml) olive oil

3 cups (330 g) carrot, coarsely grated

¼ cup (25 g) celery, grated

½ cup (120 ml) low sodium vegetable broth

1 teaspoon ginger root, grated

½ teaspoon coriander

½ cup (40 g) coconut, grated

1¼ cups (195 g) frozen spinach, thawed and drained

Sauté green onion, garlic, and turmeric in oil until scallions are soft. Add remaining ingredients, simmer for 10 minutes, and serve.

6 SERVINGS

Each with: 89 Calories (48% from Fat, 6% from Protein, 47% from Carb); 1 g Protein; 5 g Total Fat; 2 g Saturated Fat; 2 g Monounsaturated Fat; 0 g Polyunsaturated Fat; 11 g Carb; 3 g Fiber; 3 g Sugar; 42 mg Phosphorus; 40 mg Calcium; 154 mg Sodium; 313 mg Potassium; 8398 IU Vitamin A; 0 mg ATE Vitamin E; 8 mg Vitamin C; 0 mg Cholesterol

Sesame Green Beans

These beans are a perfect side dish. They taste great, are low in fat and calories, and high in fiber and nutrition. What more could you ask?

1 teaspoon sesame seeds

1 pound (455 g) green beans, thawed if frozen

½ cup (120 ml) low sodium chicken broth

2 teaspoons lemon juice

Toast sesame seeds in a heavy nonstick skillet over medium heat, about 3 minutes, shaking pan constantly until seeds are browned and have popped. Add green beans and broth. Cover skillet and cook 7 to 8 minutes or until green beans are tender and liquid is evaporated. Stir in lemon juice before serving.

4 SERVINGS

Each with: 45 Calories (12% from Fat, 21% from Protein, 67% from Carb); 3 g Protein; 1 g Total Fat; 0 g Unsaturated Fat; 0 g Monounsaturated Fat; 0 g Polyunsaturated Fat; 9 g Carb; 4 g Fiber; 2 g Sugar; 57 mg Phosphorus; 51 mg Calcium; 16 mg Sodium; 269 mg Potassium; 783 IU Vitamin A; 0 mg ATE Vitamin E; 20 mg Vitamin C; 0 mg Cholesterol

Mediterranean Fresh Green Beans and Tomatoes

Tomatoes and Greek spices give these beans a Mediterranean flavor. And like many recipes featuring fresh vegetables, you get to eat a really large portion for very few calories.

2 pounds (900 g) fresh green beans, cut into 1-inch (2.5 cm) lengths
½ teaspoon garlic, crushed
2 cups (360 g) tomatoes, chopped
1 cup (160 g) onion, chopped
½ teaspoon dried oregano
1 teaspoon lemon juice
black pepper, fresh ground, to taste

Combine all ingredients in a large covered saucepan and simmer until beans are tender, about 30 minutes.

6 SERVINGS

Each with: 69 Calories (4% from Fat, 17% from Protein, 79% from Carb); 3 g Protein; 0 g Total Fat; 0 g Saturated Fat; 0 g Monounsaturated Fat; 0 g Polyunsaturated Fat; 16 g Carb; 6 g Fiber; 3 g Sugar; 77 mg Phosphorus; 66 mg Calcium; 14 mg Sodium; 468 mg Potassium; 1359 IU Vitamin A; 0 mg ATE Vitamin E; 40 mg Vitamin C; 0 mg Cholesterol

 Tip: These are good with a grilled chicken breast flavored with Greek or Italian spices.

Italian Green Beans

This has got to be the easiest recipe ever for spicing up the flavor of green beans and lifting them out of the ordinary, bland vegetable category.

2 cups (200 g) fresh green beans
1 tablespoon (15 ml) lemon juice
¼ teaspoon dried oregano
1 teaspoon pimento, chopped
dash garlic powder

Cook green beans in boiling water until just tender; drain. Combine lemon juice, oregano, pimento, and garlic powder. Pour over beans.

5 SERVINGS

Each with: 15 Calories (3% from Fat, 19% from Protein, 78% from Carb); 1 g Protein; 0 g Total Fat; 0 g Unsaturated Fat; 0 g Monounsaturated Fat; 0 g Polyunsaturated Fat; 3 g Carb; 2 g Fiber; 1 g Sugar; 17 mg Phosphorus; 17 mg Calcium; 3 mg Sodium; 98 mg Potassium; 329 IU Vitamin A; 0 mg ATE Vitamin E; 9 mg Vitamin C; 0 mg Cholesterol

Creamy Crunchy Squash

This creamy squash casserole with crunchy panko bread crumbs is sure to be a hit with any meal.

2 cups (240 g) yellow squash
1 cup (110 g) carrot, grated
1 cup (160 g) onion, chopped
1 cup (230 g) fat-free sour cream
1 can (10¾ ounces, or 305 g) low sodium cream of chicken soup
½ cup (58 g) low fat cheddar cheese, shredded
½ cup (25 g) panko bread crumbs

Thoroughly mix all ingredients except panko bread crumbs. Pour mixture into 2-quart (1.9 L) casserole dish. Put panko bread crumbs on top. Bake at 350°F (180°C, or gas mark 4) for 45 minutes.

6 SERVINGS

Each with: 179 Calories (45% from Fat, 16% from Protein, 39% from Carb); 7 g Protein; 9 g Total Fat; 4 g Unsaturated Fat; 3 g Monounsaturated Fat; 1 g Polyunsaturated Fat; 18 g Carb; 2 g Fiber; 4 g Sugar; 150 mg Phosphorus; 135 mg Calcium; 537 mg Sodium; 315 mg Potassium; 2902 IU Vitamin A; 66 mg ATE Vitamin E; 10 mg Vitamin C; 22 mg Cholesterol

Cheesy Corn and Zucchini Bake

Low fat cheese custard lifts this corn and zucchini out of the ordinary. It's great with just about any meat and only contributes a little over 100 calories despite all that taste.

3 cups (360 g) zucchini, sliced
¼ cup (40 g) onion, chopped
1 tablespoon (15 ml) olive oil
10 ounces (280 g) frozen corn, cooked
½ cup (55 g) low fat Swiss cheese, shredded
½ cup (120 ml) egg substitute
2 tablespoons (10 g) Parmesan cheese

Cook zucchini in boiling water until soft. Drain and mash with fork. Sauté onion in oil until soft. Combine zucchini, onion, corn, cheese, and egg substitute. Turn into a 1-quart (950 ml) casserole sprayed with nonstick vegetable oil spray. Sprinkle Parmesan cheese over top. Place on a baking sheet and bake uncovered at 350°F (180°C, or gas mark 4) until a knife inserted near the center comes out clean, about 40 minutes.

6 SERVINGS

Each with: 117 Calories (32% from Fat, 28% from Protein, 41% from Carb); 9 g Protein; 4 g Total Fat; 1 g Saturated Fat; 2 g Monounsaturated Fat; 1 g Polyunsaturated Fat; 13 g Carb; 2 g Fiber; 3 g Sugar; 159 mg Phosphorus; 153 mg Calcium; 106 mg Sodium; 325 mg Potassium; 227 IU Vitamin A; 7 mg ATE Vitamin E; 12 mg Vitamin C; 6 mg Cholesterol

Rich and Zippy Corn Casserole

A creamy corn casserole is spiced up by the addition of a can of chopped green chili peppers. Fat-free cream cheese gives it a rich taste and texture but helps hold down the calories.

16 ounces (455 g) frozen corn
4 ounces (115 g) fat-free cream cheese, softened
4 ounces (115 g) green chilies, chopped

Combine ingredients and place in a 1-quart (950 ml) baking dish. Cook in a 350°F (180°C, or gas mark 4) oven until corn is tender, about 25 minutes.

6 SERVINGS

Each with: 109 Calories (29% from Fat, 14% from Protein, 57% from Carb); 4 g Protein; 4 g Total Fat; 2 g Saturated Fat; 1 g Monounsaturated Fat; 0 g Polyunsaturated Fat; 17 g Carb; 2 g Fiber; 3 g Sugar; 91 mg Phosphorus; 25 mg Calcium; 278 mg Sodium; 243 mg Potassium; 415 IU Vitamin A; 34 mg ATE Vitamin E; 15 mg Vitamin C; 11 mg Cholesterol

Mashed Better Than Potatoes

Ok, so I'm holding out on you a bit with the recipe name. But if I told you that it was mashed cauliflower would you have looked at it? The truth is we all love mashed potatoes. But they aren't the best thing in the world for us. Sure, potatoes have a lot of good nutrition, but they also have a lot of calories, even before we add the butter and milk. Mashed cauliflower actually makes a great substitute that is just as nutritious and a lot lower in calories. Give it a try, you may be surprised.

4 cups (400 g) cauliflower, cut into 1-inch (2.5 g) pieces
8 ounces (225 g) low calorie cream cheese substitute, see recipe in chapter 2

Steam or roast cauliflower until tender. Combine cauliflower and cream cheese substitute in a food processor and process until smooth and well blended.

6 SERVINGS

Each with: 45 Calories (20% from Fat, 30% from Protein, 51% from Carb); 4 g Protein; 1 g Total Fat; 1 g Saturated Fat; 0 g Monounsaturated Fat; 0 g Polyunsaturated Fat; 6 g Carb; 2 g Fiber; 4 g Sugar; 86 mg Phosphorus; 89 mg Calcium; 41 mg Sodium; 214 mg Potassium; 31 IU Vitamin A; 6 mg ATE Vitamin E; 37 mg Vitamin C; 3 mg Cholesterol

Balsamic Onions

Balsamic vinegar is good on lots of meats and vegetables, providing flavor with less acidity than other vinegars and almost no calories. It's particularly good on onions, helping to mellow their strong flavor. This simple recipe is great with grilled meat. You can even grill the onions instead of baking them.

1 tablespoon (15 ml) olive oil
4 medium onions
¼ cup (60 ml) balsamic vinegar

Preheat oven to 375°F (190°C, or gas mark 5). Lightly spray a shallow roasting pan with nonstick vegetable oil spray. Wash onions and remove any loose skins. Rub onions with olive oil. Bake until tender, about 45 minutes to 1 hour. Open onions by cutting in half; drizzle with balsamic vinegar. Serve hot.

4 SERVINGS

Each with: 83 Calories (35% from Fat, 5% from Protein, 60% from Carb); 1 g Protein; 3 g Total Fat; 0 g Saturated Fat; 3 g Monounsaturated Fat; 0 g Polyunsaturated Fat; 13 g Carb; 2 g Fiber; 6 g Sugar; 34 mg Phosphorus; 28 mg Calcium; 4 mg Sodium; 191 mg Potassium; 2 IU Vitamin A; 0 mg ATE Vitamin E; 8 mg Vitamin C; 0 mg Cholesterol

Yes You Can Have Refried Beans

Beans contain a lot of protein, fiber, and other nutrients. But traditional refried beans also contain a lot of fat, which makes them unhealthy. These contain no fat at all. The use of the slow cooker makes it easy to prepare. The flavor is still fairly traditional but not spicy at all.

½ pound (225 g) pinto beans
2 cups (475 ml) water
½ cup (120 ml) coffee
1 teaspoon garlic, minced
1 cup (160 g) onion, diced
1 tablespoon (7 g) ground cumin
2 teaspoons chili powder
1½ teaspoons dried oregano

Rinse beans and place in a large bowl covered with water overnight. Drain and place in slow cooker along with remaining ingredients. Stir well, cover, and cook 8 to 10 hours or until beans are tender. Use a potato masher or large spoon to mash the beans until desired consistency.

8 SERVINGS

Each with: 105 Calories (6% from Fat, 23% from Protein, 71% from Carb); 6 g Protein; 1 g Total Fat; 0 g Saturated Fat; 0 g Monounsaturated Fat; 0 g Polyunsaturated Fat; 19 g Carb; 5 g Fiber; 2 g Sugar; 126 mg Phosphorus; 49 mg Calcium; 14 mg Sodium; 470 mg Potassium; 208 IU Vitamin A; 0 mg ATE Vitamin E; 4 mg Vitamin C; 0 mg Cholesterol

Slim You Down Baked Beans

A picnic's not a picnic without baked beans. And beans by themselves are good nutrition, low in calories, and high in fiber. Where we usually get into trouble is adding so much sugar and other bad things to them. So we've avoided that here, giving you great flavor without the extra calories.

½ pound (225 g) navy beans
4 cups (950 ml) water
1 cup (275 g) chili sauce
¾ cup (120 g) onion, chopped
2 tablespoons (40 g) molasses
2 tablespoons (2 g) brown sugar substitute, such as Splenda
1½ teaspoons dry mustard
¼ teaspoon garlic powder
1 cup (235 ml) water

Place beans in 4 cups (950 ml) water in large saucepan. Bring to boil and cook 1 minute. Remove from heat and let stand 1 hour. Return to heat and simmer until almost done, about 1 hour. Drain. Mix together with remaining ingredients. Place in a 1½-quart (1.4 L) baking dish. Cover and bake at 325°F (170°C, or gas mark 3) 1½ to 2 hours. Add water if needed during cooking.

6 SERVINGS

Each with: 91 Calories (4% from Fat, 16% from Protein, 80% from Carb); 4 g Protein; 0 g Total Fat; 0 g Saturated Fat; 0 g Monounsaturated Fat; 0 g Polyunsaturated Fat; 19 g Carb; 2 g Fiber; 7 g Sugar; 59 mg Phosphorus; 50 mg Calcium; 450 mg Sodium; 244 mg Potassium; 670 IU Vitamin A; 0 mg ATE Vitamin E; 9 mg Vitamin C; 0 mg Cholesterol

Sweet Island Baked Beans

Sweet and just slightly spicy, with the unexpected addition of pineapple, these beans go well with any grilled meat but especially jerk seasoned meat.

2 cups (364 g) navy beans, cooked
½ cup (120 g) low sodium catsup
1 can (20 ounces, or 570 g) pineapple chunks, drained
2 tablespoons (2 g) brown sugar substitute, such as Splenda
1½ teaspoons mustard
⅛ teaspoon ground cloves

Combine all ingredients and pour into 1-quart (950 ml) casserole. Bake, uncovered, at 375°F (190°C, or gas mark 5) for 50 to 55 minutes or until beans are hot, stirring occasionally.

6 SERVINGS

Each with: 111 Calories (4% from Fat, 20% from Protein, 76% from Carb); 6 g Protein; 0 g Total Fat; 0 g Unsaturated Fat; 0 g Monounsaturated Fat; 0 g Polyunsaturated Fat; 22 g Carb; 4 g Fiber; 5 g Sugar; 103 mg Phosphorus; 48 mg Calcium; 5 mg Sodium; 332 mg Potassium; 213 IU Vitamin A; 0 mg ATE Vitamin E; 4 mg Vitamin C; 0 mg Cholesterol

More Nutritious Than Rice Pilaf

This bulgur and lentil dish makes a great side dish by itself, but it can also be the base for a vegetable rich sauce, providing a lower calorie option to rice or pasta.

1 cup (192 g) lentils

4 cups (950 ml) low sodium vegetable broth

1 bay leaf

1 tablespoon (15 ml) olive oil, unsalted

1 cup (160 g) onion, chopped

1 cup (150 g) green bell pepper, chopped

1 cup (100 g) bulgur

Rinse the lentils and put in a pot with enough broth to cover. Add bay leaf, bring to a boil, and keep covered. Turn off heat and let stand for 30 minutes. While the lentils are soaking, heat oil in a heavy pot. Add chopped onion and green bell pepper. Sauté until onions are tender and transparent. When onions are ready, keep heat at medium, stir in bulgur, and continue stirring until all the oil is absorbed. Lower heat to a simmer and add the rest of the broth and lentils in their broth. Bring to a boil, reduce heat again, cover tightly, and simmer until all the liquid has been absorbed. Add more liquid as needed until the bulgur and lentils are cooked. Remove bay leaf and serve.

6 SERVINGS

Each with: 140 Calories (39% from Fat, 12% from Protein, 49% from Carb); 4 g Protein; 6 g Total Fat; 1 g Saturated Fat; 3 g Monounsaturated Fat; 1 g Polyunsaturated Fat; 18 g Carb; 3 g Fiber; 2 g Sugar; 103 mg Phosphorus; 33 mg Calcium; 782 mg Sodium; 224 mg Potassium; 5 IU Vitamin A; 0 mg ATE Vitamin E; 5 mg Vitamin C; 0 mg Cholesterol

Perfect Under Anything Confetti Couscous

For anyone not familiar with couscous, it's very small Middle Eastern pasta. It can be used as a base for curries, tomato-based sauces, or any number of other things or by itself as a side dish.

1 cup (175 g) whole wheat couscous

1½ cups (355 ml) low sodium chicken broth

¼ cup (40 g) onion, finely chopped

¼ cup (38 g) red bell pepper, finely chopped

¼ cup (25 g) celery, finely chopped

1 tablespoon (15 ml) olive oil

Sauté all vegetables in oil until tender. Bring broth to a boil. Stir in couscous and veggies. Cover and let stand 5 minutes. Fluff with fork before serving.

4 SERVINGS

Each with: 206 Calories (16% from Fat, 14% from Protein, 70% from Carb); 7 g Protein; 4 g Total Fat; 1 g Saturated Fat; 3 g Monounsaturated Fat; 0 g Polyunsaturated Fat; 36 g Carb; 3 g Fiber; 1 g Sugar; 97 mg Phosphorus; 23 mg Calcium; 219 mg Sodium; 202 mg Potassium; 325 IU Vitamin A; 0 mg ATE Vitamin E; 19 mg Vitamin C; 0 mg Cholesterol

Lemon Herb Rice

This was just a quick stir together side dish to serve with fish. You could add additional herbs depending on the meal and your tastes. It's also a good way to use leftover rice.

2 cups (390 g) brown rice, cooked
¼ cup (60 ml) low sodium chicken broth
2 tablespoons (28 ml) lemon juice
¼ teaspoon garlic powder
½ teaspoon onion powder
1 tablespoon (4 g) fresh parsley, chopped
¼ teaspoon black pepper

Stir all ingredients together in a saucepan or microwave safe bowl and heat through.

4 SERVINGS

Each with: 105 Calories (2% from Fat, 9% from Protein, 89% from Carb); 2 g Protein; 0 g Total Fat; 0 g Saturated Fat; 0 g Monounsaturated Fat; 0 g Polyunsaturated Fat; 23 g Carb; 0 g Fiber; 0 g Sugar; 42 mg Phosphorus; 21 mg Calcium; 38 mg Sodium; 66 mg Potassium; 81 IU Vitamin A; 0 mg ATE Vitamin E; 5 mg Vitamin C; 0 mg Cholesterol

Sweet Tropical Rice

This gives you slightly sweet side dish. It works well with dishes like the *Carry Me Away to Hawaii Chicken.*

¾ cup (178 g) tropical fruit cocktail
1½ cups (285 g) brown rice, uncooked
3⅓ (780 ml) cups water
¼ cup (20 g) coconut
1 teaspoon ground ginger

Process the fruit cocktail in a food processor or blender until finely chopped. Place all ingredients in a saucepan with a tightly fitting lid. Bring to a boil, reduce heat to low, cover, and simmer until rice is soft, about 20 minutes. Stir before serving.

6 SERVINGS

Each with: 93 Calories (11% from Fat, 5% from Protein, 83% from Carb); 1 g Protein; 1 g Total Fat; 1 g Saturated Fat; 0 g Monounsaturated Fat; 0 g Polyunsaturated Fat; 20 g Carb; 1 g Fiber; 0 g Sugar; 24 mg Phosphorus; 16 mg Calcium; 5 mg Sodium; 73 mg Potassium; 41 IU Vitamin A; 0 mg ATE Vitamin E; 6 mg Vitamin C; 0 mg Cholesterol

Barley Mushroom Pilaf

Barley is a nutritious whole grain that both filling and tasty. And it will go with any kind of meat. Here is a quick and easy way to give barley some extra flavor, without adding much to the calorie count.

1 teaspoon olive oil
½ cup (35 g) mushrooms, sliced
1 cup (200 g) pearl barley
3 cups (700 ml) low sodium chicken broth
2 tablespoons (13 g) green onion, chopped
¼ teaspoon dried rosemary

Heat olive oil in saucepan; add mushrooms and sauté until limp. Add barley, broth, green onion, and rosemary. Bring to a boil. Reduce heat to low, cover, and cook 45 minutes or until barley is tender and liquid is absorbed.

6 SERVINGS

Each with: 136 Calories (14% from Fat, 18% from Protein, 68% from Carb); 6 g Protein; 2 g Total Fat; 0 g Saturated Fat; 1 g Monounsaturated Fat; 1 g Polyunsaturated Fat; 24 g Carb; 5 g Fiber; 0 g Sugar; 123 mg Phosphorus; 17 mg Calcium; 40 mg Sodium; 266 mg Potassium; 28 IU Vitamin A; 0 mg ATE Vitamin E; 1 mg Vitamin C; 0 mg Cholesterol

Bulgur Wheat with Pecans

This is a simple recipe, but the pecans give an extra flavor boost to the bulgur, which can seem plain if cooked by itself. This is a good thing because bulgur is full of whole grain nutrition.

1 cup (140 g) bulgur, uncooked
½ teaspoon dried basil
⅛ teaspoon black pepper
2 cups (475 ml) water, boiling
¼ cup (28 g) pecans, chopped

Preheat oven to 350°F (180°C, or gas mark 4). Lightly spray a 1-quart (950 ml) baking dish with a nonstick vegetable oil spray. Place bulgur, basil, and black pepper in prepared baking dish. Add boiling water and mix well. Cover tightly and bake 20 minutes. Fluff with a fork, add pecans, and mix well. Serve hot.

6 SERVINGS

Each with: 111 Calories (27% from Fat, 11% from Protein, 62% from Carb); 3 g Protein; 4 g Total Fat; 0 g Saturated Fat; 2 g Monounsaturated Fat; 1 g Polyunsaturated Fat; 18 g Carb; 5 g Fiber; 0 g Sugar; 83 mg Phosphorus; 14 mg Calcium; 6 mg Sodium; 117 mg Potassium; 12 IU Vitamin A; 0 mg ATE Vitamin E; 0 mg Vitamin C; 0 mg Cholesterol

Bulgur Wheat with Squash

Sometimes grain side dishes can be pretty plain. This one gets it flavor from butternut squash, and it turns out to be a winning combination.

1 tablespoon (14 g) unsalted butter
½ cup (80 g) onion, chopped
1 cup (140 g) butternut squash, peeled and cubed
½ cup (70 g) bulgur
2 whole cloves
½ teaspoon dried rosemary
2-inch (5 cm) cinnamon stick
1 bay leaf
1 cup (235 ml) low sodium chicken broth

Melt butter over medium heat. Add onion and squash. Cook until onion is soft. Add wheat, cloves, rosemary, cinnamon, and bay leaf. Stir until bulgur is brown. Stir in chicken broth. Cover and bring to a boil. Reduce heat and cook 15 minutes. Remove bay leaf before serving.

4 SERVINGS

Each with: 119 Calories (25% from Fat, 12% from Protein, 63% from Carb); 4 g Protein; 4 g Total Fat; 2 g Saturated Fat; 1 g Monounsaturated Fat; 0 g Polyunsaturated Fat; 20 g Carb; 4 g Fiber; 2 g Sugar; 88 mg Phosphorus; 31 mg Calcium; 23 mg Sodium; 276 mg Potassium; 3811 IU Vitamin A; 24 mg ATE Vitamin E; 9 mg Vitamin C; 8 mg Cholesterol

Mix and Match: Desserts

Desserts don't have to be a no no. On our mix and match plan, you have a number of options. There are desserts here as low as 40 calories and about ¾ of them are less than 100 calories. And there are plenty of options to choose from including pie, cake, and cookies. You might also consider fresh fruit, which is superior nutritionally and still gives you that sweet finish, all for a low calorie total. Some samples of fresh fruit calories follow.

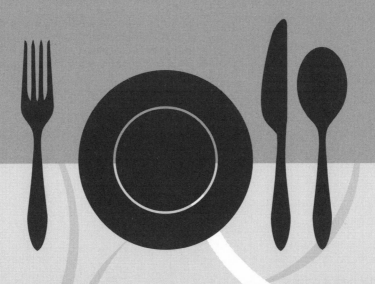

Per serving, 1 cup or 1 piece

Strawberries	49 calories
Apples	53 calories
Blueberries	89 calories
Pears	96 calories
Peaches	110 calories
Apricots	117 calories
Pineapple	131 calories
Bananas	200 calories

Honey Grilled Apples

This is a sweet treat and a great finish to your grilled meal.

4 apples
1 tablespoon (20 g) honey
2 tablespoons (28 ml) lemon juice
1 tablespoon (14 g) butter, unsalted

Core apples and cut slices through skin to resemble orange sections. Mix together the honey, lemon juice, and butter. Divide mixture and spoon into apple cores. Wrap apples in greased heavy duty aluminum foil, fold up, and seal. Grill until tender, about 20 minutes. Cut in half to serve.

8 SERVINGS

Each with: 40 Calories (2% from Fat, 2% from Protein, 97% from Carb); 0 g Protein; 0 g Total Fat; 0 g Unsaturated Fat; 0 g Monounsaturated Fat; 0 g Polyunsaturated Fat; 11 g Carb; 1 g Fiber; 9 g Sugar; 7 mg Phosphorus; 4 mg Calcium; 0 mg Sodium; 64 mg Potassium; 25 IU Vitamin A; 0 mg ATE Vitamin E; 4 mg Vitamin C; 0 mg Cholesterol

Holiday Spiced Fruit

This still makes a great holiday fruit mixture, although it may not look as much like one as the original recipe that contained the empty calories of candied cherries.

½ cup (12 g) sugar substitute, such as Splenda

¼ cup (60 ml) cider vinegar

1 tablespoon (6 g) whole cloves

4 cinnamon sticks

20 ounces (570 g) peaches, drained with juice reserved

20 ounces (570 g) pears, drained with juice reserved

20 ounces (570 g) pineapple slices, drained with juice reserved

Combine sugar substitute, vinegar, cloves, cinnamon sticks, and reserved fruit juices in large saucepan; bring to boil and boil 5 minutes. Take off stove and add fruit to syrup. Cool to room temperature. Refrigerate in covered container at least overnight before using. It keeps for 2 weeks.

8 SERVINGS

Each with: 131 Calories (2% from Fat, 3% from Protein, 95% from Carb); 1 g Protein; 0 g Total Fat; 0 g Unsaturated Fat; 0 g Monounsaturated Fat; 0 g Polyunsaturated Fat; 34 g Carb; 4 g Fiber; 27 g Sugar; 26 mg Phosphorus; 26 mg Calcium; 6 mg Sodium; 265 mg Potassium; 301 IU Vitamin A; 0 mg ATE Vitamin E; 11 mg Vitamin C; 0 mg Cholesterol

A Taste of the Islands Fruit Salad

The little extras in the dressing for this salad, such as lime juice and crystallized ginger, are what really make it special. This goes really well with the *Carry Me Away to Hawaii Chicken*, adding lots of good nutrition and still leaving room for brown rice or some other starch.

2 cups (310 g) pineapple, diced

1 cup (170 g) honeydew melon, diced

1 cup (175 g) mango, diced

2 tablespoons (28 ml) lime juice

2 tablespoons (40 g) honey

1 tablespoon (1 g) fresh cilantro, chopped

1 tablespoon (6 g) crystallized ginger, minced

½ cup (75 g) red bell pepper, minced

1 tablespoon (8 g) sesame seeds

Mix all ingredients except sesame seeds in large bowl. Let stand 10 minutes for flavors to blend. Divide fruit mixture among wineglasses and sprinkle with sesame seeds.

6 SERVINGS

Each with: 110 Calories (8% from Fat, 4% from Protein, 88% from Carb); 1 g Protein; 1 g Total Fat; 0 g Saturated Fat; 0 g Monounsaturated Fat; 0 g Polyunsaturated Fat; 27 g Carb; 2 g Fiber; 24 g Sugar; 27 mg Phosphorus; 34 mg Calcium; 8 mg Sodium; 255 mg Potassium; 679 IU Vitamin A; 0 mg ATE Vitamin E; 45 mg Vitamin C; 0 mg Cholesterol

Fresh Fruit for Anytime

Well maybe not ANYTIME, but this recipe makes a refreshing ending to just about any meal, especially in the spring when berries are in season. And the number of calories is low enough that you can work it into many meals or a smaller portion as a snack, knowing that it will satisfy your stomach and your sweet tooth without blowing your diet.

2 peaches, sliced
1 cup (145 g) blueberries
¼ cup sugar substitute, such as
    Splenda
2 cups (300 g) banana, sliced
2 cups (340 g) strawberries,
    hulled and halved
1 cup (230 g) low fat vanilla
    yogurt

Combine fruit with sugar substitute in a large bowl. Toss and transfer to a serving bowl. Serve with yogurt.

12 SERVINGS

Each with: 76 Calories (6% from Fat, 9% from Protein, 85% from Carb); 2 g Protein; 1 g Total Fat; 0 g Saturated Fat; 0 g Monounsaturated Fat; 0 g Polyunsaturated Fat; 18 g Carb; 2 g Fiber; 12 g Sugar; 49 mg Phosphorus; 43 mg Calcium; 14 mg Sodium; 277 mg Potassium; 128 IU Vitamin A; 2 mg ATE Vitamin E; 21 mg Vitamin C; 1 mg Cholesterol

Hot Spiced Fruit Dessert for Those Cold Nights

This is great for Thanksgiving or during the winter. This is easy to make ahead in the slow cooker and is best served the next day to allow the spices to blend with fruit. You can also add apricots, Queen Anne cherries, or any other fruit you like.

½ pound (225 g) peaches
½ pound (225 g) pears
½ pound (225 g) pineapple
½ cup (125 g) prunes, stewed
¼ cup (80 g) orange marmalade
¼ teaspoon cinnamon
¼ teaspoon nutmeg
¼ teaspoon ground cloves

Drain liquid from all fruit, reserving ¾ cup (175 g) to make syrup. Combine marmalade, spices, and reserved liquid. Bring to boil and then simmer 3 to 4 minutes. Gently add fruit that has been cut into chunks. Transfer to slow cooker and cook on low at least 4 hours.

6 SERVINGS

Each with: 114 Calories (1% from Fat, 2% from Protein, 96% from Carb); 1 g Protein; 0 g Total Fat; 0 g Saturated Fat; 0 g Monounsaturated Fat; 0 g Polyunsaturated Fat; 30 g Carb; 3 g Fiber; 26 g Sugar; 20 mg Phosphorus; 22 mg Calcium; 10 mg Sodium; 206 mg Potassium; 247 IU Vitamin A; 0 mg ATE Vitamin E; 7 mg Vitamin C; 0 mg Cholesterol

Nicely Spiced Grilled Fruit

We never seem to eat as much fruit as we should. This recipe makes it easy to get people to eat more. It's a great choice for dessert if you already are using the grill for the main course, but it's also worth firing up the grill just for dessert.

1 apple

1 pear

1 bananas

2 tablespoons (28 ml) unsalted butter, melted

3 tablespoons (3 g) brown sugar substitute, such as Splenda

1 teaspoon cinnamon, ground

½ teaspoon ground ginger

Cut the fruit in half or wedges. Do not peel. The banana should be cut lengthwise, then in half. Remove the cores. Combine butter, brown sugar substitute, and spices. Baste fruit with mixture. Place fruit on grill with skin up. Grill on medium 8 to 10 minutes for halves, 4 to 5 minutes for smaller wedges.

6 SERVINGS

Each with: 76 Calories (44% from Fat, 2% from Protein, 54% from Carb); 1 g Protein; 4 g Total Fat; 2 g Saturated Fat; 1 g Monounsaturated Fat; 0 g Polyunsaturated Fat; 11 g Carb; 2 g Fiber; 7 g Sugar; 12 mg Phosphorus; 9 mg Calcium; 1 mg Sodium; 138 mg Potassium; 144 IU Vitamin A; 32 mg ATE Vitamin E; 4 mg Vitamin C; 10 mg Cholesterol

Colorful Fruit Cup

A great blend of citrus and other fruit gives you a dessert that is both tasty and colorful.

20 ounces (570 g) pineapple chunks, in juice

2 pink grapefruits, sectioned

3 oranges, sectioned

2 bananas, sliced

10 maraschino cherries, quartered

1 apple, cut into small pieces

3 tablespoons (45 ml) lemon juice

2 teaspoons sugar substitute, such as Splenda

Put pineapple chunks, sectioned grapefruit, and sectioned oranges into large container. Slice the 2 bananas. Cut the apple and cherries. Mix together lemon juice and Splenda. Mix into fruit.

8 SERVINGS

Each with: 123 Calories (2% from Fat, 6% from Protein, 92% from Carb); 2 g Protein; 0 g Total Fat; 0 g Unsaturated Fat; 0 g Monounsaturated Fat; 0 g Polyunsaturated Fat; 32 g Carb; 4 g Fiber; 22 g Sugar; 34 mg Phosphorus; 55 mg Calcium; 1 mg Sodium; 454 mg Potassium; 921 IU Vitamin A; 0 mg ATE Vitamin E; 68 mg Vitamin C; 0 mg Cholesterol

Strawberry Parfait

This is a cool and creamy dessert with the added benefit of strawberries
(which is great both for taste and nutrition).

8 ounces (225 g) fat-free vanilla
  yogurt
1 cup (170 g) strawberries
½ cup (63 g) granola

Chop the strawberries. Layer the ingredients in parfait glasses
in the following order: fruit, yogurt, and granola. Repeat layers.

2 SERVINGS

Each with: 104 Calories (10% from Fat, 8% from Protein, 82% from Carb);
2 g Protein; 1 g Total Fat; 0 g Saturated Fat; 0 g Monounsaturated Fat; 0 g
Polyunsaturated Fat; 22 g Carb; 3 g Fiber; 10 g Sugar; 75 mg Phosphorus; 20 mg
Calcium; 78 mg Sodium; 174 mg Potassium; 9 IU Vitamin A; 0 mg ATE Vitamin E;
45 mg Vitamin C; 0 mg Cholesterol

Vanilla Fruit Salad

This is so easy to prepare, and fruit salads are always enjoyed. This one is particularly good with
the vanilla pudding adding flavor and the generous portion of fruit filling you up.

14 ounces (390 g) pineapple
  chunks, in juice
11 ounces (310 g) mandarin
  oranges, undrained
1 cup (150 g) bananas, sliced
1 cup (170 g) strawberries, halved
¾ cup (113 g) seedless green
  grapes, halved
1 cup (145 g) blueberries, fresh or
  frozen thawed
3½ ounce (100 g) instant sugar-
  free vanilla pudding mix
½ cup (63 g) granola

Drain chunk pineapple and orange segments, reserving liquid
in small bowl. In large bowl, combine fruits. Sprinkle pudding
mix into reserved liquid; mix until combined and slightly
thickened. Fold into fruit until well combined. Spoon into
serving dishes. Garnish with granola.

8 SERVINGS

Each with: 97 Calories (4% from Fat, 6% from Protein, 90% from Carb); 1 g Protein;
1 g Total Fat; 0 g Saturated Fat; 0 g Monounsaturated Fat; 0 g Polyunsaturated Fat;
24 g Carb; 3 g Fiber; 16 g Sugar; 34 mg Phosphorus; 20 mg Calcium; 23 mg
Sodium; 289 mg Potassium; 390 IU Vitamin A; 0 mg ATE Vitamin E; 33 mg Vitamin C;
0 mg Cholesterol

Mixed Fruit Plus

This is a sweet treat, enhanced by the flavor of sugar-free instant pudding, but it's also full of the great nutrient density of fruit.

20 ounces (570 g) fruit cocktail, undrained
20 ounces (570 g) pineapple chunks, drained
2 bananas, sliced
1 box sugar-free strawberry instant pudding

Mix all ingredients together and chill.

8 SERVINGS

Each with: 135 Calories (2% from Fat, 3% from Protein, 95% from Carb); 1 g Protein; 0 g Total Fat; 0 g Unsaturated Fat; 0 g Monounsaturated Fat; 0 g Polyunsaturated Fat; 34 g Carb; 2 g Fiber; 29 g Sugar; 108 mg Phosphorus; 20 mg Calcium; 182 mg Sodium; 293 mg Potassium; 267 IU Vitamin A; 0 mg ATE Vitamin E; 11 mg Vitamin C; 0 mg Cholesterol

Tip: You can also try other flavors of pudding.

Sweet Finish Baked Apples

This simple baked apple recipe contains no added sugar, letting the flavor of the apples come through and holding down the calories. It makes a great dessert for almost any kind of meal, but it's especially good with chicken or pork.

4 apples
¼ cup (35 g) raisins
½ cup (120 ml) apple juice, unsweetened

Preheat oven to 375°F (190°C, or gas mark 5). Wash and core apples. Pare a strip from top of each apple. Put tablespoon of raisins in each apple. Pour apple juice over apples. Bake 40 minutes or until done. Baste apples with juice during cooking. Serve warm or chilled.

4 SERVINGS

Each with: 106 Calories (2% from Fat, 2% from Protein, 96% from Carb); 1 g Protein; 0 g Total Fat; 0 g Saturated Fat; 0 g Monounsaturated Fat; 0 g Polyunsaturated Fat; 28 g Carb; 2 g Fiber; 22 g Sugar; 27 mg Phosphorus; 13 mg Calcium; 3 mg Sodium; 230 mg Potassium; 49 IU Vitamin A; 0 mg ATE Vitamin E; 6 mg Vitamin C; 0 mg Cholesterol

Balsamic Berries

A few drops of balsamic vinegar brings out the flavor of the fruit—you won't taste the vinegar, but you will taste the difference.

---

4 cups strawberries, about 1 pound (455 g)
1 tablespoon (13 g) sugar
¼ teaspoon balsamic vinegar

Wash, dry, hull, and quarter the strawberries lengthwise. Put the strawberries into a large bowl. Add the sugar and balsamic vinegar and toss gently to combine. Refrigerate 1 hour.

4 SERVINGS

Each with: 61 Calories (6% from Fat, 6% from Protein, 88% from Carb); 1 g Protein; 0 g Total Fat; 0 g Unsaturated Fat; 0 g Monounsaturated Fat; 0 g Polyunsaturated Fat; 15 g Carb; 3 g Fiber; 10 g Sugar; 37 mg Phosphorus; 24 mg Calcium; 2 mg Sodium; 233 mg Potassium; 18 IU Vitamin A; 0 mg ATE Vitamin E; 89 mg Vitamin C; 0 mg Cholesterol

Jell-O Squares

This recipe has been in the family for years. It even got included in an article in the local newspaper about kids cooking that featured some of our three children's favorite recipes. This variation has lower calories with the use of fat-free evaporated milk to replace the cream originally called for and sugar substitute to replace the sugar. The result is a low calorie finger food that looks and tastes great. One nice thing is that you can vary the colors for whatever the occasion, from the red, white and blue here to red and pink for Valentine's Day or purple and orange for Halloween.

1 large box sugar-free flavored
  gelatin, red
2½ envelopes unflavored gelatin
4½ cups (1.1 L) water
½ pint (225 g) fat-free evaporated
  milk
½ pint (225 g) fat-free sour cream
½ cup (12 g) sugar substitute,
  such as Splenda
1 teaspoon vanilla
1 large box sugar-free flavored
  gelatin, blue

In a medium sized bowl, mix one large box of sugar-free gelatin (red or blue) and ½ envelope unflavored gelatin with 2 cups (475 ml) of HOT tap water. Combine completely. Make sure gelatin is dissolved. Pour into a pan and chill for 1 hour or more. When it is set, go to the next step. In a medium sized pot, combine evaporated milk and sour cream. In a small bowl, mix unflavored gelatin and ½ cup (120 ml) COLD water. Add this mixture to cream mixture and bring mixture to boil. Remove from heat and add sugar substitute and vanilla. Pour this mixture on top of chilled gelatin mixture and chill for another hour or more. When it is set, go to the next step. Again in a medium sized bowl, mix the second large box of sugar-free gelatin (red or blue) and ½ envelope unflavored gelatin with 2 cups (475 ml) of HOT tap water. Combine completely. Make sure gelatin is dissolved. Pour on top of cream mixture and chill for 1 hour or more. When ready to serve, cut into squares.

24 SERVINGS

Each with: 59 Calories (18% from Fat, 15% from Protein, 66% from Carb); 2 g Protein; 1 g Total Fat; 1 g Unsaturated Fat; 0 g Monounsaturated Fat; 0 g Polyunsaturated Fat; 10 g Carb; 0 g Fiber; 9 g Sugar; 54 mg Phosphorus; 42 mg Calcium; 59 mg Sodium; 49 mg Potassium; 80 IU Vitamin A; 23 mg ATE Vitamin E; 0 mg Vitamin C; 4 mg Cholesterol

There's Always Room for Jell-O

Or at least there is if you have 100 calories left in your mix and match meal plan. This full of fruit dessert with its creamy topping is sure to please, but there's also a lot of nutrition packed in this sweet treat.

2 small boxes sugar-free flavored gelatin, any flavor

2 cups (475 ml) boiling water

10 ounces (280 g) frozen strawberries, with juice, defrosted

14 ounces (390 g) crushed pineapple, with juice

2 bananas, mashed

12 ounces (340 g) plain low fat yogurt

Dissolve Jell-O in boiling water. Add all fruit and juices. Pour half into large mold and set. Spread with yogurt. Pour remaining Jell-O mixture over and chill until firm.

8 SERVINGS

Each with: 100 Calories (7% from Fat, 12% from Protein, 80% from Carb); 3 g Protein; 1 g Total Fat; 0 g Unsaturated Fat; 0 g Monounsaturated Fat; 0 g Polyunsaturated Fat; 21 g Carb; 2 g Fiber; 15 g Sugar; 86 mg Phosphorus; 94 mg Calcium; 47 mg Sodium; 338 mg Potassium; 80 IU Vitamin A; 6 mg ATE Vitamin E; 22 mg Vitamin C; 3 mg Cholesterol

Sweet Treat Apple Tapioca

This makes a nice warm comfy dessert that has great nutrition and not very many calories. We like it warm with just a couple of tablespoons (28 ml) of skim milk over it, which adds about 10 calories. But it's also good cold.

4 cups apples, peeled and sliced

½ cup (8 g) brown sugar substitute, such as Splenda

¾ teaspoon cinnamon

2 tablespoons (19 g) tapioca

2 tablespoons (28 ml) lemon juice

1 cup (235 ml) water, boiling

In medium bowl, toss apples with brown sugar substitute, cinnamon, and tapioca until evenly coated. Place apples in slow cooker. Pour lemon juice over top. Pour in boiling water. Cook on high for 3 to 4 hours.

4 SERVINGS

Each with: 73 Calories (2% from Fat, 2% from Protein, 96% from Carb); 0 g Protein; 0 g Total Fat; 0 g Unsaturated Fat; 0 g Monounsaturated Fat; 0 g Polyunsaturated Fat; 19 g Carb; 2 g Fiber; 11 g Sugar; 13 mg Phosphorus; 13 mg Calcium; 1 mg Sodium; 111 mg Potassium; 44 IU Vitamin A; 0 mg ATE Vitamin E; 8 mg Vitamin C; 0 mg Cholesterol

Creamy Frozen Cherry Dessert

This frozen dessert makes a great alternative to ice cream. It has yogurt for creaminess and protein and cherry flavor both from fruit and cherry flavored gelatin. And with all that, it's still low in calories.

8 ounces (225 g) sweet cherries, undrained, pitted

1 small sugar-free gelatin, cherry flavor

1 cup (235 ml) water, boiling

8 ounces (225 g) plain fat-free yogurt

2 cups (150 g) fat-free whipped topping, such as Cool Whip

Line bottom and sides of 9 × 5-inch (23 × 13 cm) loaf pan with plastic wrap; set aside. Drain cherries, reserving syrup. If necessary, add enough cold water to reserved syrup to measure ½ cup (120 ml). Cut cherries into quarters. Completely dissolve gelatin in boiling water. Add measured syrup. Stir in yogurt until well blended. Chill until mixture is thickened but not set, about 45 minutes to 1 hour, stirring occasionally. Gently stir in cherries and whipped topping. Pour into prepared pan; cover. Freeze until firm, about 6 hours or overnight. Remove pan from freezer about 15 minutes before serving. Let stand at room temperature to soften slightly. Remove plastic wrap. Cut into slices. Cover and store leftovers in freezer.

12 SERVINGS

Each with: 49 Calories (40% from Fat, 10% from Protein, 50% from Carb); 1 g Protein; 2 g Total Fat; 2 g Saturated Fat; 0 g Monounsaturated Fat; 0 g Polyunsaturated Fat; 6 g Carb; 0 g Fiber; 6 g Sugar; 37 mg Phosphorus; 34 mg Calcium; 23 mg Sodium; 67 mg Potassium; 58 IU Vitamin A; 5 mg ATE Vitamin E; 1 mg Vitamin C; 3 mg Cholesterol

Frozen Fruit Cups

These make a delightful warm weather dessert. They are full of the nutrition
of fruit and naturally low in calories.

1 cup (235 ml) water

1 cup (25 g) sugar substitute,
such as Splenda

30 ounces (840 g) frozen
strawberries

12 ounces (340 g) orange juice
concentrate, undiluted

2 tablespoons (28 ml) lemon juice

17 ounces (485 g) apricot,
drained

20 ounces (570 g) crushed
pineapple, drained

3 cups (450 g) bananas, sliced

 Tip: Set out 5 to 10 minutes
before serving.

Heat water and sugar substitute. Add strawberries (juice and
all). Add orange juice concentrate and lemon juice. Cut up
apricots and add with pineapple and bananas. Put paper
muffin holders in muffin tin. Divide mixture among cups. Place
in freezer. After frozen, remove from pan and store in plastic
bags in freezer.

36 SERVINGS

Each with: 54 Calories (3% from Fat, 5% from Protein, 92% from Carb); 1 g Protein;
0 g Total Fat; 0 g Unsaturated Fat; 0 g Monounsaturated Fat; 0 g Polyunsaturated Fat;
14 g Carb; 1 g Fiber; 10 g Sugar; 19 mg Phosphorus; 12 mg Calcium; 2 mg Sodium;
207 mg Potassium; 283 IU Vitamin A; 0 mg ATE Vitamin E; 31 mg Vitamin C; 0 mg
Cholesterol

Extraordinarily Low Calorie Strawberry Ice

If you have an ice cream freezer, you can make a delicious frozen strawberry dessert similar to Italian ices. Made with fresh berries and sugar substitute, it has great nutrition, almost no sodium, and so few calories that you can fit it into many meals for a sweet treat.

½ cup (12 g) sugar substitute, such as Splenda
⅔ cup (160 ml) water
6 cups (870 g) strawberries, pureed
¼ cup (60 ml) lemon juice

Combine sugar substitute and water in a medium saucepan and bring it to a boil, stirring to dissolve the sugar substitute. Lower the heat and simmer for 5 minutes and then cool to room temperature and refrigerate until cold. Hull strawberries and puree them. You should have about 3 cups (696 g) puree. In a large bowl, combine the pureed strawberries, sugar syrup, and lemon juice. Pour the mixture into an ice cream maker and freeze according to manufacturer's directions.

8 SERVINGS

Each with: 60 Calories (2% from Fat, 4% from Protein, 93% from Carb); 1 g Protein; 0 g Total Fat; 0 g Unsaturated Fat; 0 g Monounsaturated Fat; 0 g Polyunsaturated Fat; 16 g Carb; 4 g Fiber; 8 g Sugar; 22 mg Phosphorus; 27 mg Calcium; 4 mg Sodium; 255 mg Potassium; 76 IU Vitamin A; 0 mg ATE Vitamin E; 72 mg Vitamin C; 0 mg Cholesterol

Cappuccino Mousse

This is great for those times when you want a fancy dessert that no one knows is low in calories. Sugar-free pudding mix helps to hold down the calorie total.

3 cups (700 ml) skim milk
1 package sugar-free chocolate pudding mix
6 teaspoons (12 g) instant coffee, decaffeinated
½ teaspoon cinnamon
2 cups (150 g) whipped topping, fat-free

Pour skim milk into 5-quart (4.7 L) mixer bowl. Add pudding mix, instant coffee, and cinnamon. Blend by hand with a wire whisk, scraping the sides of bowl to moisten completely. Whip at medium speed on machine for 3 minutes or until pudding is smooth and creamy. Fold in whipped topping. Immediately portion out ½ cup (115 g) into stemmed glasses or coffee mugs. Chill at least 1 hour. Keep refrigerated.

10 SERVINGS

Each with: 117 Calories (32% from Fat, 12% from Protein, 56% from Carb); 3 g Protein; 4 g Total Fat; 3 g Unsaturated Fat; 0 g Monounsaturated Fat; 0 g Polyunsaturated Fat; 17 g Carb; 0 g Fiber; 10 g Sugar; 178 mg Phosphorus; 110 mg Calcium; 189 mg Sodium; 180 mg Potassium; 172 IU Vitamin A; 45 mg ATE Vitamin E; 1 mg Vitamin C; 1 mg Cholesterol

Double Apple Cookies

This is a nice, soft, chewy cookie with the double nutritional bonus of apples and applesauce. It's low in calories and almost fat free.

2 cups (250 g) all purpose flour
1 teaspoon baking soda
1 teaspoon cinnamon
½ teaspoon ground cloves
½ teaspoon nutmeg
½ cup (125 g) applesauce
1¼ cups (20 g) brown sugar substitute, such as Splenda
¼ cup (60 ml) egg substitute
½ cup (60 g) chopped walnuts
½ cup (60 g) walnuts, chopped
1 cup (150 g) apple, finely chopped
1 cup (145 g) raisins
¼ cup (60 ml) skim milk

Preheat oven to 375°F (190°C, or gas mark 5). Sift flour with baking soda, cinnamon, cloves, and nutmeg. In a large mixing bowl, combine applesauce and brown sugar substitute; beat in egg substitute until well blended. Stir in half of flour and spice mixture and then stir in walnuts, apple, and raisins. Blend in skim milk, then remaining flour mixture. Drop by rounded tablespoons of dough, about 2 inches (5 cm) apart, onto greased baking sheets. Bake for 12 to 15 minutes or until done.

36 SERVINGS

Each with: 67 Calories (31% from Fat, 8% from Protein, 61% from Carb); 1 g Protein; 2 g Total Fat; 0 g Unsaturated Fat; 1 g Monounsaturated Fat; 1 g Polyunsaturated Fat; 11 g Carb; 1 g Fiber; 4 g Sugar; 25 mg Phosphorus; 10 mg Calcium; 40 mg Sodium; 69 mg Potassium; 13 IU Vitamin A; 1 mg ATE Vitamin E; 0 mg Vitamin C; 0 mg Cholesterol

Fruity, Good for You Cookies

Healthy and low in fat and calories but high in flavor, these cookies are favorites at our house. You can pick your favorite dried fruit or fruits to make these cookies your own. My personal favorites are cranberries, cherries, and pineapple. You can leave out the nuts and save another 16 calories per cookie.

2 large bananas
⅓ cup (60 ml) canola oil
1 teaspoon vanilla
1½ cups (120 g) rolled oats
½ cup (58 g) oat bran
1½ cups (270 g) mixed dried
  fruits, coarsely chopped
½ cup (60 g) walnuts, chopped

Preheat oven to 350°F (180°C, or gas mark 4). Grease 2 cookie sheets. Mash bananas in a large bowl until smooth. Stir in oil and vanilla. Add oats, oat bran, mixed fruits, and nuts. Stir well to combine. Drop by rounded teaspoonfuls on cookie sheets about 1 inch (2.5 cm) apart. Flatten slightly with back of a spoon. Bake 20 to 25 minutes or until bottom and edges are lightly brown. Cool completely and refrigerate.

24 SERVINGS

Each with: 102 Calories (42% from Fat, 6% from Protein, 51% from Carb); 2 g Protein; 5 g Total Fat; 0 g Saturated Fat; 2 g Monounsaturated Fat; 2 g Polyunsaturated Fat; 14 g Carb; 2 g Fiber; 7 g Sugar; 46 mg Phosphorus; 8 mg Calcium; 4 mg Sodium; 89 mg Potassium; 19 IU Vitamin A; 3 mg ATE Vitamin E; 1 mg Vitamin C; 0 mg Cholesterol

Granola Cookies

These cookies make a tasty treat for breakfast, perhaps with a smoothie or a snack.

1 cup (178 g) dates, firmly packed
1 cup (284 g) apple juice
  concentrate
3 tablespoons (48 g) peanut butter
3 tablespoons (60 g) honey
1 teaspoon vanilla
1 tablespoon (20 g) molasses
1 tablespoon (8 g) walnuts, chopped
½ cup (40 g) coconut
½ cup (75 g) raisins
2⅓ cups (280 g) whole wheat flour
2 cups (160 g) quick cooking oats

Blend dates and apple juice concentrate until smooth; add peanut butter, honey, vanilla, and molasses. Blend well and place in mixing bowl. Add nuts, coconut, raisins, and flour and mix well. Add rolled oats and blend, with hands if needed. Spoon onto nonstick cookie sheet and press with wet fork or fingers until ¼-inch (6 mm) thick. Bake at 300°F (150°C, or gas mark 2) for about 20 minutes.

36 SERVINGS

Each with: 86 Calories (16% from Fat, 11% from Protein, 74% from Carb); 2 g Protein; 2 g Total Fat; 1 g Saturated Fat; 0 g Monounsaturated Fat; 0 g Polyunsaturated Fat; 17 g Carb; 2 g Fiber; 6 g Sugar; 61 mg Phosphorus; 10 mg Calcium; 8 mg Sodium; 120 mg Potassium; 1 IU Vitamin A; 0 mg ATE Vitamin E; 0 mg Vitamin C; 0 mg Cholesterol

Have a Cookie for Breakfast (or Dessert)

These are good for breakfast on the run as well as dessert. They are fairly soft but can be easily eaten on the go and are fat free.

3 cups (675 g) banana, mashed
⅓ cup (82 g) applesauce
2 cups (160 g) quick cooking oats
¼ cup (60 ml) skim milk
½ cup (60 g) dried cranberries
1 teaspoon vanilla
1 teaspoon cinnamon
1 tablespoon sugar

Preheat oven to 350°F (180°C, or gas mark 4). Mix all ingredients in a bowl really well. Let this mixture stand for at least 5 minutes to let the oats become good and hydrated. Heap the dough by teaspoonfuls onto a greased cookie sheet. Bake for 15 to 20 minutes and let cool.

20 SERVINGS

Each with: 108 Calories (10% from Fat, 11% from Protein, 79% from Carb); 3 g Protein; 1 g Total Fat; 0 g Saturated Fat; 0 g Monounsaturated Fat; 0 g Polyunsaturated Fat; 22 g Carb; 3 g Fiber; 7 g Sugar; 93 mg Phosphorus; 16 mg Calcium; 3 mg Sodium; 198 mg Potassium; 29 IU Vitamin A; 2 mg ATE Vitamin E; 3 mg Vitamin C; 0 mg Cholesterol

Carrot Cookies

This is kind of like a carrot muffin, only smaller so it doesn't blow your diet. These cookies are almost fat free and full of nutrition. Use them as dessert or as part of a breakfast with fruit and yogurt.

1 cup (110 g) carrot, grated
½ cup (115 g) nonfat plain yogurt
¼ cup brown sugar
2 tablespoons (28 ml) canola oil
1 teaspoon vanilla
1½ cups (267 g) dates
1½ cups (180 g) whole wheat
  pastry flour
¼ cup (29 g) grape-nuts cereal
½ teaspoon baking soda

Tip: You can substitute raisins or other dried fruit for the dates.

Preheat oven to 350°F (180°C, or gas mark 4). Spray baking sheets with nonstick vegetable oil spray or line with parchment paper or silicone sheet. In medium mixing bowl, stir carrot, yogurt, sugar, oil, vanilla, and dates. Let stand 15 minutes. Stir in remaining dry ingredients until well blended. Drop tablespoons of mixture onto baking sheets, spacing 1½ inches (3.8 cm) apart. Reduce to teaspoon drops for mini-size cookies. Bake 15 minutes or until cookie top springs back when lightly touched. Let cool.

30 SERVINGS

Each with: 69 Calories (14% from Fat, 8% from Protein, 78% from Carb); 1 g Protein; 1 g Total Fat; 0 g Saturated Fat; 1 g Monounsaturated Fat; 0 g Polyunsaturated Fat; 14 g Carb; 2 g Fiber; 8 g Sugar; 36 mg Phosphorus; 16 mg Calcium; 34 mg Sodium; 115 mg Potassium; 530 IU Vitamin A; 1 mg ATE Vitamin E; 0 mg Vitamin C; 0 mg Cholesterol

Don't Tell Anyone That They Are Zucchini Cookies

No one will ever guess the secret ingredient in these super moist cookies. But we'll know that's its zucchini, which adds not only the moisture but also a lot more nutrition than a typical cookie has.

½ cup (123 g) unsweetened
  applesauce
¾ cup (18 g) sugar substitute, such
  as Splenda
¼ cup (60 ml) egg substitute
½ teaspoon vanilla
1½ cups (180 g) whole wheat
  pastry flour
1 teaspoon cinnamon
½ teaspoon baking soda
1 cup (80 g) quick cooking oats
1½ cups (180 g) zucchini,
  shredded
1 cup (125 g) granola
12 ounces (340 g) chocolate chips

Mix all ingredients in a large bowl. Drop by heaping teaspoons onto cookie sheet. Bake at 350°F (180°C, or gas mark 4) for 10 to 12 minutes.

48 SERVINGS

Each with: 67 Calories (32% from Fat, 10% from Protein, 58% from Carb); 2 g Protein; 2 g Total Fat; 1 g Saturated Fat; 1 g Monounsaturated Fat; 0 g Polyunsaturated Fat; 10 g Carb; 1 g Fiber; 5 g Sugar; 44 mg Phosphorus; 18 mg Calcium; 28 mg Sodium; 69 mg Potassium; 26 IU Vitamin A; 3 mg ATE Vitamin E; 1 mg Vitamin C; 2 mg Cholesterol

Low Fat, Low Calorie Devil's Food Cake

Yes, it is possible to make a real cake and keep the calories low. In this recipe, the applesauce takes the place of most of the fat, and the sugar is replaced by a sugar substitute that has the same volume as sugar, such as Splenda. The result is a fairly heavy, very moist cake—almost like brownies.

2 cups (250 g) all purpose flour
1¾ cups (43 g) sugar substitute, such as Splenda
½ cup (43 g) unsweetened cocoa powder
1 tablespoon (13.8 g) baking soda
⅔ cup (163 g) unsweetened applesauce
⅓ cup (80 ml) low fat buttermilk
2 tablespoons (28 ml) oil
1 cup (235 ml) coffee

Preheat oven to 350°F (180°C, or gas mark 4). Spray a 9 × 13-inch (23 × 33 cm) pan with nonstick vegetable oil spray and then dust with flour, shaking out the excess. In a large bowl, mix together flour, sugar substitute, cocoa, and baking soda. Stir in applesauce, low fat buttermilk, and oil. Heat coffee to boiling. Stir into batter. Mixture will be thin. Pour into pan. Bake 35 to 40 minutes until a toothpick inserted in the center comes out clean.

24 SERVINGS

Each with: 59 Calories (22% from Fat, 10% from Protein, 68% from Carb); 2 g Protein; 2 g Total Fat; 0 g Unsaturated Fat; 0 g Monounsaturated Fat; 1 g Polyunsaturated Fat; 11 g Carb; 1 g Fiber; 0 g Sugar; 28 mg Phosphorus; 8 mg Calcium; 164 mg Sodium; 55 mg Potassium; 2 IU Vitamin A; 0 mg ATE Vitamin E; 0 mg Vitamin C; 0 mg Cholesterol

Easy, Low Calorie Pumpkin Cupcake

Do you think that you can't a cupcake now and again? Think again. The pumpkin ups the nutrition of these sweet little treats. There is no added fat. And the use of a cake mix and canned pumpkin pie filling make these tasty cupcakes quick and easy to prepare.

1 package yellow cake mix
2 cups (490 g) pumpkin pie filling
½ cup (120 ml) egg substitute
6 ounces (170 g) butterscotch chips

Mix all ingredients together and place in greased or lined cup cake pan. Bake at 350°F (180°C, or gas mark 4) for 15 to 20 minutes.

24 SERVINGS

Each with: 63 Calories (8% from Fat, 6% from Protein, 86% from Carb); 1 g Protein; 1 g Total Fat; 0 g Saturated Fat; 0 g Monounsaturated Fat; 0 g Polyunsaturated Fat; 14 g Carb; 2 g Fiber; 7 g Sugar; 17 mg Phosphorus; 14 mg Calcium; 96 mg Sodium; 49 mg Potassium; 1893 IU Vitamin A; 2 mg ATE Vitamin E; 1 mg Vitamin C; 1 mg Cholesterol

Almost Pumpkin Pie

This is basically a pumpkin pie without the crust. It gives you the same great flavor and nutrition, without the fat and carbohydrates of the crust.

---

2 eggs
1 tablespoon (13 g) sugar
1 cup (235 ml) skim milk
2 cups (490 g) pumpkin, cooked or canned
1 teaspoon cinnamon
1 teaspoon ground ginger

Beat the eggs and combine with the sugar. Add the skim milk and mix well. Add the pumpkin and the spices and pour into an 8-inch (10 cm) pie pan. Bake in a moderate oven, 350°F (180°C, or gas mark 4), for 50 to 60 minutes. Test by inserting a knife near the edge. When it comes out clean, the custard is finished. Cut into 6 equal portions when chilled. This custard will keep the pie wedge-shape without a crust.

6 SERVINGS

Each with: 82 Calories (24% from Fat, 23% from Protein, 53% from Carb); 5 g Protein; 2 g Total Fat; 1 g Saturated Fat; 1 g Monounsaturated Fat; 0 g Polyunsaturated Fat; 11 g Carb; 3 g Fiber; 5 g Sugar; 112 mg Phosphorus; 95 mg Calcium; 55 mg Sodium; 272 mg Potassium; 12 888 IU Vitamin A; 52 mg ATE Vitamin E; 4 mg Vitamin C; 83 mg Cholesterol

Easy Apple Pie Substitute

The microwave preparation makes this dessert especially quick and easy. And it contains the whole grain of the crackers and apples for nutrition.

½ cup (84 g) graham crackers, crushed
5 apples, cored and peeled
½ teaspoon cinnamon
¼ teaspoon allspice
¼ cup (35 g) raisins
⅓ cup (80 ml) apple juice

Spray a microwave-safe pie plate with nonstick vegetable oil spray. Spread the graham cracker crumbs in the plate. Cover with apple slices. Sprinkle with spices. Sprinkle raisins over top. Pour juice over. Cover and microwave for 15 minutes.

8 SERVINGS

Each with: 81 Calories (7% from Fat, 3% from Protein, 90% from Carb); 1 g Protein; 1 g Total Fat; 0 g Unsaturated Fat; 0 g Monounsaturated Fat; 0 g Polyunsaturated Fat; 20 g Carb; 1 g Fiber; 14 g Sugar; 20 mg Phosphorus; 11 mg Calcium; 33 mg Sodium; 132 mg Potassium; 31 IU Vitamin A; 0 mg ATE Vitamin E; 3 mg Vitamin C; 0 mg Cholesterol

Mix and Match: Bread

I know what you've been thinking, that you can never have bread again if you start on our diet plan. But you are wrong. In our mix and match world, there are actually quite a few bread options you can fit in. This chapter contains a variety of yeast breads and quick breads that will go with different kinds of meals. There are also a number of low calorie commercial breads available as more and more bakers realize that people want to be able to have a good tasting slice of bread without completely blowing their diet. A couple of examples are as follows:

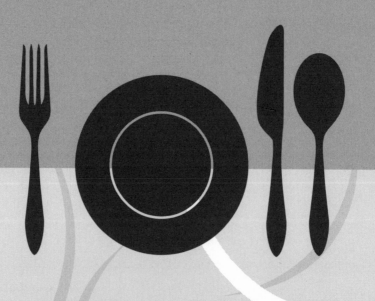

Per serving, 1 slice or 1 roll

Nature's Own 100% Whole Wheat	50 calories
Pepperidge Farms Carb Style 7 Grain	60 calories
Nature's Own Honey Wheat Rolls	130 calories

There are also now a number of brands of thin rolls and bagels that are 100 calories. They include Thomas' Bagels and rolls from Pepperidge Farms and Arnold. I sometimes toast half of one of those for a 50 calorie addition to breakfast.

Don't Blow Your Diet 100% Whole Wheat Bread

This recipe is based on one that came with my bread machine. We've reduced the amount of fat originally called for and eliminated any saturated fat or trans fats. We've also replaced the sugar with sugar substitute. Sliced fairly thin, 14 slices to a loaf, it gives you a mix and match a bread option that is only 100 calories.

1¼ cups (285 ml) water
2 tablespoons (28 ml) olive oil
3 cups (360 g) whole wheat flour
¼ cup (4 g) brown sugar
    substitute, such as Splenda
1¾ teaspoon yeast

Place ingredients in bread machine in order specified by manufacturer. Process on whole wheat cycle.

14 SERVINGS

Each with: 106 Calories (20% from Fat, 13% from Protein, 67% from Carb); 4 g Protein; 2 g Total Fat; 0 g Saturated Fat; 1 g Monounsaturated Fat; 0 g Polyunsaturated Fat; 19 g Carb; 3 g Fiber; 0 g Sugar; 95 mg Phosphorus; 10 mg Calcium; 2 mg Sodium; 114 mg Potassium; 2 IU Vitamin A; 0 mg ATE Vitamin E; 0 mg Vitamin C; 0 mg Cholesterol

Buttermilk Wheat Bread

This is another great bread with a nice hot bowl of soup or stew for dinner.
The buttermilk gives it an almost sourdough flavor.

1 cup (235 ml) low fat buttermilk
¼ cup (60 ml) water
1 tablespoon (15 ml) canola oil, unsalted
1½ cups (180 g) whole wheat flour
1½ cups (206 g) bread flour
1 tablespoon (1.5 g) sugar substitute, such as Splenda
1 teaspoon yeast

Place ingredients in bread machine in order specified by the manufacturer. Process on the whole wheat cycle.

14 SERVINGS

Each with: 113 Calories (13% from Fat, 15% from Protein, 73% from Carb); 4 g Protein; 2 g Total Fat; 0 g Saturated Fat; 1 g Monounsaturated Fat; 1 g Polyunsaturated Fat; 21 g Carb; 2 g Fiber; 1 g Sugar; 78 mg Phosphorus; 27 mg Calcium; 20 mg Sodium; 99 mg Potassium; 6 IU Vitamin A; 1 mg ATE Vitamin E; 0 mg Vitamin C; 1 mg Cholesterol

Crusty Italian Rolls

These makes good dinner rolls, but you could also use one for a sandwich, maybe with grilled veggies.
Like all good Italian breads, they are simple, but tasty.

1 cup (235 ml) water
2¾ cups (240 g) bread flour
1 tablespoon (13 g) sugar
1½ teaspoons yeast
2 tablespoons (28 ml) egg substitute
2 tablespoons (28 ml) water

Place ingredients in bread machine in order specified by the manufacturer. Process on dough cycle. Remove from pans and separate into 12 balls. Place in greased 9 × 13-inch (33 × 23 cm) pan, cover, and allow to rise until doubled, about 30 to 40 minutes. Mix egg substitute and water and brush over top of rolls. Bake at 375°F (190°C, or gas mark 5) until golden brown, about 12 to 14 minutes.

12 SERVINGS

Each with: 121 Calories (5% from Fat, 14% from Protein, 81% from Carb); 4 g Protein; 1 g Total Fat; 0 g Saturated Fat; 0 g Monounsaturated Fat; 0 g Polyunsaturated Fat; 24 g Carb; 1 g Fiber; 1 g Sugar; 40 mg Phosphorus; 7 mg Calcium; 6 mg Sodium; 50 mg Potassium; 10 IU Vitamin A; 0 mg ATE Vitamin E; 0 mg Vitamin C; 0 mg Cholesterol

Sun-Dried Tomato Rolls

These are great tasting rolls to serve with Italian meals.

¾ cup (175 ml) skim milk
2 cups (274 g) bread flour
¼ cup (28 g) sun-dried tomatoes,
  drained and 1 tablespoon oil
  (15 ml) reserved
1 tablespoon (1.5 g) sugar
  substitute, such as Splenda
1½ teaspoons yeast

Place all ingredients in bread machine pan in the order recommended by the manufacturer. Select dough cycle. Remove dough from pan; place on lightly floured surface. Cover and let rest 10 minutes. Lightly grease cookie sheet with cooking spray. Gently push fist into dough to deflate. Divide dough into 12 equal pieces. Shape each piece into a ball. Place 2 inches (5 cm) apart on cookie sheet. Cover and let rise in warm place 30 to 45 minutes or until almost double. Heat oven to 350°F (180°C, or gas mark 4). Bake 12 to 16 minutes or until golden brown. Remove from cookie sheet to wire rack.

12 SERVINGS

Each with: 93 Calories (5% from Fat, 16% from Protein, 79% from Carb); 4 g Protein; 0 g Total Fat; 0 g Unsaturated Fat; 0 g Monounsaturated Fat; 0 g Polyunsaturated Fat; 18 g Carb; 1 g Fiber; 0 g Sugar; 50 mg Phosphorus; 27 mg Calcium; 33 mg Sodium; 99 mg Potassium; 42 IU Vitamin A; 9 mg ATE Vitamin E; 1 mg Vitamin C; 0 mg Cholesterol

Yes, I Did Say Carrot Bread

I know that it sounds a bit strange for a yeast bread. But the carrot color and flavor make this a great bread to serve with a bowl of veggie laden soup or stew.

½ cup (120 ml) water, boiling
¼ cup (30 g) wheat, cracked
1¾ teaspoon yeast
¼ cup (60 ml) water
2⅔ cups (228) bread flour
⅓ cup (80 ml) skim milk, warm
¼ cup (55 g) butter, unsalted
¼ cup (4 g) brown sugar
  substitute, such as Splenda
1 cup (110 g) carrot, shredded
¼ cup (60 ml) egg substitute
⅔ cup (77 g) oat bran

In small bowl, pour boiling water over cracked wheat; let stand 15 minutes. Drain excess water. Place ingredients in bread machine pan in order specified by manufacturer. Process on the white bread cycle.

14 SERVINGS

Each with: 143 Calories (26% from Fat, 13% from Protein, 62% from Carb); 4 g Protein; 4 g Total Fat; 2 g Saturated Fat; 1 g Monounsaturated Fat; 0 g Polyunsaturated Fat; 22 g Carb; 1 g Fiber; 1 g Sugar; 59 mg Phosphorus; 23 mg Calcium; 50 mg Sodium; 101 mg Potassium; 1251 IU Vitamin A; 37 mg ATE Vitamin E; 1 mg Vitamin C; 9 mg Cholesterol

Make It a Meal with Brown Bread

This is a hearty bread, great with full flavored soups or chili. It also makes great toast.

¼ cup (60 ml) egg substitute
1 cup (235 ml) water
2 tablespoons (28 g) margarine, unsalted
2 tablespoons (40 g) molasses
1 tablespoon (1 g) brown sugar substitute, such as Splenda
1½ cups (206 g) bread flour
1 cup (120 g) whole wheat flour
½ cup (40 g) oats, rolled or quick cooking
⅓ cup (47 g) cornmeal
1½ teaspoons yeast

Place ingredients in the bread machine in the order specified by the manufacturer. Process on the wheat bread cycle.

14 SERVINGS

Each with: 130 Calories (7% from Fat, 15% from Protein, 78% from Carb); 5 g Protein; 1 g Total Fat; 0 g Saturated Fat; 0 g Monounsaturated Fat; 0 g Polyunsaturated Fat; 26 g Carb; 2 g Fiber; 2 g Sugar; 88 mg Phosphorus; 17 mg Calcium; 11 mg Sodium; 146 mg Potassium; 24 IU Vitamin A; 0 mg ATE Vitamin E; 0 mg Vitamin C; 0 mg Cholesterol

Whole Wheat Naan

This Indian bread is traditionally made by sticking the dough to the inside of the clay tandoor oven that the chicken is cooked in. In looking for a recipe, I found alternatives ranging from grilling to cooking it on unglazed tiles in the oven. I opted for the one that called for cooking it on a griddle, and it turned out just fine. I've made the breads a little smaller than usual to hold down the calorie count, but it would still fit in under 400 calories in a meal containing the *Indian Chicken* and one of the curried vegetables.

¾ cup (175 ml) water
1 cup (230 g) plain yogurt
1 tablespoon (1.5 g) sugar substitute
3½ cups (420 g) whole wheat flour
1½ teaspoons yeast

Place ingredients in bread machine in order specified by manufacturer and process on dough cycle. When finished, remove dough, punch down, and divide it into 12 equal pieces. Roll each piece out with a rolling pin or flatten using the heel of your hand into a smooth oval about 3 by 6 inches (7.5 to 15 cm). Place the ovals or rounds on a greased baking sheet and let rise 25 to 30 minutes until doubled in bulk. Transfer the bread to a preheated griddle. Check the bread in 3 minutes, lifting them to check the color of the bread on the underside. Flip each oval when golden brown and crusty and then cook another 3 minutes.

12 SERVINGS

Each with: 133 Calories (6% from Fat, 17% from Protein, 77% from Carb); 6 g Protein; 1 g Total Fat; 0 g Saturated Fat; 0 g Monounsaturated Fat; 0 g Polyunsaturated Fat; 27 g Carb; 4 g Fiber; 2 g Sugar; 157 mg Phosphorus; 50 mg Calcium; 17 mg Sodium; 200 mg Potassium; 14 IU Vitamin A; 3 mg ATE Vitamin E; 0 mg Vitamin C; 1 mg Cholesterol

Whole Wheat Biscuits

This is a variation of the standard biscuit recipe using whole wheat pastry flour and reduced fat that gives you a biscuit that is higher in nutrition and lower in calories. But it's still flaky and has an even better flavor than those made with white flour. These are great with soup and the leftovers can be frozen and reheated as needed.

1½ cups (188 g) all purpose flour

½ cup (69 g) whole wheat pastry flour

2 teaspoons sugar substitute, such as Splenda

3 tablespoons (41.4 g) baking powder

2 tablespoons (28 g) unsalted butter

⅔ cup (160 ml) skim milk

Stir together dry ingredients. Cut in butter until mixture resembles coarse crumbs. Add skim milk. Stir until just mixed. Knead gently on floured surface a few times. Press to ½-inch (1.3 cm) thickness. Cut into rounds with 2½-inch (6.4 cm) biscuit cutter or cut into squares with a knife. Transfer to ungreased baking sheet. Bake at 450 for 10 to 12 minutes or until golden brown.

10 SERVINGS

Each with: 118 Calories (20% from Fat, 11% from Protein, 69% from Carb); 3 g Protein; 3 g Total Fat; 2 g Saturated Fat; 1 g Monounsaturated Fat; 0 g Polyunsaturated Fat; 21 g Carb; 1 g Fiber; 0 g Sugar; 151 mg Phosphorus; 272 mg Calcium; 450 mg Sodium; 76 mg Potassium; 105 IU Vitamin A; 29 mg ATE Vitamin E; 0 mg Vitamin C; 6 mg Cholesterol

Cornbread

Cornbread goes well with a lot of things. Our version holds down the calories by using sugar substitute and reducing the amount of fat. (Yes, I know if I made southern style cornbread I wouldn't need to worry about the sugar, but I like this recipe better.) I prefer to make it in a preheated cast iron skillet because it makes the crust so nice and crispy, but you could also use a 9-inch (23 cm) square baking pan.

3 tablespoons (45 ml) canola oil, divided
1 cup (140 g) cornmeal
1 cup (125 g) all purpose flour
¼ cup (6 g) sugar substitute
1 tablespoon (13.8 g) baking powder
1 cup (235 ml) skim milk
¼ cup (60 ml) egg substitute

Place 1 tablespoon oil (15 ml) in a cast iron skillet and place it in oven while it preheats to 425°F (220°C, or gas mark 7). Mix together dry ingredients. Stir skim milk, egg substitute, and remaining oil together. Add to dry ingredients, stirring until just mixed. Swirl oil in pan to coat the bottom and sides. Place batter in pan and bake 20 to 25 minutes until golden brown.

12 SERVINGS

Each with: 124 Calories (29% from Fat, 11% from Protein, 60% from Carb); 3 g Protein; 4 g Total Fat; 0 g Saturated Fat; 2 g Monounsaturated Fat; 1 g Polyunsaturated Fat; 18 g Carb; 1 g Fiber; 0 g Sugar; 75 mg Phosphorus; 102 mg Calcium; 144 mg Sodium; 85 mg Potassium; 85 IU Vitamin A; 13 mg ATE Vitamin E; 0 mg Vitamin C; 0 mg Cholesterol

Parmesan Pepper Breadsticks

These contain a little more fat than most of the recipes, but the serving size is small, so you can still enjoy them with soup or an Italian meal from chapter 13. And being made will baking powder rather than yeast means that they are quick to prepare.

2 cups (247 g) whole wheat pastry flour
1 tablespoon (13.8 g) baking powder
¼ cup (55 g) unsalted butter
½ cup (120 ml) cold water
½ teaspoon black pepper, cracked
⅓ cup (33 g) Parmesan cheese
1 tablespoon (14 g) unsalted butter, melted

Stir together flour and baking powder. Cut in butter until mixture resembles crumbs. Stir in water, black pepper, and 2 tablespoons (10 g) of the cheese until soft dough forms. Place dough on lightly floured surface. Roll to 10 × 8-inch (25 × 20 cm) rectangle. Brush with butter. Sprinkle with remaining cheese. Cut crosswise into 14 strips. Place ½-inch (1.3 cm) apart on lightly greased cookie sheet. Bake at 450°F (230°C, or gas mark 8) until light golden brown, 10 to 12 minutes.

14 SERVINGS

Each with: 103 Calories (41% from Fat, 12% from Protein, 47% from Carb); 3 g Protein; 5 g Total Fat; 3 g Saturated Fat; 1 g Monounsaturated Fat; 0 g Polyunsaturated Fat; 13 g Carb; 2 g Fiber; 0 g Sugar; 96 mg Phosphorus; 89 mg Calcium; 138 mg Sodium; 74 mg Potassium; 141 IU Vitamin A; 36 mg ATE Vitamin E; 0 mg Vitamin C; 12 mg Cholesterol

Pepper Jack Cheese Bread

Slightly spicy with the pepper cheese and very good, this bread is made for Mexican meals, but it serves well with just plain grilled meat too.

2 cups (250 g) all purpose flour

1 cup (115 g) low fat Monterey Jack cheese, with jalapeño peppers, shredded

1 teaspoon sugar

1 teaspoon baking powder

¼ teaspoon baking soda

1 cup (235 ml) low fat buttermilk

¼ cup (55 g) unsalted butter, melted

½ cup (120 ml) egg substitute, slightly beaten

Preheat oven to 350°F (180°C, or gas mark 4). Lightly grease bottom only of loaf pan, 9 × 5 × 3-inch (23 × 13 × 7.5 cm) or 8½ × 4½ × 2½-inch (21.5 × 11.4 × 6.4 cm), with nonstick vegetable oil spray. Stir together flour, cheese, sugar, baking powder, and baking soda in medium bowl. Stir in remaining ingredients just until moistened (batter will be lumpy). Spread in pan. Bake for 35 to 45 minutes or until golden brown and toothpick inserted in center comes out clean. Cool 5 minutes; run knife around edges of pan to loosen. Remove from pan to wire rack. Cool 30 minutes before slicing.

16 SERVINGS

Each with: 110 Calories (33% from Fat, 19% from Protein, 48% from Carb); 5 g Protein; 4 g Total Fat; 2 g Unsaturated Fat; 1 g Monounsaturated Fat; 0 g Polyunsaturated Fat; 13 g Carb; 0 g Fiber; 1 g Sugar; 87 mg Phosphorus; 76 mg Calcium; 131 mg Sodium; 72 mg Potassium; 138 IU Vitamin A; 30 mg ATE Vitamin E; 0 mg Vitamin C; 10 mg Cholesterol

Fresh Berry Muffins

These sweet muffins are made with real berries. And they are low in calories, so you can work them into your diet.

2 cups (274 g) whole wheat pastry flour

¼ cup (60 ml) egg substitute

2 tablespoons (28 ml) canola oil, melted

2 teaspoons baking powder

2 tablespoons (3 g) sugar substitute, such as Splenda

1 cup (235 ml) skim milk

1 cup (170 g) strawberries, sliced

Stir together the dry ingredients. Mix together the rest of the ingredients and stir into dry, stirring until just moistened. Spoon into greased or paper lined muffin tins. Bake at 350°F (180°C, or gas mark 4) for 20 to 25 minutes until done.

12 SERVINGS

Each with: 105 Calories (24% from Fat, 15% from Protein, 61% from Carb); 4 g Protein; 3 g Total Fat; 0 g Saturated Fat; 1 g Monounsaturated Fat; 1 g Polyunsaturated Fat; 17 g Carb; 3 g Fiber; 1 g Sugar; 118 mg Phosphorus; 86 mg Calcium; 104 mg Sodium; 155 mg Potassium; 64 IU Vitamin A; 13 mg ATE Vitamin E; 8 mg Vitamin C; 0 mg Cholesterol

Cooking Terms, Weights and Measurements, and Gadgets

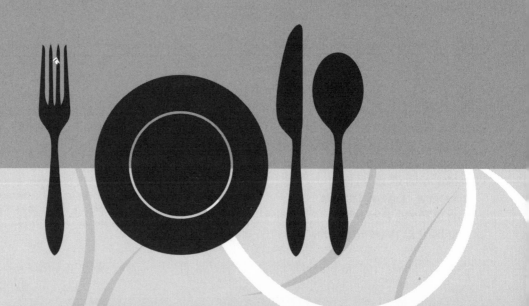

Cooking Terms

Are you confused about a term I used in one of the recipes? Take a look at the list here and see if there might be an explanation.

Al dente

This means *to the tooth*, in Italian. The pasta is cooked just enough to maintain a firm, chewy texture

Bake

To cook in the oven—food is cooked slowly with gentle heat, concentrating the flavor.

Baste

To brush or spoon liquid, fat, or juices over meat during roasting to add flavor and to prevent it from drying out

Beat

To smoothen a mixture by briskly whipping or stirring it with a spoon, fork, wire whisk, rotary beater, or electric mixer

Blend

To mix or fold two or more ingredients together to obtain equal distribution throughout the mixture

Boil

To cook food in heated water or other liquid that is bubbling vigorously

Braise

This cooking technique requires browning meat in oil or other fat and then cooking slowly in liquid. The effect of braising is to tenderize the meat.

Bread

To coat the food with crumbs (usually with soft or dry bread crumbs), sometimes seasoned

Broil

To cook food directly under the heat source

Broth or Stock

A flavorful liquid made by gently cooking meat, seafood, or vegetables (and/or their by-products, such as bones and trimming) often with herbs and vegetables, in liquid, usually water

Brown

A quick sautéing, pan/oven broiling, or grilling done either at the beginning or end of meal preparation, often to enhance flavor, texture, or visual appeal

Brush

Using a pastry brush to coat a food such as meat or bread with melted butter, glaze, or other liquid

Chop

To cut into irregular pieces

Coat

To evenly cover food with flour, crumbs, or a batter

Combine

To blend two or more ingredients into a single mixture

Core

To remove the inedible center of fruits such as pineapples

Cream

To beat butter or margarine with or without sugar, until light and fluffy; This process traps in air bubbles, later used to create height in cookies and cakes

Cut In

To work margarine or butter into dry ingredients

Dash

A measure approximately equal to $\frac{1}{16}$ teaspoon

Deep Fry

To completely submerge the food in hot oil; This is a quick way to cook some food, and as a result, this method often seems to seal in the flavors of food better than any other technique

Dice

To cut into cubes

Direct Heat

Heat waves radiate from a source and travel directly to the item being heated with no conductor between them; Examples are grilling, broiling, and toasting

Dough

Used primarily for cookies and breads; Dough is a mixture of shortening, flour, liquid, and other ingredients that maintains its shape when placed on a flat surface, although it will change shape once baked through the leavening process

Dredge

To coat lightly and evenly with sugar or flour

Dumpling

A batter or soft dough, which is formed into small mounds that are then steamed, poached, or simmered

Dust

To sprinkle food lightly with spices, sugar, or flour for a light coating

Fold

To cut and mix lightly with a spoon to keep as much air in the mixture as possible

Fritter

Sweet or savory foods coated or mixed into batter, then deep-fried

Fry

To cook food in hot oil, usually until a crisp brown crust forms

Glaze

A liquid that gives an item a shiny surface; Examples are fruit jams that have been heated or chocolate that has been thinned

Grease

To coat a pan or skillet with a thin layer of oil

Grill

To cook over the heat source (traditionally over wood coals) in the open air

Grind

To mechanically cut a food into small pieces

Hull

To remove the leafy parts of soft fruits such as strawberries or blackberries

Knead

To work dough with the heels of your hands in a pressing and folding motion until it becomes smooth and elastic

Marinate

To combine food with aromatic ingredients to add flavor

Mince

To chop food into tiny irregular pieces

Mix
To beat or stir two or more foods together until they are thoroughly combined

Pan-fry
To cook in a hot pan with small amount of hot oil, butter, or other fat, turning the food over once or twice

Poach
Simmering in a liquid

Pot Roast
A large piece of meat, usually browned in fat, cooked in a covered pan

Puree
Food that has been mashed or sieved

Reduce
To cook liquids down so that some of the water they contain evaporates

Roast
To cook uncovered in the oven

Sauté
To cook with a small amount of hot oil, butter, or other fat, tossing the food around over high heat

Sear
To brown a food quickly on all sides using high heat to seal in the juices

Shred
To cut into fine strips

Simmer
To cook slowly in a liquid over low heat

Skim
To remove the surface layer (of impurities, scum, or fat) from liquids such as stocks and jams while cooking; This is usually done with a flat slotted spoon

Smoke
To expose foods to wood smoke to enhance their flavor and help preserve and/or evenly cook them

Steam
To cook in steam by suspending foods over boiling water in a steamer or covered pot

Stew
To cook food in liquid for a long time until tender, usually in a covered pot

Stir
To mix ingredients with a utensil

Stir-fry
To cook quickly over high heat with a small amount of oil by constantly stirring; This technique often employs a wok

Toss
To mix ingredients lightly by lifting and dropping them using two utensils

Whip
To beat an item to incorporate air, augment volume, and add substance

Zest
The thin, brightly colored outer part of the rind of citrus fruits; It contains volatile oils, used as a flavoring

Weights and Measurements

Here is a quick refresher on measurements.

3 teaspoons = 1 tablespoon
2 tablespoons = 1 fluid ounce
4 tablespoons = 2 fluid ounces = ¼ cup
5⅓ tablespoons = 16 teaspoons = ⅓ cup
8 tablespoons = 4 fluid ounces = ½ cup
16 tablespoons = 8 fluid ounces = 1 cup
2 cups = 1 pint
4 cups = 2 pints = 1 quart
16 cups = 8 pints = 4 quarts = 1 gallon

Metric Conversions

There are some measurements that I can give you an easy conversion for, such as Fahrenheit to Celsius oven temperatures. Other things are not so easy. The information below is intended to be helpful to those readers who use the metric system of weights and measures.

Measurements of Liquid Volume

The following measures are approximate, but close enough for most, if not all, of the recipes in this book.

1 quart = 950 milliliters
1 cup = 235 milliliters
¾ cup = 175 milliliters
½ cup = 120 milliliters
⅓ cup = 80 milliliters
¼ cup = 60 milliliters
1 fluid ounce = 28 milliliters
1 tablespoon = 15 milliliters
1 teaspoon = 5 milliliters

Measurements of Weight

Much of the world measures dry ingredients by weight, rather than volume, as is done in the United States. There is no easy conversion for this, as each item is different. However the following conversions may be useful.

1 ounce = 28 grams
1 pound (455 g) = 455 grams (about half a kilo)

Oven Temperatures

Finally, we come to one that is relatively straightforward, the Fahrenheit to Celsius conversion.

100°F = 38°C
150°F = 66°C
200°F = 93°C
225°F = 107°C
250°F = 120°C
275°F = 140°C
300°F = 150°C
325°F = 170°C
350°F = 180°C
375°F = 190°C
400°F = 200°C
425°F = 220°C
450°F = 230°C
475°F = 240°C
500°F = 250°C.

Gadgets I Use

The following are some of the tools that I use in cooking. Some are used very often and some very seldom, but they all help make things a little easier or quicker. Why are some things here and other not? There is no reason except that most of these are things I considered a little less standard than a stove, oven, grill. and mixer.

Blender

Ok, so everyone has a blender. And it's a handy little tool for blending and pureeing things. I don't really think I need to say any more about that.

Bread Machine

When I went on a low sodium diet, I discovered that one of the biggest single changes that you can make to reduce your sodium intake is to make your own bread. Most commercial bread has well over 100 mg per slice. Many rolls and specialty breads are in the 300–400-mg range. A bread machine can reduce the amount of effort required to make your own bread to a manageable level. It takes at most 10 minutes to load it and turn it on. You can even set it on a timer to have your house filled with the aroma of fresh bread when you come home. Even if you're not watching your sodium, there is nothing like the smell of bread baking and the taste right out of the oven.

Canning Kettle

If you are planning on making batches of things such as pickles and salsa in volume so you don't have to go through the process every couple of weeks, then you are going to need a way to preserve things. Most items can be frozen of course, if that is your preference. But some things just seem to me to work better in jars. What you need is a kettle big enough to make sure the jars can be covered by water when being processed in a boiling water bath. There are also racks to sit the jars in and special tongs to make lifting them in and out of the water easier. I've had a porcelain covered kettle I use for this for a lot of years and it also doubled as a stockpot before I got the one described below. It's better for canning than for soup because the relatively thin walls allow the water to heat faster (and the soup to burn).

Deep Fryer

Obviously, if you are watching your fat intake, this should not be one of your most often used appliances. I don't use it nearly as often as I used to, but it still occupies a place in the appliance garage in the corner of the kitchen counter. It's a Fry Daddy, big enough to cook a batch of fries or fish for 3 to 4 people at a time.

Food Processor

I'm a real latecomer to the food processor world. It always seemed like a nice thing to have, but something I could easily do without. We bought one to help shred meat and other things for my wife's mother, who was having some difficulty swallowing large chunks of food. I use it now all the time to grind bread into crumbs or chop the peppers and onions that seem to go into at least 3 meals a week. It's a low-end model that doesn't have the power to grind meat and some of the heavier tasks, but I've discovered it's a real time saver for a number of things.

Contact Grill

The George Foreman models are the most popular example of this item. My son's girlfriend gave me this for Christmas a few years ago. (And he didn't have the good sense to hang onto her . . . but that's a different story). I use it at fairly often. When we built our house we included a Jenn-Air cooktop with a built-in grill and for years that was used regularly. It still is for some things . . . I much prefer the way it does burgers or steak when it's too cold to grill them outside, but it's difficult to clean and doesn't do nearly as nice a job as the Foreman at things like grilled veggies and fish. And the design allows the fat to drain away, giving you a healthier, lower fat meal.

Grinder

MANY years ago we bought an Oster Kitchen Center. It was one of those all in one things that included a stand mixer, blender (the one we still use), food chopper, and a grinder attachment. The grinder was never a big deal that got any use . . . until I started experimenting with sausage recipes. Since then I've discovered that grinding your own meat can save you both money and fat. Buying a beef or pork roast on sale, trimming it of most fat, and grinding it yourself can give you hamburger or sausage meat that is well over 90% lean and still less expensive than the fattier stuff you buy at the store. So now the grinder gets fairly regular use.

Hand Chopper

My daughter got this gem at a Wal-Mart in North Carolina while she was in school there. It was from one of those guys with the podium and the auctioneer's delivery and the extra free gifts if you buy it within the next 10 minutes. Neither of us has ever seen one like it since. The food processor has taken over some of its work, but it still does a great job chopping things like onions as fine as you could want without liquefying them.

Pasta Maker

I bought this toy after seeing it on a Sunday morning TV infomercial. It's a genuine Ronco/Popiel *As Seen on TV* special, but try not to hold that against it. Unlike the pasta cutters that merely slice rolled dough into flat noodles, this one mixes the whole mess then extrudes it through dies with various shaped holes in them. The recipes say you can use any kind of flour, but I've found that buying the semolina flour that is traditionally used for pasta gives you dough that's easier to work with, as well as better texture and flavor. The characterization of it as a *toy* is pretty accurate. There aren't really any nutritional advantages over store bought pasta. If you buy the semolina, the cost is probably about the same as some of the more expensive imported pasta. But its fun to play with, makes a great conversation piece, and the pasta tastes good.

Salad Shooter

We seem to end up with a lot of these gadgets, don't we? This is another one that's been around for a while, but it's still my favorite implement for shredding potatoes for hash browns or cabbage for coleslaw.

Sausage Stuffer

This is really an addition to the Kitchen Center grinder. I found it at an online appliance repair site. It is really just a series of different sized tubes that fit on the end of the grinder to stuff your ground meat into casings. I do this occasionally to make link sausage, but most of the time I just make patties or bulk sausage.

Slicer

This was a close out floor model that I bought years ago. Before going on the low sodium diet I used to buy deli meat in bulk and slice it myself. Now its most often used to slice a roast or smoked piece of meat for sandwiches.

Slow Cooker

I've tried to avoid calling it a Crockpot, which is a trademark of Rival. Anyway, whatever the brand, no kitchen should be without one.

Smoker

This was another pre-diet purchase that has been used even more since. I started with a Brinkman that originally used charcoal. Then I bought an add-on electric heat source for it that works a lot better in cold weather. Last year the family gave me a fancy MasterChef electric one that seals like an oven and has a thermostat to hold the temperature.

Not only do I like the way it does ribs and other traditional smoked foods, but we also use it fairly regularly to smoke a beef or pork roast or turkey breast to use for sandwiches.

Springform Pan
This is a round, straight-sided pan. The sides are formed into a hoop that can be unclasped and detached from its base.

Steamer (Rice Cooker)
I use this primarily for cooking rice, but it's really a Black and Decker Handy Steamer Plus that does a great job steaming vegetables too. It does make excellent rice, perfect every time. So I guess the bottom line is that those of you who have trouble making rice like me (probably because like me you can't follow the instructions not to peek) should consider getting one of these or one of the Japanese style rice cookers.

Stockpot
The key here is to spend the extra money to get a heavy gauge one (another thing I eventually learned from personal experience.). The lighter weight ones not only will dent and not sit level on the stove, but they will burn just about everything you put in them. Mine also has a heavy glass lid that seals the moisture in well.

Turbocooker
This was another infomercial sale. It is a large dome-lidded fry pan with racks that fit inside it. You can buy them at many stores too, but mine is the Plus model that has two steamer racks and a timer. It really will cook a whole dinner quickly, *steam frying* the main course and steaming one or two more items. The only bad news is most of the recipes involve additions and changes every few minutes, so even if you only take a half hour to make dinner, you spend that whole time at the stove.

Waffle Maker
We don't use this often, but it makes a nice change of pace for breakfast or dinner.

Wok
This is a round-bottomed pan popular in Asian cooking.

About the Author

After being diagnosed with congestive heart failure, Dick Logue threw himself into the process of creating healthy versions of his favorite recipes. A cook since the age of twelve, he grows his own vegetables, bakes his own bread, and cans a variety of foods. He currently has a website www.lowsodiumcooking.com and weekly online newsletter with more than 21,000 subscribers world-wide. He is the author of *500 Low Sodium Recipes*, *500 Low-Cholesterol Recipes*, *500 High-Fiber Recipes*, *500 Low-Glycemic-Index Recipes*, and *500 Heart-Healthy Slow Cooker Recipes*. He lives in southern Maryland.

Index